RELIGION IN
GLOBAL HEALTH
AND DEVELOPMENT

RELIGION IN GLOBAL HEALTH AND DEVELOPMENT

The Case of Twentieth-Century Ghana

BENJAMIN BRONNERT WALKER

McGill-Queen's University Press

Montreal & Kingston • London • Chicago

ISBN 978-0-2280-1052-4 (cloth)
ISBN 978-0-2280-1169-9 (paper)
ISBN 978-0-2280-1159-0 (ePDF)
ISBN 978-0-2280-1160-6 (ePUB)
ISBN 978-0-2280-1366-2 (open access)

Legal deposit first quarter 2022
Bibliothèque nationale du Québec

Printed in Canada on acid-free paper that is 100% ancient forest free
(100% post-consumer recycled), processed chlorine free

The open access edition of this book was funded by the Wellcome Trust.

Library and Archives Canada Cataloguing in Publication

Title: Religion in global health and development : the case of twentieth-century Ghana /
Benjamin Bronnert Walker.
Names: Walker, Benjamin Bronnert, author.
Description: Includes bibliographical references and index.
Identifiers: Canadiana (print) 20210350962 | Canadiana (ebook) 20210351047
 | ISBN 9780228010524 (cloth) | ISBN 9780228011699 (paper) | ISBN
 9780228011590 (ePDF) | ISBN 9780228011606 (ePUB) | ISBN 9780228013662
 (Open access PDF)
Subjects: LCSH: World health—History—20th century. | LCSH: Health—Religious
 aspects—Christianity. | LCSH: Missions, Medical—Ghana—History—20th century.
 | LCSH: Public health—Ghana—History—20th century.
Classification: LCC RA441 .W35 2022 | DDC 362.109667—dc23

This book was typeset in 10.5/13 Sabon.

Contents

Figures and Tables

FIGURES

TABLES

Abbreviations

AIC	African-initiated Church
AME Zion	African Methodist Episcopal Zion
BELRA	British Empire Leprosy Relief Association
CCGC	Christian Council of the Gold Coast
CDC	Centers for Disease Control (USA)
CDU	Christian Democratic Union (West Germany)
CDWA	Colonial Welfare and Development Act
CHAG	Christian Health Association of Ghana
CIDA	Canadian International Development Agency
CMC	Christian Medical Commission
CMS	Church Missionary Society
CPP	Convention People's Party (Ghana)
CRS	Catholic Relief Services
DFL	Dutch florins
DM	deutsche marks
EMMS	Edinburgh Medical Missionary Society
FBO	faith-based organisation
FIDES	Fonds d'Investissement et de Développement Economique et Social
FRG	Federal Republic of Germany (West Germany)
ICRC	International Committee of the Red Cross
IPPF	International Planned Parenthood Federation
KVP	Catholic People's Party (Netherlands)
LSTM	Liverpool School of Tropical Medicine
MFU	medical field units (Gold Coast/Ghana)
MMS	Medical Mission Sisters
NC	national cedis

NGO	non-governmental organisation
NLM	National Liberation Movement (Ghana)
NPP	Northern People's Party (Ghana)
OS	Oversea Service
PCG	Presbyterian Church of Ghana
PHC	Primary Health Care
PNDC	Provisional National Defence Council (Ghana)
PRAAD	Public Records and Administration Department (Ghana)
SDA	Seventh-day Adventist
SOAS	School of Oriental and African Studies
UMCA	Universities' Mission to Central Africa
UNICEF	United Nations Children's Fund
UP	United Party (Ghana)
USAID	United States Agency for International Development
VSO	Voluntary Overseas Service
WAMS	West African Medical Service
WCC	World Council of Churches
WHO	World Health Organization

Preface

The dominant historical narratives of global health are strikingly narrow when it comes to religion. In many sub-Saharan African countries the amount of religious health assets (clinics, hospitals, and dispensaries affiliated with or run by religious organisations) can be up to 40 or 50 per cent.[1] Yet, frequently, global health histories are overly instrumentalist and, in focusing solely on high-level institutions like the World Health Organization (WHO), exclude religion.[2] The diverse, long-term, multi-layered, and contingent formations that created global health (and in which the WHO operates) are squeezed out, along with many non-European and non-American practitioners.[3] By exploring the historical role of religion in global health and development, using previously unexplored or underexplored archives, this book breaks new conceptual ground. It offers new ways of imagining transnational collaborations, adding to the increasing efforts to decolonise our health histories both nationally and internationally.

Honing our studies of what global health is and where it comes from requires looking closely at the history of how religious groups – small and large – have jostled for power in communities, colonial states, emerging decolonising nations, and regional governments. It also demands better attention to the battles for supremacy over the meaning of medical care at different spatial scales and to the consequences of delivery, which have been some of the most intractable and far-reaching of the twentieth century. This book interrogates these competing actors and, by using a case study of colonial and postcolonial Ghana, it explores the sometimes slow and sometimes rapid processes of religious transformation that have informed what global health has become. It emphasises how some of the greatest triumphs of global health practice – smallpox eradication, Primary Health Care, disease crisis management – make little sense without understanding the role of medical missionaries, faith-based organisations, and religious communities.

A historical approach focused on religion can offer the chance for improved categories as well as a better picture of who made global health and which various long-term processes factored in its creation. As a political category 'global health' has been useful to its practitioners partly because, under its umbrella, a variety of interests can join together while masking deeper conflicts.[4] Joseph M. Hodge and Gerald Hödl have conceptualised development as 'a conscious process of ideas, interventions and practices – one filled with contradictions and fueled by crises, but also amorphous enough to encompass a wide spectrum of expressions and experiences'.[5] The concept of 'global health' has similar qualities. Organisations and individuals that want to empower particular interpretations of health, to eradicate specific diseases, or even to create wholesale social engineering have united within narratives of universal human endeavour. Yet, it is also within specific cultural encounters between diverse groups that the meanings and the interpretative communities that could practise development and global health took shape. Crucially, both terms were formed and contested in local contexts and traditions, in conjunction with international communities and networks.[6]

Developing a coherent debate about how religion, development, and global health relate historically is especially important for understanding fragile and fragmented states. This was abundantly clear during the 2014–16 Ebola crisis in Liberia, Sierra Leone, and Guinea. As Sally Smith and Katherine Marshall argue: 'Despite religions' deep-rooted health and social roles ... national governments and international actors were late to appreciate the vital roles of religious actors in addressing Ebola and supporting health systems'.[7] Not only in this specific instance but across the world, the spread of disease and the absence of well-being can be challenged by better attention to religion, its cultures, its relation to power, and its role in the state.[8] Notably, in contexts where health care is made up of a patchwork of humanitarian interventions, weak or hollowed-out state services, multi-lateral development financing, and local community medical pluralism, the role of religion can be critical – socially, culturally, and in the basis of governance. Continuing to neglect the historical complexities of religion in our definitions of global health and development will mean further harm to those living at the sharp end of national and international agendas.

Acknowledgments

Writing and researching a global history has incurred debts of gratitude that cross continents. I was helped by many Ghanaians to whom I am very thankful: Fred Sai, Mary Grant, Anna Mary Grant, Francis Grant, the Bediako Family, Felix Konotey-Ahulu, George Ossom-Batsa, Peter Yeboah, Michael Baddoo, the staff at Korle Bu Library, the staff at the National Catholic Secretariat, the staff at the George Padmore Research Library, and the staff at the libraries and bookshops of the University of Ghana. For his friendship, guidance, and inspiration, Jake Obeng Bediako deserves a special mention. I was also supported and directed by many other medical missionaries, health workers, hospital administrators, anthropologists, historians, and global health leaders, especially: the Medical Mission Sisters (Philadelphia), Anne Louise van Hoening, Suzanne Maschek, Mary Ann Tregoning, David Newberry, Naomi Forbes, Doris Hodds, Louise Duncan, Mwai Makoka, Shiva Murugasampillay, Marissa Mika, Hannah-Louise Clark, Stephanie Newell, Sjaak van der Geest, Ted Karpf, Bill Foege, Aliko Ahmed, Ralph H. Henderson, Natasha Gray, Paul Jenkins, Walter Bruchhausen, Donald Henderson, Arthur Hibbles, Nathan Grills, Fawzia Rasheed, and Mimi Kiser. Archivists and librarians in Italy, Germany, the Netherlands, the United Kingdom, and the United States have also been vital to this research, and although there are too many to name, their assistance has been invaluable.

I am sincerely grateful to the Wellcome Trust for their generosity in funding the Medical Humanities PhD Studentship (108593/Z/15/Z), and with it the extensive travel – to archives, interviews, and conferences – that made this book possible. The main research was based at the Centre for Global Health Histories (CGHH) – a World Health Organization Collaborating Centre at the University of York. Thank you to the director of the CGHH and my PhD supervisor, Sanjoy Bhattacharya, for his insight, expertise, diligence, and encouragement. Thank you to the CGHH members and university colleagues for reading drafts and discussing ideas: Margaret Jones, Alex Medcalf, Arnab Chakraborty, Suranga Dolamulla, Monica Saavedra, Sarah Hartley, Tara Alberts, Gerard McCann, Sabine Clarke, Shaul Mitelpunkt, Joshua Cockayne, and David Efird. As well as at the University of York, opportunities to present the arguments in this book were provided by international conferences, seminars, and lectures, where I met many fascinating and able scholars: Peking University, Johns Hopkins University, Hughes Hall, Cambridge, African Studies Association UK, UK Libraries and Archives Group on Africa (SCOLMA), Wellcome Witness Seminar on the Worldwide Antimalarial Resistance Network (WWARN) at the University of Oxford, European Social Science History Conference at Queen's University Belfast, Socialist International Health workshop at the University of Exeter, the 'Inspiring Communities in Global Health' event at the Wellcome Collection, the BBC History Magazine Weekend, the 'Christian Missions in Global History' event at the Institute of Historical Research, University of London, Global Health Histories Seminar 112 at the World Council of Churches (WCC) in Geneva (with WHO Euro, the University of York, and the Wellcome Trust), and, lastly, the roundtable on the spiritual dimension of health at the WCC organised by the University of Zurich.

The initial ideas and research that gave a foundation for this book were drawn from conversations, lectures, and seminars during my BA and MPhil at the University of Cambridge. The Newton Trust and Peterhouse funding I received, with further grants for travel to Ghana, facilitated the privilege of postgraduate study. I was supervised by David Maxwell and taught by Emma Hunter, who launched my work on Africa, mission, and development. I am also grateful for the fellows of Gonville and Caius College who taught me the practice of history and have given me support along the way, particularly Melissa Calaresu, Annabel S. Brett, Peter Mandler, Robert Priest, Ruth Scurr, and Sujit Sivasundaram.

In writing the book I have benefitted from many helpful reviews, comments, and feedback. Thank you especially to Richard Baggaley, Stephen Taylor, Emma Wild-Wood, Shane Doyle, Joel Isaac, Jesse

Boardman Bump, Henning Grunwald, Scott Howard, and the editors and reviewers of McGill-Queen's University Press.

Thank you to the communities, teams, and staff at St Aidan's and St John Fisher Associated Sixth Form (Harrogate), Holy Trinity Church (Cambridge), G2 (York), and the Diocese of York. For their love and support, thank you to my parents, Ruth and Andy Walker, my brother Jamie, my grandparents Gwen and Geoff Walker, and John and Freda Bronnert. Thank you to all my family, to Debbie Whitehead and Phil Whitehead, Ann and Andrew Bronnert, Derek and Jo Ward, and Alexandra Ward. Thanks also to Josiah Judson and Richard Braham.

Lastly, thank you to a talented and dedicated health service leader, my wife Holly, for her kindness, patience, laughter, and continuous support over the many years of researching and writing this book.

RELIGION IN
GLOBAL HEALTH
AND DEVELOPMENT

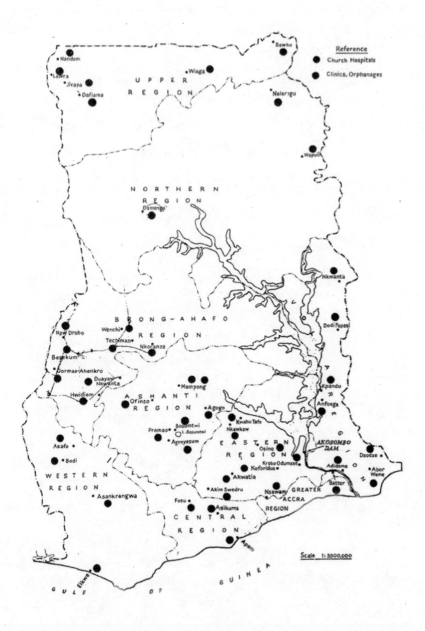

Figure I.1 | 'CHAG Member Institutions (1976)':
The Growth of Medical Mission in Ghana

Introduction

The history of global health needs to begin at the bottom. Histories of global health often start with high-level policy making and work their way down to the effect of those policies on the ground. Most of the time they do not extend beyond institutional leadership in Washington, DC and Geneva. In these histories the WHO becomes a celestial body – everything either is drawn into its orbit or is born out of it. In many cases power seems to start at some particular middle and then emanates outwards. For example, in their influential work, Theodore Brown, Marcos Cueto, and Elizabeth Fee oversimplify the shift from 'international health' to 'global health' in terms of elites struggling to carve out a role in a fight with forces outside their control.[1] This limits the frame through which the transition between 'international health' and 'global health' can be historicised and periodised. Theirs is a diffusionist model and one further bolstered by their institutional history of the WHO, which, though full of important detail and a key reference for scholars, has the tendency to suggest that the WHO is the centre of global health.[2] Such histories are certainly valuable, but they make it sound like global health happens in the offices of director-generals and departmental heads. Of course, there are key decisions made in these places; management and coordination of campaigns on an international scale are vital work. Nevertheless, this is not all that constitutes global health. Power in global health moves in lots of different directions and comes from transnational, regional, local, national, and international sources.

Taking this call to action seriously, this history of global health starts not in Geneva but in the Gold Coast (Ghana from independence in 1957); not in the meeting rooms of WHO HQ but in the small clinics and dispensaries of a mostly rural colonial state. Tracking from here in the 1920s to the expansion of health infrastructure in the 1950s, to the disintegration of the state in the 1970s and the impoverished 1980s, allows us to see global health policies and practices differently. It shows that global health is a diverse and decentralised process that is constantly being remade in local contexts in parallel with international communities and networks.[3] Understanding global health fully must start at this ground level and from there feel where international health was part of a patchwork of other forces – competing for space, certainly, but on a multi-layered landscape.

By drawing out the longer processes in Ghana that have helped to create contemporary global health, a central claim of this book is that the role of religion cannot be viewed as a minor or optional addition. Global health does not make sense without understanding its colonial missionary past, and this work is only in its infancy. In recent years, historians of global health have been interrogating Africa as a site of international public health interventions and continued experimentation. Incursions have increased since the 1990s, though actual health outcomes often have not, and these have strong continuities with colonial pasts. Ruth Prince describes Kisumu in Kenya as a place in which bodies and health are tied to 'global assemblages of medicine' where 'a grid of services, resources and opportunities interlock with government, and deepen dependence'. She argues that this connection to development and the global is imagined 'not as a process encompassing the national collective but as an opportunity for individual social and geographic mobility'.[4] Tamara Giles-Vernick, L.A. James, and J.R. Webb's edited volume *Global Health in Africa* shows how the issues that Prince discusses have roots in long-term, persistent interventions by NGOs, international health organisations, and medical researchers.[5] Yet, these forms of deepening dependence are not only the short-term product of a mixed set of interventions, but also a continuous track of structural and cultural change in which the global has been a constant feature of the grid of medical services, resources, and opportunities since the 1920s. Religious providers and agents, across the twentieth century, were a vital part of this much longer-term process.

The postcolonial state has not been able or has not wanted to uproot the legacies of colonial health and medical missionary interventions. Paul Wenzel Geissler argues that the African state is at times an ephemeral figure, not monolithic and predictable but weak amidst other forms of global governmentality.[6] This is strikingly apparent when assessing the longevity of medical mission and colonial health. Global health may try to project homogeneity, but ultimately medical missions, in terms of data collection, surveying, and service delivery, have long been creating alternative sites of citizenship with global imaginaries, by offering alternatives to secular provision. These global imaginaries have their roots in historic mission traditions and colonial identities. The colonial past continues to shape the way in which development is practised and how modern medical care, and the healthy and unhealthy body, are envisaged in the present. The raging conflicts for priority in global health agendas can easily become uncoupled from the realities of health systems, detached from the long-term experiences of local communities with foreign interventions, and ignorant of how internal organisational cultures have informed what is imaginatively possible for current debate. Histories, those that are not in thrall to the interests of a particular national or organisational narrative, provide an opportunity for global health to know better where it came from and therefore have a more grounded plan for where it is going.[7]

Crossing the colonial and postcolonial divide, this book will focus on unpacking and analysing how religious health care became so vital to national development, international health, and global health in Ghana.[8] It will look carefully at the forerunners of contemporary global health practice in medical missions and in the religious health assets which began to develop rapidly during the middle of the twentieth century. It will detail how transnational organisations and foreign states over the last century – Britain, West Germany, the Netherlands, Switzerland, Canada, and the United States – all played a part (with finance, labour, ideas, food, medicine, and resources) in the creation of large-scale Christian health in Ghana. Moreover, it will show how these processes occurred unevenly, inconsistently, and often detached from the 'global community'.[9] It will also show how local African leaders, Ghanaian religious figures, and postcolonial nationalists drove and shaped global initiatives from 'below'. All this will contribute to posing a key question: how have religious health actors contributed to the creation of global health in the twentieth and twenty-first centuries? This book offers a critical starting point in answering this vital question. For it to be answered completely will require new studies of religious health assets encompassing a range of religion organisations, beliefs, and believers. Crucially, this book adds to the growing voices urging such work to be undertaken.[10]

Throughout these changes, what happened on the ground in Ghana reshaped what was possible for global health and also how global health campaigns were pioneered. Ghanaians themselves made global health happen and eventually would be key figures in running international organisations; one Christian Ghanaian – Kofi Annan – became the secretary-general of the United Nations.[11] Many leaders at the highest echelons of global organisations since the 1950s have been Africans. In 2016 the WHO elected its first African director-general. This did not emerge from nowhere, but rather from a long history of increasing African medical interventions and the creation of health assets. Many of the ways in which global health organisations understand their role has come out of experiences in colonial and postcolonial African encounters between communities, health workers, and government. Unsurprisingly, Tedros Adhanom Ghebreyesus was a champion of rural strengthening when he was the Ethiopian health minister (garnering him some Chinese support). Global health, to be understood fully, needs a multi-layered, multi-focal, and non-Eurocentric narrative.

In showing how global health emerged alongside and in strategic coordination with medical mission, the hope is to challenge how we define global health. However, this book is not promoting a form of global health ruled by religious believers. Part of decolonising the history of mission has included attention to the destructive power embedded in missionary work; not simply in its direct ability to convert but also its ability to impose foreign categorizations, systems of knowledge, and subjectivities.[12] As Achille Mbembe puts it: 'the act of conversion is also involved in the destruction of worlds … the abandonment of familiar landmarks, cultural and symbolic. The act means, therefore, stripping down to the skin'.[13] The diplomatic status of global health, an arena in which there is more than enough space for a variety of perspectives on the purpose of natural life and its destiny afterwards, is something to be lauded. Yet, a presumably accidental byproduct of the postcolonial critique of missionary proselytism has been losing an understanding of mission's significance in the creation of global health.

Providing a wider lens will give global health some less restrictive options for how it chooses to approach its current problems. The focus of this book will not be on the narrow language of debate in Geneva but on the much larger landscape of global health work across the world. The WHO is not only in Europe, and its sites around the globe have as significant a bearing on practice as the director-general's office does. The optic of this book will not be framed by certain types of global health organisation, nor simply those that have been able to lay claim to more international media attention and glory (or opprobrium). A key benefit of this critical historical approach is, as Sanjoy Bhattacharya and Carlos Eduardo D'Avila Pereira Campani recently put it, to inform 'those charged with public health leadership that their work cannot be based on an inflexible, top-down enforcement of narrow sets of ideas and practices'.[14] The policy implications of this analysis for the changing pattern of tension, neglect, and cooperation between global health organisations and religious providers will be addressed in the conclusion. Overall, critically looking at global health history can help present-day actors answer some of the fundamental questions about when certain health structures emerged, how they have been changed, who moulded global health into its current shape, and, ultimately, why global health operates in this state at all.

In order to form this argument, the first chapter will disrupt traditional accounts of the periodisation of international health and global health by examining the colonial foundations of development. It was in the context of newly independent states, negotiating with and pushing at the boundaries of imperial infrastructure, that global health was formed. Building on a proliferation of missionary health providers between the 1930s and 1950s, the majority of the basis of the health-care system in Ghana was constructed by the late colonial state using a network of medical missionary hospitals. This was decided over and against funding preventative forms of public health. Instead, a voluntary sector was financed by the colonial state and staffed by missions, creating a legacy for postcolonial Ghana that could not be uprooted. This chapter will also show how some forms of mission were empowered over others in this process, and how diverse conceptions of development and voluntarism operated across the various layers of the sector.

The second chapter will then examine the early independent Ghanaian state and show how battles over the religious meanings of development and the actors within it were central to making 'modern' health. Rather than dismantling the late colonial voluntary sector, Ghanaian nationalist leaders added to it, financed it, and fought over its significance. Medical mission became a feature of attacks on the colonial legacy and also a necessary part of the postcolonial modernisation project. The institutional ways in which medical missionaries imagined Africanisation will be contrasted with the more complex notions of 'African-ness'. The chapter will examine how medical mission was reconceptualised and reclaimed by high-level politicians such as Kwame Nkrumah, Joseph Emmanuel Appiah, Jambaidu Awuni, and Alhaji Mumuni Bawumia (a prominent Muslim lawyer and one of the founding members of the Northern People's Party). Their constructions of the relationship between religion and development in this period cast backward to the 1920s and forward to an African modernity. Amidst tumultuous changes, medical missions grew larger but were becoming a publicly silent feature of postcolonial health. This had ramifications for later secularised understandings of global health, and it simultaneously established a context in which medical mission could expand through new forms of international support.

The third chapter will reframe postcolonial international health by showing how West Germany and the Netherlands financed and staffed large-scale medical mission work in Ghana between the 1950s and 1990s. Without the global community or international health organisations, without previous recent colonial connection to Ghana or a South-South development relationship, the old colonial powers of West Germany and the Netherlands established health development in a postcolonial state. Part of the reason for this aid in Ghana was to create a 'reverberation' of humanitarian development that, by using transnational Catholic identities, would help to unite modern Germany. Detached from older colonial patterns or the emerging global community, this was fresh development work in a decolonised setting where renewed European nationalism could be performed and embodied. This chapter will show the limits of these transnational networks to create identities, and the complex experiences of missions and health in particular medical sites. However, it will show how the overall effect of this process was to create further long-term sustainability for missions and their continued growth across the twentieth century.

The fourth chapter will examine the variety of actors and voices that make up 'international' and 'global' health, challenging their restricted usage as historical concepts. Extending beyond elite policy makers, it will detail the wide array of participants involved in small-pox control and eradication, as well as in food aid, in Ghana. As a result of the foundational infrastructure of medical mission in the 1950s and increased support in the 1960s and 1970s, international health campaigns relied on missionary networks in Ghana to function. Moreover, Ghanaian Christian doctors emerge in this period as a form of postcolonial 'Africanised' medical missionary, laying claim to earlier missionary models. Medical missionaries and Ghanaian Christian doctors figured as negotiators, intermediaries, and advocates, who drove and empowered health campaigns which used USAID (United States Agency for International Development) and the WHO for their own ends. This chapter will emphasise that international and global health are shaped by the historical networks and institutions in a given country, and that supposed externally led interventions rely on internal infrastructure. In the case of Ghana, religious medical assets are absolutely vital in controlling disease and making health.

The fifth chapter will examine how medical missions in the 1960s and 1970s had strategic roles in creating international and global health policy, and how they continued to create health even as they grew less visible to global organisations in the 1980s and 1990s. How missions navigated the changing pressures of international and global health will be unpacked. The significant contribution of religious actors to the creation of key international movements, such as Primary Health Care and Universal Health Coverage, will be detailed. The chapter will disaggregate the various layers of medical mission and global health; it will show how, in Ghana, health workers on the ground could continue longer-term patterns of missionary health care and disregard international policy changes. All this will be set in the context of missionaries weathering the storms of the disintegration of the Ghanaian state from the mid 1970s and across the 1980s. Regardless of the truncating of global imaginaries, religion continued to play a central role in the meanings, practices, and future of health and development across the world.

Finally, this book concludes by showing how the history of the relationship between religion, global health, and development can offer new ways of imagining the postcolonial state and its emergence. It will indicate the fresh historical questions that these conclusions open up, as well as map some of their implications for future policy making in global health.

METHODOLOGY

Histories of global health which are largely drawn from the archives of WHO and prioritise its narrative can produce too-narrow perspectives on how global health was formed and performed. Challenging the elite-focused histories of institutions which more easily impose themselves in archives and in memory can provide alternative, broader historical narratives of global health. This book will produce a particular kind of in-depth history of health, politics, religion, and mission in Ghana, and show the importance of a variety of transnational, international, and global connections and interactions in global health. In doing so it will push away from the commanding presence of large institutions like states and international organisations. Changes in medical mission, Ghanaian national health, and international health are not represented in the records of high-level organisations like the WHO or national government stores like the US National Archives. By not relying on high-level archives like these, it is possible to reframe the historical concepts of international health and development by attending to their layers and to parts that cut in directions different from the 'hegemonic' or more visible global imaginaries of the time.

Triangulating historical sources – simultaneously using written and spoken, public and private, ephemeral and published medias – can offer a course which does not rest on official narrative but can be critiqued for reliability. The problem with the focus on official records, published documents and statistics, or institutional reports is that they can privilege the perspective of elites, of the colonial state and of those who are able to print, disseminate, and store their output in archives. Using only national public archives and private institutional ones can steer historians toward repeating the narratives of the powerful or those of a small, visible minority who had an interest in posterity. For African Studies, Jan Vansina challenged this sort of history in 1965 with his work on oral tradition, which offered the opportunity to include a wider range of actors in histories by arguing that orality should be permissible historical evidence.[15]

To piece this history together has required going beyond reports and policy documents. This study will utilise a plethora of types of media and literary genres which recorded and expressed medical missionary encounters and interactions. These include but are not limited to: inspirational writing, autobiography, correspondence, funeral brochures, unpublished anthropology and ethnography, documentaries, magazine and journal articles, and travel diaries. Such sources offer contrasting and new perspectives, angles, and performances into key historical processes. With regard to newspapers, as Emma Hunter writes for East Africa, they were 'spaces in which new identities and new political formations were imagined and critiqued'.[16] In the long-running free Gold Coast presses, Africans could articulate challenges to the state, which offers insight into literate nonelite Africans who were outside of political power but could voice critique in the public sphere. These newspapers include critiques of which missions and types of development were seen as legitimate and which were not. In the first era of postcolonial Ghana these spaces were used to reconstruct Christian liturgy for the purposes of Ghanaian nationalism. Mission newspapers and magazines also gave missionaries a platform for reading and writing their transnational identities within ecclesiastical and eschatological narratives. Finally, in postwar Germany, regional newspapers provided a context for the construction of national identities and suffering bodies in relation to mission, development, and Ghana.

Alongside a variety of sources, much of the evidence for this study was found in written reports retrieved from public and private archives. Including government and institutional reports ensures that inequalities in colonial and postcolonial systems are shown alongside more fluid forms of networks. Analysing structures is an important part of showing the interrelationship between the centre and the margins, between institutional structures and fluid aspects of networks. As Simon Potter has argued, assessing 'informal, integrative, competing and constantly shifting interconnections' is vital, but it must be accompanied by 'more formal, entrenched, and limited patterns of interconnection' in order that the inequalities of power in 'institutional terms' are not missed for over-regard to 'contingent networks'.[17] Markku Hokkanen's work on medical networks in Nyasaland builds on these insights, arguing for a distinction between 'hubs' as fluid points in a network and a 'nodal point' to represent a 'localised site of encounter, exchange and transmission'. Mission stations for Hokkanen could operate as 'nodal points' or 'nexuses', whereas other groups, such as the 'bioprospecting' of the Zambesi expedition which had far more mobility, can be defined as 'hubs'. This framework provides one way of understanding how mobility informed the creation of types of knowledge, without losing how the benefits of this process

were 'unevenly distributed between patients and practitioners', as well
as how colonial powers increasingly attempted to contain fluidity
'through permits and control measures'.[18] Crucially, medical missions
could be loose and informal, and they could also be a feature of more
formal national and transnational systems. Where different missions
fit in this framework could significantly affect their ability to endure
or not, over the long term.

Furthermore, the role of colonial and postcolonial governance
will be consistently assessed alongside more contingent international
networks. The legislative council debates, parliamentary assemblies,
and annual health reports of the Gold Coast and Ghana are all currently under-explored by historians. These sets of documents are
available in Balme Library at the University of Ghana, the library
of Korle Bu Teaching Hospital in Accra, the Liverpool School of
Tropical Medicine, and the British Library. They give a detailed picture of how political and national changes were experienced and
acted on by the colonial and postcolonial state.[19] Interrogating parliamentary records shows how there were changing faces of state
power which were in coordination with the varying fluidity and
rigidity of international networks. The complexity of the colonial
and postcolonial state over time can emerge from this more nuanced
analysis. So too can the diversity of missions' experience of shifts in
authority, hierarchy, and state control.

Various other historians, sociologists, and anthropologists have
written on the history of Ghanaian religion and health, which
this book will build on with a focus that is both more specific and
more broad. First, an important foundation is the work of Patrick
Twumasi, who produced varied and important medical sociological
research, particularly on indigenous/African medicine and medical
pluralism.[20] Far less well known are Twumasi's detailed local reports
on Catholic health in the early 1980s which will feature in chapters
3 and 5, and the appendix, of this book. Second, Barbra Mann Wall's
work on the Holy Family Hospital at Berekum in Ghana published in
2015 has described some of the hospital's hierarchies, the diseases it
had to treat, its maternal health aims, its nurse training programmes
for Ghanaians, and how Holy Family hospital was financed.[21] Yet
all this remains disconnected from what these low-level processes
meant within the local, regional, national, and international context, or within longer-term changes in medical mission. Third, Pascal
Schmid's work on the Protestant Basel Mission's Agogo Hospital

shows how the institution changed from its inception in the 1930s and pushed ahead with PHC reforms in the 1970s.[22] Schmid's focus provides important evidence and discussion from which can be built more extensive and broader analyses of mission, the Ghanaian state, and global health.[23] Fourth, a significant foundation can be found in the recent work of Jill Olivier and Annabel Grieve, who have charted the development of the Christian Health Association of Ghana (CHAG) with detailed maps showing the distribution of church hospitals since 1957 and their resilience to the present day.[24]

A foundational text in the history of Ghanaian health is K.D. Patterson's history from 1978 and 1981, which drew together state records and statistics to map how Ghanaian health changed.[25] Patterson built on the work of David Scott, the director of the medical field units (MFUs) in Ghana in the 1950s and early 1960s, which collated the incidence of disease in Ghana since the early 1900s.[26] Drawing on these early histories, Stephen Addae, a Ghanaian physician, compiled a three-volume history which was completed in 2012 for a Ghanaian press. Recently, Addae's work has become the most widely referenced history of Ghanaian medicine. It aims at recording the basic history of the MFUs, diseases, sanitation, health surveys, colonial medical policies, and medical staff. This is combined with a simple history of the 'principal' Ghanaian medical personalities and events, as well as a history of a variety of key institutions. While his history is certainly useful and detailed, Addae focuses generally on state health care and mission, ignoring the role of culture, theology, or politics. In his account, medicine operates in isolation from such dynamics, in a sphere of rationality and technocratic innovation.[27] As medical historians (including those of Ghana) have continually shown, medical culture changes over time due to factors that are not only the result of rational decision making but also the result of politics, economics, identities, materiality, and ideas. In medical mission especially, the categories of medicine and theology could be transcended and their boundaries blurred. In the Gold Coast and Ghana, medical missionary culture operated at many levels and had a variety of layered norms, ideas, politics, encounters, and financial choices. These all shaped the kind of medicine and mission that were produced and the kinds of national and international health that were possible.[28]

The overall historical picture of religion, development, and global health in Ghana that emerges reflects the fragility of the postcolonial nation-state, which has not been able to exert the same kind of technologies of rule over information as that of European nation-states.[29] The Ghanaian parliamentary records are largely complete for the 1950s and 1960s when the state was functioning fairly effectively, but trail off in the 1970s and are entirely absent for most of the next decade, not returning until the 1990s. Coups, revolutions, and the loss of archival stores meant that the Ghanaian state has struggled to impose much of a narrative on historical accounts. The effect of this incomplete record is that the early parts of this study can analyse in more depth government policies, missions, and the processes of statecraft; whereas in later parts of the research this is more difficult. Thus, only certain kinds of arguments can be made about the 1970s and 1980s, and these rely more on missionary and international records than on the nation-state's perspective itself. However, combined with the archives of medical missions and international organisations, these incomplete parliamentary papers remain a rich but neglected repository for historical enquiries to carve fresh paths and challenge older categories.

MAKING DEVELOPMENT:
EARLY TWENTIETH-CENTURY GOLD COAST

A theme that runs throughout this book and across the century covered, beginning in the early twentieth-century Gold Coast, is that medical missions were vital in the creation of the meanings, embodiment, and performance of development. Before moving on to the main chapters, this section will elucidate that early formational framework of development and the initial intimacy of mission and government which set the stage for later articulations of (and conflicts over) the concept. Missions in the 1920s were proactive in ensuring that the government conceptions of development were aligned with their own ways of viewing African advancement. This decade was a key period, a crucible of the creation of longer-term ideas and culture of development, and it was one in which medical mission was informing and defining the terms of operation. Christian human development and its temporal, racial framework was directly influential in the creation of high-level medical education and in the foundations of wider medical provision across the colony. Much of this occurred through collaboration between the African educator J.E.K. Aggrey, the Phelps Stokes Commission, Governor Gordon Guggisberg, and Scottish Presbyterian missionaries.

In the Gold Coast, a series of alliances resulted in the concept of development being framed in lasting ways by a particular religious tradition. The concept of development has been variously defined: for example, as the trajectory of human progress and civilisation, or as environmental and industrial productivity. Development has been seen as a spontaneous process, a structural driving force for change, or a programme of government intervention. Conflicting meanings did sometimes operate together; the term 'development' could provide an all-encompassing umbrella to allow diverse interests space to work in combination.[30] Yet, crucially, as Richard Drayton has shown, the concept of development was also imagined differently in specific imperial contexts depending on how colonists themselves were shaped by cultural encounters with non-Europeans.[31] It is not only its breadth of use that formed development as a concept – it was also its specific traditions of use and contexts of ideas and practice, such as the context of religion.[32] In its early phases, the colonial development encounter drew together a set of mission, state, and African interests under the label of 'development' in ways that created a specific and durable (though later contested) tradition of its practice.

As the Scottish Presbyterian mission grew rapidly from 1919, it became intimately aligned with the state and personally with Governor Guggisberg. Contrary to many other colonies, medical mission began in the Gold Coast in the nineteenth century but it was minimal in professional terms and it was almost entirely created to provide care for the missionaries themselves.[33] By 1900, there was some in-patient accommodation at a mission house at Aburi, but formal medical work was not the key feature of Protestant missionary practice and evangelism that it was in other areas of nineteenth-century colonial Africa.[34] On the eve of the First World War, Aburi had been consistently visited by Europeans and Africans and there were plans to turn it into a major hospital. However, this progress was arrested by the evictions of the Swiss Germans, leading to an overall drop in missionary numbers as the Scottish Presbyterians who were invited to plug the gap struggled to staff even this small facility.[35] The Presbyterians had to be given financial support from the government in order to send two women mission doctors to the Gold Coast mission.[36] With this backing they were able to grow. The two initial missionaries became part of a wider shift amongst mission and state toward the creation of child welfare clinics, as well as more widespread schools and hospitals.

Table I.1 Fluctuating missionary numbers in the Gold Coast
between 1908 and 1951

Year	1908	1919	1927–28	1935	1946	1951
Total missionaries in the Gold Coast	162	66	152	274	499	658

Sources: *Government of the Gold Coast: Medical and Sanitary Report for
the Year 1908* (Gold Coast: Government Printer, 1909), 6, Korle Bu Teaching
Hospital Library (Accra, Ghana); *Government of the Gold Coast Report on
the Medical Department for the Year 1920* (Gold Coast: Government Press,
Accra, 1921), 9, Korle Bu Teaching Hospital (Accra, Ghana); *Gold Coast
Colony Report on the Medical and Sanitary Department for the Financial
Year 1928–1929* (Gold Coast: Government Press, Accra, 1929), 15, Korle Bu
Teaching Hospital (Accra, Ghana); *Report on the Medical Department for the
Year 1947* (Accra: Government Printing Office, 1948), 12, Korle Bu Teaching
Hospital (Accra, Ghana); *Report on the Medical Department for the Year
1951* (Accra: Government Printing Office, 1952), 2–3, Korle Bu Teaching
Hospital (Accra, Ghana).

Quickly, Guggisberg's relationship with the Scottish Presbyterian
mission became close. Unlike in interwar Ceylon, for example
(where the state produced health-care development without missionaries), in the Gold Coast Protestant ideals and staff were a
critical feature of Guggisberg's vision of development in a model
colony in the 1920s.[37] In 1919, A.W. Wilkie became the head of
the Scottish Presbyterian mission in the Gold Coast that took over
from the Basel Mission. Guggisberg, Wilkie, and A.G. Fraser (who
oversaw educational development) became allies. In Wilkie's diary
he describes several dinners and even a bedside meeting with the
governor discussing medicine. Wilkie also joined the board of visitors for the colonial hospitals – this in addition to his more formally
ecclesiastical duties travelling widely to assess disease outbreaks and

standards in mission schools.[38] In the first chapter of this book the wider consequences for health care of this alliance will be analysed in more detail. For example, chapter 1 will show how the intimacy of Guggisberg and the Presbyterians ultimately led to the government attempt at the total handover of all maternal and child health to the missions in 1926.

Between 1919 and 1927, when Guggisberg stepped down, there was huge spending on hospital, dispensary, and public health improvements. From 1 January 1920 to 31 March 1927 there were nineteen new hospitals. Sixteen of these facilities were built by the Public Works Department and they ranged in size from the massive 220-bed Gold Coast Hospital in Accra (costing £254,343) to the smallest form which had 'a ward of from 4 to 12 beds, operating theatre, dispensary, offices, stores, and mortuary'. Additions (in many cases the doubling of accommodation) were also made to twelve of the old hospitals, such as in Kumasi, where the extension was so large that it effectively amounted to a new hospital. An extra twenty dispensaries were also built.[39]

In 1915, £25,118 16s. 5d. was spent by the Public Works Department on sanitation, with an additional £53,117 2s. 5d. by the head of sanitation and £1570 4s. 9d. on sleeping sickness prevention.[40] By 1927, sanitation spending had risen greatly. Between 1925 and 1927 spending on water supplies, town improvements, special anti-plague measures, electric light, hospitals, and dispensaries amounted to between 16.2 and 17.7 per cent of total revenue. This was estimated at £670,000 for 1926–27 and then £755,000 for 1927–28.[41] By the end of Guggisberg's tenure, the health-care infrastructure in the Gold Coast had well more than doubled and there were about thirty-seven hospitals with around 800 beds.[42]

For the Gold Coast government, in the context of limited financial backing from the Colonial Office, local Europeans, medicals missionaries, Africans, and the West African Medical Service (WAMS) were more significant than those in the metropole. Up to the 1930s there were loans and funds being created for colonial development, especially in the poorer areas of East Africa; however, there was not a root change from West African supervisory model of pre-First World War policy.[43] Instead, governors like Guggisberg had considerable room to make their own agenda through local taxation, private investment, and raising loans on the London stock market (a source far bigger than British imperial government expenditure).[44]

Table I.2 Gold Coast Medical, Sanitation, and Research Department
spending between 1919 and 1927

Year	1919	1926	1927
Medical, Sanitation and Research Department Spending (£)	121,000	294,000	305,000

Sources: 'Review of Public Health Work, 1920–1927', 3 March 1927, *Gold Coast Colony Legislative Council Debates No. 1 Session 1927–8*, 185–6, Balme Library, University of Ghana (Accra).

There were also immediate improvements in export revenue at the outset of Guggisberg's tenure.[45]

Guggisberg borrowed large sums to pay for roads, harbours, schools, and hospitals to create his own model colony – but he needed local support.[46] On the eve of the Second World War, the administrative division of the African colonial service (including district officers and the central secretariat) only numbered around 1,200 men.[47] Colonies could not administratively spread much beyond their capitals, or, in the Gold Coast, much beyond the South and Asante. With the Gold Coast colonial government stretched across a large land mass, relations with non-European and non-state actors were vital. How Guggisberg conducted and imagined these communities could shape how development was managed and executed, and who was involved. First, relations with chiefs were particularly significant because the Gold Coast followed an 'indirect rule' system, as made famous by Lord Lugard in northern Nigeria where resources were scarce and Islamic communities sizeable.[48] Second, Guggisberg had to negotiate with local Europeans who resisted when he tried to add more African doctors to their notoriously racist health-care service.[49] Third were medical missions.

Allying with missionaries, Guggisberg formed his own Christian agenda for human development which, using his model colony, he performed to a wider English imperial audience. In 1929 Guggisberg published a book on the 'development of a race' with Gold Coast

Table I.3 Gold Coast exports and imports between 1919 and 1920

Year	Total Exports and Imports (£)	Value of imports (£)
1919	26,000,000	8,000,000
1920	17,500,000	14,000,000

Sources: *Government of the Gold Coast: Medical and Sanitary Report for the Year 1908* (Gold Coast: Government Printer, 1909), 6, Korle Bu Teaching Hospital Library (Accra, Ghana); *Government of the Gold Coast Report on the Medical Department for the Year 1920* (Gold Coast: Government Press, Accra, 1921), 9, Korle Bu Teaching Hospital (Accra, Ghana); *Gold Coast Colony Report on the Medical and Sanitary Department for the Financial Year 1928–1929* (Gold Coast: Government Press, Accra, 1929), 15, Korle Bu Teaching Hospital (Accra, Ghana); *Report on the Medical Department for the Year 1947* (Accra: Government Printing Office, 1948), 12, Korle Bu Teaching Hospital (Accra, Ghana); *Report on the Medical Department for the Year 1951* (Accra: Government Printing Office, 1952), 2–3, Korle Bu Teaching Hospital (Accra, Ghana).

missionary teacher A.G. Fraser, and referred to A.W. Wilkie. In this work, Guggisberg and Fraser laid out a vision for universal develop- ment in which Africans would be incorporated into the worldwide Christian church. From there the 'race' would be re-engineered by the terms of the 'abundant' life offered in Christ, as described in the Gospel of John. Guggisberg envisaged this form of Christian human development to be the true outworking of policies of 'trusteeship' and the colonial civilising mission. He wrote that:

> Accepting trusteeship as our policy, it is advisable to have a clear idea of what the development of a people means. In the highest sense the development of a people should be based on the Christian ideal ... A. W. Wilkie, the experienced missionary and educator said ... 'in the words of our Lord: "I am come that they might have life, and that they might have it abundantly ..."' Nothing could more adequately express the highest and widest meaning of the word development as applied to the people.[50]

In this description, development as 'applied to the people' is
expressed in terms of the highest ideals of Christian evangelism, to
invite the stranger into the fold of the church. Little was said about
the outworking of this development for direct economic progress; the
aim was for the creation of a racial leadership in Christ. Guggisberg
went on to write: 'Our task today is infinitely more difficult, including as it now does moral and intellectual as well as material, development. It is precisely because we have this dual task that we want
more and more the best that England can give us; not only the best
in science and professions, but men and women imbued with the real
Christian spirit – the spirit of the life and teachings of Jesus, love of
mankind and a desire for service ... there is no greater work that an
Englishman can do for mankind'.[51]

For the leading missionary statesmen J.H. Oldham (who wrote
extensively on Christianity, race, and colonialism), economic development and Christian human development were tied together in 1920s
and 1930s British imperialism.[52] For Guggisberg there was similar
coordination, but he went further to foreground morality over technology. Material progress, technological advancement, and professional aid were only part of the role of English colonialism in his
vision. More than economic, technocratic, or scientific expertise, colonialism required 'moral and intellectual' teaching. In this regard, such
human progress would be modelled by 'men and women imbued with
the real Christian spirit' whose lives were embedded in biblical teaching and in the outworking of the love found through a life in Christ.
Guggisberg wanted a specific type of Christian developmentalist colonial state. These statements were directly disseminated to the wider
imperial audience in order to bolster the moral image of his colony, as
well as to entice further colonisers with opportunities for performing
certain muscular Christian identities in the Gold Coast. This dissemination can be registered in the book's positive contemporary reviews
from the International African Institute and the *Journal of the African
Society*.[53] Moreover, it was given wide coverage amongst potential
recruits to both medical missions and the Colonial Service by being
published by the Student Christian Movement, which between 1890
and the 1960s was Britain's largest student religious body.[54]

This Christian vision for human development was bound up
with the improvement of health care in the colony. The book's
authors wrote that the elusive power of Christian character
might be imbibed by teaching sanitary hygiene and thus 'moral

hygiene'. This had social power to change the character of the race, in Guggisberg's eyes, as well as the individual African believer or citizen. Importantly, the authors wrote that all this could be as much the hallmark of government schools and hospitals as of mission ones. This was because missions often suffered by becoming the 'battle-ground of denominational enthusiasms'. Again, for Guggisberg, development meant spiritual as well as material growth, and he wanted practising and believing Christian staff to fill education and medicine in the Gold Coast:

> Some people would prefer to deal with character training and religious teaching separately; others to omit the latter entirely. Neither of these courses can be followed if successful results are to be achieved. The character of a child, in whatever degree it may be inherited, cannot be developed unless religion forms the basis of character training. By religion, I mean Christian habits of life and thought. However much some may hold the view that Christianity had failed to maintain peace and goodwill in the world, the fact remains that it is the highest practical system of life that the world has known ... I wish to emphasize that character training, unlike the Scriptures, cannot be a subject of instruction; but, like real Christianity, it can unconsciously be imbibed by the pupil in every act of school life if opportunities are made.[55]

Both in clinics and in schools, the vision for human development was that it would be 'imbibed' in an unconscious way, by the 'real' Spirit of Christianity. In this section the authors were laying out a way of developing the race through the development of 'habits of life and thought'. Godly character would emerge through the 'highest practical system of life'. Importantly for health care, Guggisberg conceived of human development in terms of the non-material power of Christ on the unconscious mind. Thus, clinics with the atmosphere of the Holy Spirit could be as powerful in the human development of the race as schools and direct 'religious teaching'. Moreover, Fraser made the connection even more explicit arguing that 'mission hospitals and welfare centres can be run at far less cost than Government institutions. But their greatest advantage is that in them the spirit of service is eager and constant ... Mission control, too, generally allows much more adaptability to local circumstances and gives more time to the doctor to do his real job, and by long continuance in one place, to know and be known by the people. Thus he becomes a trusted friend'.[56] In this description of the advantage of medical missions over those of government, Fraser depicts mission in the classic terms of long-term 'continuance', trust, and relationship in one place. This would both allow the missionaries to be in control and adapt to local culture, and also show through the spirit of 'eager and constant' service the truth of the gospel.

In high-level medical education, the government and mission worked closely with international partners to advance their Christian vision for human development in the Gold Coast and more widely.[57] As with Gold Coast developmentalism generally, the drive for elite medical education included Guggisberg, Presbyterian missionaries, and Fraser. These key figures in Gold Coast development were brought together and promoted by an international organisation, the Phelps Stokes Commission. The Phelps Stokes education survey between 1920 and 1921 provided a platform and funding in the Gold Coast for colonial government, mission-educated Africans, Protestant missions, American education philanthropy, and African Americans to work together on high-level medical education, among other things. A central figure in this process was J.E.K. Aggrey, who had been funded by the A.M.E. Zion Church (the first American mission church in the Gold Coast) to return to the United States to study at the church's Livingstone College, where he spent two decades as a student and teacher. Through this, Aggrey had been drawn into Phelps Stokes by its educational director Jesse Jones, whom Aggrey met when Jones was a preaching as a chaplain at Hampton Institute. Aggrey became one of Phelps Stokes's key speakers around Africa because of his passion for racial harmony based on cooperation and the Tuskegee model of education led by Booker T. Washington.[58]

Through the first Phelps Stokes education survey in Africa, Aggrey developed a close relationship with Guggisberg and the Gold Coast mission leaders.[59] As Guggisberg wrote in the first commission report, the education survey and Aggrey's visit to the Gold Coast 'was productive of great good' and showed that 'our educational progress is proceeding steadily in the right direction'. Wilkie was also quoted extensively. In spite of its challenges to imperial rule, the survey's conclusions became influential for the Colonial Office who suggested they produce a second education survey of Africa because the first was so successful.[60] They did, and the second in 1924 was partly funded by the Rockefeller Commission, another international organisation embedded in mission networks and one which would later develop international health campaigns.[61] The Phelps Stokes Commission brought together diverse actors in the mid-1920s under similar ideas with aims of building an elite college and medical school. In the Gold Coast, the suggestions became a new education ordinance in 1925, taking effect two years later.

In conceiving of elite medical education, African American accommodationist theory intersected with older colonial ideas of race and Christian character. For the Gold Coast the key effect of the Phelps Stokes Commission was to form a mission and government team which would build and staff the college of Achimota along the Christian accommodationist lines of Washington and Aggrey, shaping for generations the nation's vision for developing health care.[62] The Gold Coast government aimed to ensure that aspiring medical students did not have to leave the Gold Coast because, as the legislative council put it in 1927:

> owing to the absence of suitable hostels in Great Britain,
> it was impossible for Africans there to develop character
> satisfactorily ... [The conditions are] in the majority of cases
> injurious to his character. His previous education in the Gold
> Coast has not prepared him to meet them ... the only remedy
> was for the Gold Coast to start a medical school of its own ... it
> was probable that during the first few years of the school's exis-
> tence it might be necessary for African students to complete their
> training in Great Britain; but that there would be less harmful
> result owing to the opportunities for developing character that
> would be given both at Achimota and in the Medical School.[63]

As already described in Guggisberg's development theorising, Christian 'character' was at the centre of these plans. Guggisberg had also written of his concerns about the dangerous influence of foreign travel on elite Africans in a 'Review of 1920' for the Gold Coast Pioneer, in which he argued:

> A few of our citizens, unfortunately only a few, have received a
> higher education. As this, however, has usually been received in
> Europe it by no means follows that it does not bring with it a
> certain danger, for it must be dangerous to send a youth away to
> a foreign country during the most impressionable time of his life

when he incurs the risk of becoming so impressed with European
institution as to run a grave change of losing touch with his
people ... a race must learn to think before it can cope with the
great rush of a civilisation which is alien to it.[64]

Here Guggisberg and the Presbyterian missionaries' conception of
racial development directly impinged on the way in which development spending was focused. Given his elitist model, a higher education was vital to ensuring that Christian character drove the African
leaders who were increasingly taking a key role within government.
For example, between 1921 and 1922 there were fifty-seven 'Special
Native Appointments' to the government, compared with twenty-six
in 1919. These were within technical departments, but the role of
native authorities and the power of chiefs within the Legislative
Assembly was also growing.[65]

For Guggisberg, human development in the Gold Coast was imagined in terms of the interaction between leaders and the people, and
framed by his temporal understanding of racial progress. In the view
of Guggisberg and other like-minded groups, education had to ensure
that there were not irreparable socio-political divisions created by
training Africans abroad and severing them from their roots before
sending them back to their homelands. Guggisberg's conception of
African development had protectionist and conservative underpin-
nings about the speed of change for African character, and its pater-
nalism was expressed through concern for not dismantling 'the race'
through rapid civilization. As Christopher Clark has elucidated, the
operation of power in statecraft bears significantly on conceptions
of time: 'As gravity bends light, so power bends time'. In the Gold
Coast, conceptions of racial time, and the relationship between past,
present, and future, were being determined by the state in dialogue
with Christian ideas about character. As Clark argues for different
German political regimes, there were 'temporal textures', and the
'sequence that results is more oscillating, recursive, and nonlinear
than a strongly sequential and modernisation-based theory would
allow'.[66] This way of historicising the relationship between time and
modernisation figures importantly in the creation of imperial models of civilisation. Guggisberg envisioned a specific temporal texture
to the way health, education, race, and civilisation were intercon-
nected. These were held together and aligned in a temporal framework. This was not linear but recursive and oscillating in dialogue

with nineteenth-century ways of viewing Christian eschatology or racial progress. Crucially, these attempts to construct time and race emerged in this very particular context of rapid development, government-linked religion, and emerging colonial statecraft. They were also particular to a commonly repeated West African concern about male development and sexuality.

It may have been that Guggisberg and Aggrey were concerned about the pace of change within African men. They were not alone in being anxious about how progress might detach educated African men from their communities and traditions. The popular moralising tract *Marita or the Folly of Love* serialised in a newspaper in the Gold Coast in 1886 challenged colonial legal marriage as unsuited to the civilisational position of the African man. Crucially, the text navigated divisions in literacy and the risk that the latter might lead to undue domination within male-female relations. For example, there was particular concern that men who could read should not run Bible study groups where they could control women. *Marita* provided a script for an African civilised masculinity which was not too detached from past norms.[67] These concerns had been shared by Fantes like Aggrey in 1902 who, through the Aborigines Rights Protection Society, argued that they wanted 'educated Fantis not Europeanised natives'. Guggisberg's concerns about racial development, in addition to making certain that traditional norms were included in development, may have been related to these older models of a careful pace of change, which aimed not to disrupt racial unity but to map out a civilised African masculinity. His trade schools at Kyebi, Asante-Mampong, Asuantsi, and Yendi in the 1920s aimed to ensure that educated Africans also could still work with their hands, rather than thinking manual labour to be a 'disgrace'.[68]

For Guggisberg, development funding in the interwar Gold Coast was also divided up based on a model of extraction of labour from the South, facilitating the transition to cash crops in Asante and civilisational human development (schools and universities) on the coast. Guggisberg's vision for human development in the capital was structured around a geography of exploitation and capitalist progress in Asante, where cocoa and mineral exports such as gold were largely produced. In order to secure the necessary labour for gaining tax revenues on income and on exports, the Northern Territories were viewed as a labour reservoir that should not be developed too much. As John Nott's path-breaking work on the spatial aspects of nutritional health has shown, education was actively held back in the North to all but the most exceptional boys.[69] Instead, fighting yaws and trypanosomiasis was focused on ensuring stability in the animal population and health in labouring men. By contrast, measles, which probably was one of the biggest killers in the North even in this period, was almost completely ignored. The Gold Coast Ministry of Health report in 1953 noted that the disease had not been discussed in previous annual reports.[70] In Asante, much medical mission work was begun in the interwar years. Only with determination and some conflict could missionaries set up any health institutions in the North before the mid-1940s; the real expansion had to wait until the wider agenda of the first central national development plans in the 1950s. In the South, there were extensive discussions about the extent of development. However, the major concern for the South and Accra was to produce a cadre of Christian leadership which could manage the other regions. Guggisberg's human development relied on extraction and coercion in the North and high-level leadership development in Accra, and the extent of his funding was shaped by geographies of neglect.

For Aggrey, a Cape Coast Fante, Christianity, mission, and the medical school also figured in disputes over authority within colonial governance and how the sacral space of 1920s Accra was mapped. There were divisions within regions and between ethnic groups, as well as across the colony. For Aggrey, the medical school work was linked to harmony between the races on the lines of gradual training programmes at Tuskegee. It may also have been linked to the long-term attempts of the Cape Coast Fante elite to push for political power and status within the capital since the early twentieth century. For decades, the Fante elite (which counted Aggrey as a member) had despised the role of the Ga ethnic group in Accra, and challenged it with a modernising Christian discourse of access to education and rejection of traditional culture. Frustrated at being away from the centre of power, in 1903 the Cape Coast Fante elite had fulminated in their paper the *Gold Coast Leader* at the 'fetish' dances that were allowed in Accra and argued that these should not be tolerated by any 'civilized and Christian government'.[71]

Power inequalities on the coast were being repeated in battles over elite medical education in the 1920s. The Cape Coast elite wanted to secure their place in the increasing inclusion of Africans in the Legislative Assembly and technical advisory roles. It was not new to utilise concepts of civilised Christianity in government to support claims to ethnic power. Still, this was not simply pragmatic. Ethnic disputes intersected with religious battles for Accra – a landscape considered sacral by the Ga-Adangme tribes whose ancestral and ritual topography continued to matter in the capital in the 1920s. As John Parker has shown, there were a variety of competing visions of the city in 1920s Accra, with Christianity 'gradually form(ing) a new moral community and offering an alternative vision of the future'.[72] At stake here was not simply financial and political power but also ritual power. Placing the medical school on this landscape was for Aggrey and Guggisberg a part of the ongoing conflict between civilising Christian mission, traditional religion, and government over who had spiritual authority within the colonial capital. These represented overlapping geographies of ritual and modernisation.[73]

In spite of colonial intentions, a medical school did not materialise in Accra until the 1960s, but through the Phelps Stokes Commission, missionaries, and the colonial government, Achimota College did embody ideals of elite Christian human development. Most of the Phelps Stokes suggestions were unable to be put into practice; their standards were simply too high and in the Gold Coast by 1930, 150 'bush schools' had to close, at a time when only 10 per cent of the children in the colony had any education.[74] In 1924 Achimota was set up by Aggrey, Guggisberg, and Fraser, who had met Aggrey at J.H. Oldham's home in Surrey.[75] It was financed originally with £607,000, which was around 85 per cent of the entire 1920s development budget, and then in the 1940s it was given another £127,000 through the Colonial Welfare and Development Act.[76] Achimota became the school which produced the majority of the politicians, lawyers, and doctors of independent Ghana who began their careers in the 1950s and 1960s. These figures imbued the school and its pupils with an international Christian vision of race, development, and health.

Along with Guggisberg and the missionaries, Aggrey disseminated and embodied a very specific kind of Christian development culture within Achimota which had implications for health care – in ways that lasted across many decades. After his death in 1927, Aggrey was consistently cited and his memory battled over as a symbol of African development, internationalism, modernity, progress, and religion. As Guggisberg said of him at the memorial service: 'he had two incalculably valuable assets – faith in God and faith in his people ... Only the real faith that lifted him above himself could

have sustained through the last three years and he had that faith –
the real faith of a real Christian ... Aggrey indeed was the finest
interpreter which the present century has produced of the white man
to the black'.[77] Fraser added: 'He was one of the purest men I have
ever met ... He it was who persuaded me to go out to Achimota'.[78]
Alongside these articles were numerous tributes in the *Gold Coast
Leader* by Africans. In spite of his death, Aggrey's alliance with the
missions and Guggisberg in the 1920s framed how development
would be imagined as it expanded hugely in the ensuing decades.
The combined role of this group was to forge a set of religious meanings and practices for health and development which were fought
over consistently by a diverse array of individuals and organisations
during the next seventy years. Notably, it was at Achimota, when he
was a pupil and teacher, that Kwame Nkrumah was introduced to
the thought and writing of W.E.B. Du Bois and Marcus Garvey – by
Aggrey himself.[79] Ultimately, in the crucible of ideas about development in the 1920s, through the construction of a model colony,
an agenda and an imaginative landscape were created for the Gold
Coast and Ghana, in which religion and health were bound up with
one another for the long term.

The Colonial Foundations of Global Health:
Britain, Gold Coast, and Ghana, 1919–61

Twenty-first-century global health governance is not newly pushing up against national sovereignty or distinct from international
health – a more historically nuanced narrative is needed to challenge these overly simplistic dividing lines. International health was
formed in the context of nations redefining themselves politically
on the basis of imperial infrastructures that they could not dismantle. Former colonies are structured in ways that only make sense in
the wider imperial context of their creation. It was in the context
of determining the limits of national sovereignty and creating collaborations to stave off former colonial powers' control that much
of modern international governance was formed. Global health is
no different in this from international health. There are significant
continuities between global health and international health; the line
subdividing them has unhelpfully placed them within analytical
frameworks that distort the long histories of their emergence. Both
require a more historically detailed narrative of the infrastructure,
culture, and ideas that make up the local and regional contexts to
which they relate.

This chapter will detail how between 1919 and 1961 missionary
health infrastructure in the Gold Coast and Ghana grew at a rapid
and extraordinary rate. The foundations created in a network of
hospitals, clinics, and dispensaries formed the core around which
the rest of health provision would grow over the rest of the century.
Between 1951 and 1960, across the divide of independence won in
1957, the government would build four hospitals. Missionaries built
twenty-three.[1] As a result of a combination of factors, medical mission grew rapidly in the 1950s and ensured that their institutions,

beliefs, and culture would remain long after the formal end of colonialism in 1957. The ramifications of this change were widespread and repeated across Sub-Saharan Africa in francophone as well as anglophone contexts. It is necessary to understand this infrastructure if we are to comprehend the health campaigns of the 1950s and 1960s, the declines in medical provision in the 1970s and 1980s, and the restorations of the 1990s onwards.

This chapter will look first at the dominating role of the Scottish Presbyterians on health in the 1920s and their declining power in the 1930s. The second section will then explore the denominational diversification of medical mission and the growing 'voluntary sector' in the 1940s and 1950s. Focusing on the mid-1950s to the early 1960s, the final section will then analyse the contrasts between the Seventh-day Adventists (SDAs) at Kwahu who benefitted from the voluntary sector, the Pentecostals and Scottish Presbyterians at Sandema in the North who navigated its boundaries, and the Roman Catholic missions who turned down its funding. Ultimately, across these processes no single mission was normative; medical missions were heterogenous and there was a variety of ways in which they imagined their work. The chapter closes by assessing the disconnects in expectations and narrative between missions, African communities, medical officers, and government officials that coincided with increasing formalised structure.

MEDICAL MISSIONARIES AND THE EXPANSION OF THE COLONIAL STATE

Missions were laying the groundwork in the 1930s for what would become a huge part of Ghanaian health infrastructure and a network of health practitioners, clinics, and dispensaries that was necessary for international health campaigns to be possible from the 1950s onwards. In conceptual terms and in logistical ones, this period was critical for setting in motion international health policies in the twentieth century. It is in these battles for local and national supremacy that global health acquired the conditions in which it could function. Though the role of the Scottish Presbyterians declined after 1927 and the government's relationship with missions became more diffuse, the close connection between development and religion in the Gold Coast remained significant. Much like networks of colonial science that informed international health, networks of colonial medical mission were influential for what would later emerge in global health.

In the 1920s mission and colonial efforts at development had led to the growth of maternal and child health care in the Gold Coast. Child welfare work was begun by the Scottish mission in January 1921 by Dr Jessie Beveridge, who, according to government reports, 'opened a clinic and dispensary for the treatment of minor ailments of school children and infants at Christiansborg, Accra'. It was a roaring success and quickly led to the government 'supplying drugs and paying the salary of an interpreter'. Amidst a death rate of 400 per 1,000 births in some areas, the clinic was seen as an oasis by the government, and between 1923 and 1924 the government extended its own efforts by setting up temporary infant welfare centres in Christiansborg and James Town under Dr Mary Magill and other female medical officers. By 1926 the government built the Princess Mary Louise Hospital for children, with a woman European medical officer, 'African subordinate staff', and two nurse midwives. In addition, a dispensary was set up to carry on Beveridge's work and the medical officer was posted to Sekondi to begin a welfare centre and weekly clinic in Chama. In the first eight months of the 1926 financial year, the Princess Mary Louise Hospital had 8,444 attendances, the clinic at Christiansborg had 2,987, and the centre at Sekondi had 4,964.[2]

In public health too, when efforts extended beyond Accra, particularly into rural areas, missionaries were crucial.[3] This was the case in maternal and child health, and the dissemination of hygiene messages particularly. For example, in the eastern Gold Coast, the British Togoland Report of 1924 to the League of Nations wrote that 'the presence of a qualified woman doctor on the staff of the mission, concentrating on Infant Welfare, has been a benefit to some outlying districts beyond the regular scope of Government Medical Officers. In her dispensary at Amedjope, and at many villages on tour she has, by individual treatment and general instruction, and by the circulation of appropriate literature among the more intelligent people, secured the confidence of the community, and she is now endeavouring to bring about a necessary improvement in the health conditions of mothers and children and to check the heavy infant mortality'.[4]

Mission contacts could also be vital in sanitation and vaccination campaigns.[5] In A.W. Wilkie's diary he consistently notes his own inspection of sanitation and standards across the mission schools across the Gold Coast, and details the outbreak of yellow fever in August 1926. Although, as A.G. Fraser wrote, the separation of the government medical and education department meant that schools were under-utilised in their capacity to help hookworm campaigns and antenatal care, Wilkie shows how in the 1920s they were used as sites for vaccinations.[6] Where missionary education was more sporadic, for example in the Northern Territories, the colonial government had far less information or capacity to extend. Wilkie describes the significance of travelling medical missionaries such as Helen Russell, surveying a range of outposts and clinics.[7] Beyond maternal and child health work, missionary networks both medically trained or otherwise were critical for the state to be able to extend their health work into new areas.

Missionaries became such a key feature of Gold Coast colonial health that there were (unsuccessful) attempts by Guggisberg to hand over the entire maternal and child health-care system to the Presbyterians. Simultaneously with large expansions in colonial infant welfare work, in April 1926, government officials met with a Presbyterian committee 'to consider the taking over by the Missions of the Welfare work in the large centres in the Gold Coast' and 'the transfer of all welfare work including the existing work in Accra and Sekondi' to the missions. The conclusions were in favour of considerable cooperation:

> It was the opinion of the Director of Medical and Sanitary Services of that period that such work could only be successful if carried out by the Missionary Societies ... the success and development of the work can only be guaranteed if the original suggestion is adopted of asking the Missions to become responsible for all welfare work for women and children. The object of the Government is not primarily to secure economy but success ... The recommendations were approved generally by the Governor who name the Scottish Mission as the Mission to be asked to initiate the scheme ... A letter from the Colonial Secretary, of 14th April, was read conveying the thanks of the Governor to the members of the Committee and noting with pleasure the willingness of Mr Wilkie to refer the matter to headquarters; also asking, in the event of the Secretary of State approving the transfer, if the Scottish Mission is prepared to take over the present work

at Sekondi, and to advise, in consultation with the Director of
Medical and Sanitary Services, as to priority of further building
at Sekondi or Akwapim ... Council records its sense of the high
honour conferred on the Mission by the request to undertake
this responsible work for women and children.[8]

What came of these committee meetings and experiments has not
been recorded. However, the Presbyterian Mission did not fully gain
the monopoly over maternal and child health that Guggisberg seems
to have been planning for it in 1926. When Guggisberg handed over
to Slater who became governor in 1927, the stage was set for the
expansion of maternal and child health in mission work – but from
a wider set of practitioners. Not only did new governors and the lift-
ing of the papal ban in the following five to ten years draw Roman
Catholics in, they allowed back the Bremen and Basel missionaries,
and they facilitated the emergence of the International Committee
of the Red Cross as one of the top three largest actors in Gold Coast
infant welfare, alongside government and mission.

At the same time as he was empowering the Presbyterian missions,
Guggisberg had been restricting Catholic missions until convinced of
their loyalty. Up to 1926 there was struggle and negotiation between
Guggisberg and the Presbyterians on one side, and the Catholic missions on the other. In 1906 a White Fathers Catholic mission post
in the Northern Territories of the Gold Coast had been founded by
the 'Vicarde Apostolique du Soudan' (later Ouagadougou) but had
since not developed independently.[9] Tension grew in 1924 when
the Gold Coast government decided to set up schools in the North
with Protestant missions, which Leonide Barsalou noted would have
been harmful to the already financially struggling Catholic mission. In order to stop this 'invasion protestante' the White Fathers
attempted to expand their schools and missions in spite of a lack
of finances and personnel. Immediately they encountered opposition from the government, who, according to Barsalou, were concerned that French missionaries might be spies in the service of the
neighboring colony. Thus, the White Fathers appealed to Rome to
separate them from the Haute Volta diocese and create an autonomous mission at Navrongo. The Gold Coast government responded
immediately to this, offering to send £100 in a grant when it had
been completed. In June 1927 the White Fathers Catholic mission
became the 'Prefecture Apostolique de Navrongo'. After this there

were few conflicts with the government, who were described by the Catholics as assuring their liberty of conscience.[10] It was only in non-religious training that the governor demanded 'final control'. By 1930 the mission had expanded and put a medical dispensary in every mission station, which gave government employees free treatment. The Catholic mission had also been able to set up a special leprosy centre at Navrongo. Nevertheless, the Presbyterians still had power over the French missions. A.G. Fraser was deployed to inspect the Catholic mission schools – though he was very positive about the progress that was being made.[11]

Yet there were limits to the power of the Presbyterians before 1927, too – actual experiences, effects, and interpretations of religious visions for development were varied and cut in directions that its architects could not always control. The upheaval of the government expulsion of the Basel Mission and its replacement with the Scottish caused considerable protest from African Christians in the colony. For example, the Scottish Presbyterians may have seamlessly replaced the Basel Mission in the eyes of the colonial government, but indigenous Abokabi Christians were far less amenable to such a sudden change enacted by the state, especially as it resulted from diplomatic issues external to the colony. Many towns and congregations of African Christians desperately wanted the Basel missionaries to return, as can be seen in several articles and letters in the African-run newspaper the *Gold Coast Independent* in the early 1920s. The Scottish were regularly denounced. In one article subtitled 'The Essence of the Basel Mission Spirit and the Failure of the Scottish Mission Bluff', the writer attacked the newcomers' superficiality: 'Whatever you do, you cannot vie with the Originators. In theirs, was no superficiality. And, most unfortunately, this keynote happens to underrun the whole system. Upwards of four years tutelage has failed to scottishfy our well seasoned mentality. If we keep intact our wind and limb, it is the Basel Mission Spirit that still sustains us; but what, when says its last as it surely must?'[12]

Another article suggested that ten thousand full communicants had 'evinced great interest in the return of the Basel Missionaries'. While a later piece denounced any statistical claims without evidence and a letter from the congregation in Akropong defended the 'rescue' of the mission by the Scottish, there was a considerable amount of bitterness at the forced departure of the Basel missionaries.[13] Furthermore, while missions often aimed to reformulate domestic structures and produce paragons of Christian motherhood through hygiene practices and the rituals of child and maternal health, these efforts were contested and challenged. Missions could not always structure their encounters or the way they were interpreted by local communities.[14]

In practice, amidst local tensions, missionaries often prioritised their own survival over reforming communities. In some instances, the simplifying categories that missionaries used to classify the non-Christian world were put aside in the lived experience of intimacy and exchange in the cultural encounters of the mission field.[15] For example, in 1926 in the Scottish medical and educational mission at Abokabi on the Southern Gold Coast, Wilkie wrote in his diary of how the missionaries had to rely on help from the chief to force local African Christians into providing labour for sanitary improvements to the school, otherwise the mission would be 'lost'. Negotiation with and reliance on traditional authority was sanitised in Guggisberg and Fraser's heroic development narratives, but adaptability and shrewdness were vital to the survival of a mission. Wilkie's diary shows that in practice missionaries prioritised their own long-term survival by negotiating with local traditional authorities, even if that meant using the power of the chieftaincy to bully local African Christians.[16] Robert Rothberg has emphasised how Ugandan missions were reliant on chiefs in their early and fledgling stages in the nineteenth century, but even missions such as that of Abokabi, which had been running since 1854 under the Basel Mission, could be vulnerable to local community power.[17]

Though they remained influential, the close Scottish Presbyterian relations with the government began to decline after Guggisberg left in 1927. An ecumenical organisation, the Christian Council of the Gold Coast (CCGC), was formed in 1929 following the 1926 Le Zoute conference.[18] The first joint secretary of the CCGC from 1929–31 was the Scottish Presbyterian mission leader – Wilkie. However, in the 1930s, the number of actors and groups in Gold Coast health care expanded and grew, especially empowering Catholic missions, the Basel Mission (for a short time), the Red Cross, and the Bremen mission. In the 1930s Catholic medical mission was being widely financed by the government and Sisters were empowered by the papacy to acquire formal medical training. Already there was a dispensary being set up at Kpandu in 1926 and extended to Djodje under the Sisters of Mercy.[19] By 1934 grants were being given to

Catholic medical missions at Kpandu, Oeikwe, Akim Swedru, Asankrangwa, and Djodji in the central, western, and eastern provinces of the colony.[20] In 1934 the mission in Djodje saw 6,560 children attend, in Eikwe it was 22,143, and in Kpandu it was 20,710.[21] In 1931, the Basel Mission, restored to the Gold Coast from 1926, opened a hospital at Agogo near Kumasi – though in 1940 this was closed and the staff detained. The Basel Mission's attempts to set up at Mampong and Juaso were blocked by the Scottish mission and the government, much to the chagrin of Agogo's doctors.[22] By the 1940s the Red Cross had gone from being a minor player to one of the largest actor in maternal and child health centres.[23]

Along with government officers, the Red Cross dealt with 22,789 attendances in Accra and 19,702 in Kumasi. Moreover, a Red Cross Sister was in charge of the Kumasi weighing centre and domiciliary. Even at this point the government report stated that 'a wide future would appear to lie before the (Red Cross) Society in the continuation and extension of this valuable side of their field activities'.[24] Last was the Bremen mission, which returned to the Gold Coast and set up an infant welfare clinic at Amedzope, where, in 1935, 2,363 children were attending.[25] With this work the government approved a scheme for twenty-eight midwives-in-training to have hostel.[26]

Campaigns against leprosy, increasingly funded by the government, became the focus of possible interdenominational cohesion in the 1930s.[27] In the Gold Coast, the government had been interested in leprosy work since the 1910s, and in possibly working with Catholic missionaries in this regard.[28] In 1918 there was some consideration by the government's principal medical officer of training the White Fathers around Navrongo in professional medical work because of their utility in describing the incidence of leprosy cases in the Northern Territories. In 1930, this sort of state support was furthered with Dr Seth-Smith who arrived from Lawra with medical supplies and trained the White Fathers in treating common illnesses.[29] As with child and maternal health, by the mid-1930s the government was considering giving missionaries control of all leprosy work, and in the early 1940s the director of Medical Services proposed that it all could be 'safely entrusted to missionary societies' – but this did not materialise. Some of the missionary societies would not consider the proposal until after the Second World War, and those that would wanted money that the Colonial Office would not provide. Though the new governor Alan Burns wanted

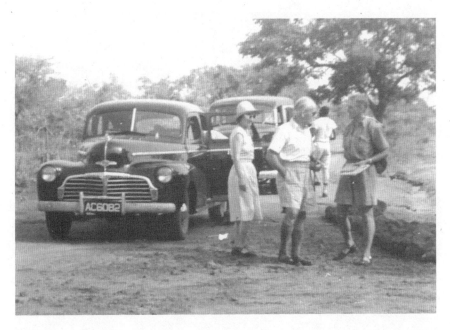

Figure 1.1 | 'Kenneth Stacey Morris in the Northern Territories (early 1940s)'.

to pay the missions, the secretary of state for the colonies rejected the suggestion, stating that overhaul of the Nigerian system was the priority. It was not until after the war that missionary leprosy work was properly institutionalised as part of a government and international organisational plan with Colonial Welfare and Development Act funding.[30]

Overall, government relations by the 1940s were more diffuse across the missions; the close relationship of the Scottish Presbyterian mission and the colonial state had been completely disrupted and major rifts emerged in the 1950s. The Gold Coast colonial state's relationship with the Scottish Presbyterians had some similarities with contemporaneous relations in Malawi, where, between the 1900s and the 1930s, the Scottish Presbyterians and the state had been closely aligned. According to John McCracken, by the 1920s, with their networks of schools and hospitals, the missions at Blantyre and Livingstonia had been 'drawn into an intimate, though, at times, strained, relationship with the government'.

Building on the work of Karen Fields on the Watchtower movement, McCracken argues that in Central Africa the early colonial
state 'had more than a passing resemblance to medieval European
states, with the spiritual and material resources of the Church being
used to bolster state authority'. However, by the 1940s and into the
1950s this had broken down, and new rifts had emerged in response
to a wider reappraisal of relations with the state by the church. In
Blantyre, the Scottish mission even became 'genuinely self-govern-
ing' by transferring financial responsibility to the synod and dis-
tancing themselves from the developmentalism of the colonial state.
Instead, the Presbyterians focused on concerns about the spiritual-
ity of their parishioners which they feared had been abandoned for
the sake of social improvement. Missions, though divided, generally
went into open opposition regarding the creation of the Federation
of Nyasaland and Rhodesia.[31] As will be analysed further in the final
section of this chapter, in the 1950s in the Gold Coast the Scottish
Presbyterians also departed from their close role with the state,
in favour of independent, synod-run missions. Often their efforts
resulted in far less support from the emerging state voluntary sector
than other medical missions received.[32]

    In the late 1940s and 1950s there was a proliferation of types of
denomination that were backed by government and majorly collaborating in medical work, such as the SDAs, the Methodists, and the
Salvation Army.[33] A symbolic turning point was in 1948 when the
Catholic Medical Mission Sisters built their hospital at Berekum.[34]
This postwar expansion was related to the huge increase in Colonial
Office provision for development which, in the ten years following
1945, provided £120 million (which was then raised to £140 million
by the 1950 Colonial Welfare and Development Act).[35] The colonial
state was beginning to create a new system and infrastructure of
liberal, voluntary sector-run health care. While there were variations
in how this was expressed, the overall outcome was an attempt to
institutionalise a variety of types of medical mission within a system
of hospitals, partly financed by the state. These could not necessarily
be controlled by colonial officials, and nor could they effectively per-
ceive the full breadth of medical mission, but they were very effective
in consolidating a network of mission hospitals that would form the
basis of a sustained voluntary sector that has survived even its partial nationalisation in the twenty-first century.

THE POSTWAR VOLUNTARY SECTOR

The emergence of the postwar voluntary sector in colonial Africa was a revolution in statecraft that is still being worked out in many African national contexts. As Ruth J. Prince and Hannah Brown have shown in their wide-ranging work, volunteerism in Africa is key to understanding states' relationships with development, and with transnational and global partners such as NGOs.[36] Moreover, the relation to formal needs such as state recognition and more diffuse identity concerns such as social obligations and gender norms all create structures in which the agency of individual volunteers is considerably constricted.[37] In the late colonial Gold Coast and early postcolonial Ghana, meanings of 'the volunteer' were consistently remade in dialogue with the expanding 'voluntary sector' which was an emerging part of the state.[38] Medical missions were central to this voluntary sector.

The process that defined the formal character of the 1950s voluntary sector began under Alan Burns, the governor of the Gold Coast in 1941 and then between 1942 and 1947. Burns was keen to promote gradual Christianisation through medical mission.[39] He wrote in his *History of Nigeria* (1929) that for a 'real Christianity' to be introduced into Africa, the work must be 'slow and patient'. Vital to this steady pace, he claimed, were 'medical missions to gain the confidence of the people, without which nothing will be accomplished'.[40] Burns quoted two of the main architects of the formal government-mission alliance in the 1920s British Empire: the missionary statesman J.H. Oldham and one of his mentors, Lord Frederick Lugard. From Oldham's notable publication *Christianity and the Race Problem*, Burns further bolstered his complaint against Christian division, echoing Oldham's claim that 'unless the Christian Church can exhibit a brotherhood as real as that of Islam, we cannot be surprised if the latter is more successful in winning the allegiance of pagan people'.[41]

Burns linked this to his disappointment about the 'friction that has existed in the past between the Government and the missionaries' because of their interference in political and judicial matters. He cited Lugard's issues with missions who were looking to the government for support when they were thrown out by a paramount chief. Burns's message was that Christianity could flourish by focusing on building trust over the long term, especially through medical mission, with government assistance in 'pagan areas', and by avoiding the tensions resulting from government challenges to Islamic authority. Burns's book linked to key debates around Oldham and mission-government cooperation, and it was successful, being republished in five editions, the last in 1955.[42] Through this academic work, several gubernatorial terms, and a stint as the assistant under-secretary of state for the colonies in the early 1940s, Burns became a major contributor to the discussion of how mission would function until the end of colonialism.[43]

As a result of his gradualist understanding of Christianity and colonialism, Burns was especially keen on hospitals, and blocked the dominance of 'preventative health'. Given the missiological and imperial culture in which Burns debated and received his ideas, his main focus was on hospital building. These were bastions of modern medicine in which over a long, sustained, and protected period of time, missionaries could build trust with local communities and display order, expertise, cleanliness, and bodily difference in biomedical clothing and equipment. As Fraser had put it, the aim was 'to know and be known by the people'.[44] Missions could also directly convert locals while they were ensconced in hospital beds, as Megan Vaughan argued: 'a lengthy stay ... provided a medical and spiritual training', it was a kind of 'rite of passage'.[45] In consequence, as Pascal Schmid details, Burns clashed with his head of medical services, James Balfour Kirk, leading to the latter's early retirement in 1944. Balfour Kirk wanted to establish a 'Policy of Preventative Medicine' which would emphasise immunisation and sanitary improvement to lower the incidence of disease. Balfour Kirk wrote that the Gold Coast needed 'a general clean up of the country by means of mass survey and treatment campaigns, combined with the provision of water supplies and other essential sanitary apparatus and improvements'.[46]

As Deborah Neill has shown, tropical medicine specialists like Balfour Kirk were equipped by their 'transnational epistemic communities' to 'influence policy making by collectively identifying problems and solutions ... circumscribing the boundaries and delimiting the options'.[47] However, while Balfour Kirk might have been supported at the transnational level by imperial medical networks, at the national level, Burns reigned. Burns's spread of options was rooted in the networks and organisations of knowledge production in British interwar mission which surrounded Oldham, not in those of imperial medicine. Just as medicine could shape missionary theology, here theological ideas were considerably shaping medicine. Burns also justified the focus on hospitals by arguing that 'while there can be no doubt of the great importance of preventive medicine, public opinion will not be satisfied if those who are actually sick are neglected in keeping well those who have so far been fortunate in escaping illness'.

This he noted especially with regard to 'primitive tribes' and people with family in hospital, both of whom needed to be inspired with 'belief in the good intentions of the Government'.[48]

Burns was able to spend more on hospitals, and development generally, because of high cocoa prices and increased revenue from the landmark 1940 Colonial Welfare and Development Act. Based on high revenue of mineral exports such as gold (which in 1938 had fetched £484,200) and cocoa (which had gained £9,990,000 in 1937 for 236,000 tonnes), Burns initiated a policy throughout the 1940s of hospital building where possible.[49] He also collected around £800,000 annually in income tax, bringing total revenue to an average of £4,469,000 annually, as opposed to the £3,669,000 annual revenue before the war. In 1944 Burns proposed £924,000 to be spent on new district hospitals, £400,000 on a new central hospital in Kumasi, and £250,000 on a mental hospital. This was out of a total of £3,789,000 spent on development, including roads, housing, water, and electric lighting, as well as harbour and railway improvements and agricultural credits which totalled £1,400,000. Hospitals therefore comprised 30.33 per cent of development expenditure. To pay for this, Burns also defrayed £1,000,000 over five years from the Colonial Welfare and Development funds, which had risen significantly in 1940. The annual expenditure on development in 1935–36 to 1939–40 was around £2,690,000 annually; under Burns this rose to around £4,250,000 annually.[50] Burns set the terms of the huge medical mission expansion in the Gold Coast which started shortly after he left office in 1947. He ensured that for the next decade hospital construction was the priority.

Burns's lack of funding for rural health projects, especially in the Northern Territories where there was a high incidence of preventable disease, frustrated rural health workers. The entomologist Kenneth Stacey Morris wrote in a letter to his mother from the Northern Territories in 1939 explaining how little his tsetse control would cost:

Our team working through a strip of Lawra district only, in six months covered 1,000 sq miles of country, visited 52 villages and towns, examined 15,000 people and found and treated over 500 cases of sleeping sickness ... This is a team of semi or un-educated local native trained by Saunders and I, none of whom gets more than £3 per month, mostly getting £1 to 35/- - The whole team of about 15 people, for diagnosis and treatment, costs only £25 per month in salaries, and works perfectly without our supervision from one month to another.[51]

Morris complained that the annual costs of his team were what 'some of the doctors will draw in allowances and perks, quite apart from salary, + quite certainly they don't do as effective work [sic]'. His three teams, he ranted to his mother, would cost £900 with £500 in drugs and other expenses and 'shall save up to 3,000 lives per year ... Cheap as life may be rated out here, or when enclosed in a black skin. I don't think the authorities could boggle at that'. The government concern for hospital provision and Christianisation clashed with Morris's aims:

here sit I, responsible for all this, and capable of its vast expansion had I but the chance, listening to the echoes of our wonderful 20th century civilisation blowing each other to bits to the tune of God knows how many hundreds of millions of pounds, and wondering, with very real doubts, if I shall be allowed, kindly graciously permitted by our wonderful human-itarian system, to spend 10/- a time saving the lives of these poor wretches who have a thing enough time of it anyway - + yet keep smiling - And above all - have given up killing each other for some time now![52]

However, Morris did eventually get part of what he wanted. In December 1949 he was offered £100,000 a year for a national tse-tse control unit, a considerable amount given that overall medical expenditure for the colony was only £1,161,250 in 1950.[53] Even upon this offer, Morris still felt the Gold Coast government's focus on such official institutions fell far short of the mark, describing the administration as content with him becoming one of the 'dull pompous cogs ... [who] kid themselves that they are doing a man's job'.[54]

In the late 1930s and 1940s, African newspapers in the Gold Coast were also complaining bitterly about poor sanitation. The *African Morning Post* provided space for 'Provincial Items' which community spokespersons mostly used to highlight unsanitary conditions, changes in chieftaincy, and church building work. On 12 January 1939 a news report for Cape Coast demanded that the 'attention of the local Medical Officer of Health' be 'called to the insanitary condition of the Castle Yard Latrine' which served officials and prominent people using the post office and the court. This 'pity' the writer blamed on the latrine being used by the public, as a result of which it had become 'very filthy'.[55] The following week the writer for Nkawkaw described how the latrines had become full and even 'when they were in use they were found to be insufficient for the inhabitants of the town'. For this, they chastised the 'indifference of the authorities concerned with the affairs of the town' who indulged in 'unnecessary litigation', and the columnist advised the sanitary inspector to ask for the chief's cooperation in helping improve the area.[56] This was the same for Kokofu, about which the author went into detail, explaining that 'the sanitary conditions here leave much to be desired. Goat and sheep's excrement abound in the streets, thus producing an unpleasant smell. This is detrimental to the health of the inhabitants. We strongly appeal to the Omanhene and M. O. H. in charge of the Bekwai district to solve the situation'.[57]

There was more in the next day's newspaper. On Wednesday the 18th the correspondent for Mepom wrote that the 'sanitary conditions of this town leave much to be desired', but this time the inhabitants themselves were blamed for ignoring the dictates of the chiefs: 'Refuse is freely thrown on streets. The outskirts of the town are weedy, thereby mosquitoes are bred and poisonous reptiles sheltered. The inhabitants do not care to carry out the orders of the Odi. kro ... This town needs special attention as there had once broken out yellow fever here'.[58] Across Gold Coast villages and market towns, the unsanitary conditions were proclaimed in a variety of appalling, illustrative examples.[59]

In 1938 seven new dispensaries were opened in Abomosu, Attabubu, Prang, Yeji, Grube Fian, and Ketiu in order to reduce the incidence of disease such as yaws and malaria 'in the poor and more remote areas'. The predominant aim for the subsequent years was to improve 'conditions in the mining health areas ... rural sanitation ... congested slums ... [and] the extension of health education'.[60] Village

Table 1.1 Gold Coast child and maternal health providers in 1942 and 1943

	Red Cross (1942)	Govern-ment (1942)	Missions (1942)	Red Cross (1943)	Govern-ment (1943)
Children attending	38,402	39,990	59,074		
Mothers attending	27,742	19,046	2,929		
Total	66,144	59,036	63,003	71,417	71,017

Source: *Gold Coast Colony Report on the Medical Department for the Year 1942* (Gold Coast: Government Printer, Accra, 1943), 4–7, Liverpool School of Tropical Medicine (Liverpool, UK).

dispensaries were the focus because, as the Legislative Council stated, 'we are fully aware that Government cannot build hospitals in every state'.[61] Moreover, as one of the African chiefs, Nana Hima Dekyi XII, stated in the legislative debates in 1940, not only had the fees become too high for the poor to visit hospitals, the council itself had 'no money' to help.[62] Moreover, there were 'severe' epidemics of cerebro-spinal meningitis and outbreaks of smallpox during the Second World War, and the training of dispensers and nurses that had been planned became impossible.[63] In 1941, R.S. Blay told the council that more than 70 per cent (and in some areas more than 90 per cent) of applicants had been rejected from the army because of poor health, particularly yaws and guinea worm, because there were few dispensers and government doctors' fees were too high.[64] By 1943, Nana Nyarko VII, the representative of the Ewe-speaking people, was complaining that 'the poorer parts of the country have little or no medical service … instead of having a few well-equipped hospitals at a few centres there should be many dispensaries all over the country, so that it should not be difficult for any one in need of medical aid to obtain same at the time he needs it ... Too much is spent at great centres, and too little is spent in vast areas'.[65]

In spite of all this, it was a hospital network where money was targeted in late colonial Gold Coast, and thus in early colonial Ghana. From 1944 onwards, hospital building had become the colony's main aim, though it was not until 1950 that this became rapid; the pathway had been chosen. In 1944, £83,000 was provided by the Legislative Council for building two new hospitals, out of a total council expenditure of £5,055,764.[66] In 1946 a nurses' training school and hospital were constructed for £46,000 using funds from the £3,500,000 allocated to the Gold Coast through the Colonial Welfare and Development Act. The only issue holding back more hospital development was staff shortages, so nurses' colleges aimed at filling the gaps. In March 1945, there was a further large outbreak of smallpox and an epidemic of cerebrospinal meningitis which recorded 1,052 deaths and had to be contained by the army. Nevertheless, the Takoradi-Sekondi hospital was renovated and in the following year a ten-year plan was laid out for 'building new hospitals and for major works in connection with existing ones'.[67] Moreover, £31,000 for a leprosy survey and £94,650 for constructing and initially staffing three leper colonies was allocated from the Colonial Welfare and Development Fund.[68]

As the colonial government increased spending on medicine after 1947 largely it was funneled into previous state and mission infrastructure channels, formalising and institutionalising them. Of a total £10,964,604 spending in 1947–48, 599,597 was spent by the medical heads. In the following year, 1948–49, there was a further increase to £11,487,703 in total and £814,616 by the medical heads.[69] By 1950, medical heads expenditure had grown to £932,831, which amounted to an overall medical service expenditure of £1,161,250 with an extra £45,210 for tsetse control and £172,333 for rural water development.[70] By 1948 plans had been passed for extensions to the hospitals at Oda, Winneba, Ho, and Keta, as well as a new dispensary on the hospital grounds at Axim.[71] By 1950, there were twenty-eight private and mission hospitals with 878 beds, and thirty-three government hospitals (twenty-seven of which had medical officers) with 1,572 beds. A further mission hospital was planned for Worawora in Southern Togoland. This was in addition to widespread clinic work by the missions and international organisations. In 1949 the International Red Cross Society had five weekly mobile clinic serving over forty towns and villages, and in 1950 they treated 60,000 patients in mobile and static clinics (suggesting some decline from the heights of their provision in the early 1940s, perhaps because of increased strains on resources during the Second World War). In 1949, two mission dispensaries were opened by Europeans and Americans in the Northern Territories.[72] In 1950, the French-Canadian Catholics began the first maternity and child welfare clinic in Jirapa, a leprosy clinic was opened at Banda in the Gonja district, and a missionary maternity clinic was being built at Nakpanduri in the Mamprusi district.[73]

While there was some innovation in health care, generally the trend was towards continuing the mission-state development consensus. In addition to the clinics, the medical field units – which formalised and unified government immunisation efforts particularly regarding yaws in the Northern Territories – had £56,190 set aside for them and were in operation by the end of the decade.[74] Much was now being spent on medical services, made possible through loans, rises in export taxes, London stocks, the Colonial Welfare and Development Fund, and the global post-1948 boom in cocoa prices.[75] Increased funding also resulted from Colonial Office change; as Joseph Hodge shows, between 1947 and 1951 there was the one and only 'full blown Chamberlainite "colonial development offensive" ... to serve the direct interests of the British national economy'.[76] However, in the Gold Coast these changes served to formally consolidate earlier local patterns of health service, not innovate fundamentally.

There was concerted government response to epidemics of yaws and smallpox from 1946, but this was nothing compared to the effort in hospital construction. In 1946 the government returned to large-scale vaccination campaigns of smallpox as they had done in Accra in the 1920s. By 1947 there was already a clear effect, with most cases confined to the Navrongo-Nangodi area; by 1948 a population of 3,962,692 had a high proportion of people vaccinated.[77]

As across Africa, these campaigns in the Gold Coast were 'a model for further public health efforts, including the WHO eradication campaign'.[78] Mass treatment of yaws also increased in the Dagomba region of the Northern Territories, in which twelve teams were able to treat 20,609 cases.[79] This work continued into the next year under the direction of trypanosomiasis staff and with the help of the French authorities over the northern border.[80] This benefitted from Colonial Welfare and Development fund money: yaws treatment

Table 1.2 Smallpox vaccinations, deaths, and cases in the Gold Coast between 1945 and 1948

Year	1945	1946	1947	1948
Smallpox vaccinations	113,361	512,939		1,377,827
Smallpox deaths		330	173	120 (61 in the Winneba-Swedru epidemic)
Smallpox cases		1646	838	651

Source: 'Chapter VII: Social Services: 1. Health', *Colonial Office: Annual Report on the Gold Coast for the Year 1948* (London: His Majesty's Stationery Office, 1950), 43–5.

gained £8,000 between 1948–49, to which the colonial government added £2,240.[81] However, in spite of these renewed efforts, communicable diseases remained huge killers with little investment to stop them; cerebrospinal meningitis recorded 11,002 cases and 868 deaths in 1948 alone.[82]

The culmination of the tying together of medical mission and government in the Gold Coast was the government report in 1951 and the Maude Commission in 1952, which together ensured that 'voluntary agencies' became institutionalised. The *Report of the Commission of Enquiry into the Health Needs of the Gold Coast* was a landmark document in colonial and mission health which produced a detailed survey of the colony's medical provision. It followed on the heels of the government's publication of a 'Statement of Principles Regulating Financial Assistance to Voluntary Agencies Undertaking Medical Work' in 1951. The statement of principles formally declared the desire to obtain 'assistance of non-Government agencies, particularly the missionary organisations, in the expansion of health service, especially in the field of maternity and child welfare work'. Following this, the statement offered capital grants and contributions toward recurrent expenditure for hospitals under the administration of combined mission-government committees. The Maude Commission supported the statement wholeheartedly: 'We are strongly in favour of a policy designed to elicit a fuller contribution from the missionary societies and other voluntary agencies ... if the maximum advantage is to be taken of these agencies whose objects are charitable and not profit-making, it is worth while having, if necessary, a careful negotiation with each without attempting to force the arrangements into a single mould'.[83]

The latter sentiment challenging the uniformity of a formal 'non profit-making' sector is noted to have emerged from 'experience' with such relations within the UK. Maude himself was one of the major proponents of voluntary-state partnership in the NHS; he was concerned about the effect of government power on voluntarism and had gained significant control during his time as the permanent secretary of the Ministry of Health in the war.[84] In his concluding Gold Coast development estimates, Maude made provision for £140,000 of grants to medical missions to be expended by the end of the year.[85] However, Maude was also arguing here that such a voluntary sector should not be in a 'single mould'. Instead, he wanted to empower the diversity and independent energy of missions *through* formalising their role within increasingly nationalised health systems. In the government's response to the report, they fully backed Maude's recommendations.[86] In doing so they proclaimed the start of a decade of very high government spending on missions, in which twenty-four medical mission hospitals would be built.[87]

In contrast to Burns, for Maude the defence of medical missionary agency was not only to bolster government efforts or missionary work, but also to ensure the survival of democracy in British societies – and of liberalism everywhere – through a vibrant culture of voluntarism. Maude's hope was to ensure a culture of liberal voluntarism, around the missions in the Gold Coast, that would provide the lifeblood of a national health-care system which otherwise could be turned into an instrument of coercion by the government. Voluntary associational life was conceived by Maude as critical to ensuring the flourishing of modern society.[88] In his 1948 address to the British Hospitals

Contributory Scheme Association on 'The Place of Voluntary Effort in the National Health Service', Maude argued that 'voluntary effort (has) the enormous advantage of elasticity and freedom of action. In pioneering and experimental work there are risks which it is right and proper for voluntary agencies disbursing voluntary funds to take, but which a Minister and public Department as trustees of public fund would be perfectly justifiable in refusing'.[89]

Moreover, Maude argued that this pioneering spirit could not only prevail in voluntary associations, but also challenge the overbearing power of the state:

> It is almost a truism to say in these days that modern inventions – the development of instruments of physical coercion and perhaps even more instruments such as a government-controlled press ... have vastly increased the scope and powers of the state ... 'You will always have a totalitarian State unless you do a great many energetic things to prevent it ...' [A]ny useful public activity carried on by voluntary workers (as Mr T. S. Eliot has recently put it, the fulfilment of a public need by a private enterprise) has a value as a counterpoise to these ever increasing activities of the State.[90]

In the context of Europe shortly after the war with the Nazis, Maude set his argument for the flourishing of the voluntarist spirit amidst the threat of totalitarianism and the 'physical coercion' which seemed abundantly possible for a state to use against its citizens. For Maude, it was in combination with the equalising powers of an interventionist state that the 'fulfilment of public need' was possible.[91] Thus, his work emphasised their combination: a formal voluntary sector which operated in the loose reigns of a nationalised system. The kind of organisations where this liberal, elastic, and private culture could take root were 'the Churches, the Universities, professional bodies, Trade Unions, Friendly Societies and many others'. These had 'a part to play in providing this counterpoise not less but rather more valuable because the nature of their work brings them into close contact and collaboration with the public services'.[92]

As the Gold Coast colonial government stretched out health services beyond the South, their decisions were informed by this vision for a progressive and lively voluntarist liberal culture, with voluntary agencies like medical missions taking risks in coordination with more restricted public services and pioneering the frontiers of the state. In their statement on Maude's recommendations, the Gold Coast government welcomed the endorsement of their policy and emphasised that 'greater flexibility' would be introduced into their financial arrangements with missionary societies and voluntary agencies.[93] This dovetailed well with the kind of voluntarism which John Stuart has argued that missionaries were trying to promote in late colonial Africa. It also fit well into the developmentalist visions already prominent within the Gold Coast, from Guggisberg and Fraser through to Burns.[94] The result was that Maude had been successful not only in encouraging the application of public funds to voluntary agencies, but also in convincing the colonial government that the national health system could be tailored to enable a liberal voluntarist state.

More widely, the emergence of the formal voluntary sector in Africa was linked to the visions for the success of postwar state welfarism. Given their lack of democratic accountability and their linkages with the 'structural adjustment' reforms of the 1980s, NGOs and FBOs have been viewed as aberrations of state health systems; however, they were actually a fixed part of these systems from the 1940s onwards. Michael Jennings has shown in his work on postwar Tanganyika that a public-private, state and non-state contract was produced through grants-in-aid provision. Nationalisation of the health-care system in the 1970s served to reinforce this formal position of voluntary agencies by 'preventing "non-authorised" alternative actors from operating in the country'. The 'NGOisation' of African health care was, therefore, not a later product of neoliberalism but a long-term legacy reflecting 'fragility, fragmentation and structural weakness'. As Susan Reynolds Whyte puts it, the projectified landscape of the global includes many vertical programmes but not many horizontal.[95] NGOs did not create the problem, they exacerbated the issues attendant on a 'franchise state' that had so few resources that it needed to outsource much of its health care to non-profit actors in order to prove that it could provide for the welfare of its citizens.[96] As Jose Harris has argued, by 1950 there had been a general shift to seeing the voluntary sector as a means to the end of 'controlling ... the sphere of public provision'. William Beveridge in his 1948 report was concerned that the Labour government was rejecting voluntary sector provision, but in fact it was seen as a component in achieving state welfarism. As Emma Hunter has shown, the visions of the Beveridge Report were repeated in the Colonial Office Social Welfare Advisory Committee and shaped the emergence of state welfarism in East Africa. Within this were concepts of duty carried over into postcolonial Tanzania state-building.[97] Voluntarist ideas as well as formal structures were a part of the shift in state health-care provision to formally incorporate medical missions.

The growth of a contracted and formal voluntary sector was happening across a variety of contexts in postwar Sub-Saharan Africa. In francophone as well as anglophone Africa, the formal voluntary sector was produced on a large scale, with colonial offices funding medical missions extensively through grants-in-aid in the late 1940s and 1950s. Part of the shift to formalise the relationship with missions that had been growing for decades was caused by the creation of massive development funds from Colonial Offices. In Cameroon in the 1950s, medical missions were funded extensively by subventions (grants) from the FIDES (Fonds d'Investissement et de Développement Economique et Social), a central French imperial fund created in 1946.[98] Much of this was Baptist medical missionary work from America, alongside older Catholic work.[99] Certainly, the drive for development can be seen in earlier prewar initiatives, and this was often with voluntary agencies' support. However, in the postwar era, development planning as a systematic, internationally centralised programme affected African health care differently. As with FIDES, from Britain the Colonial Welfare and Development Act (CWDA) of 1940 ensured far greater provision than earlier grants. In both French and British development, the process was less piecemeal, less ad hoc, and more widely distributed to national infrastructure. Postwar funding also increasingly focused on large buildings, partly because it was too difficult to commit to recurrent expenditure. In Kenya, there were grants-in-aid to medical missions for maternity services in 1925, but generally funding for hospitals was not systematically given across East Africa until the 1950s.[100] In 1954, Zambia missions were receiving 50 per cent of their recurrent expenditure.[101] From 1940, the Zimbabwean colonial government was funding many mission hospitals and by 1977 sixty-three of Zimbabwe's mission hospitals were still funded by government grants-in-aid.[102] Similarly, there were huge amounts of subventions given from FIDES to many missions in 1950s Senegal.[103] This was the case in a variety of other Sub-Saharan African contexts too (with the exception of northern Nigeria).

Crucially, while there was more formalised and systematic pro-vision after the war, still a variety of local actors had significant power in the timing and type of voluntary sector that emerged – particularly medical missionaries. A key aim of the FIDES and CWDA programmes was to ensure closely matched funding within colonial governments.[104] The postwar imperial welfarism was not defined simply by top-down control of central colonial offices but, as with the 1920s and 1930s, by local administrations and local politi-cal conflicts. Moreover, though there was connection with 1940s British welfarism, the African context was very different. In colonial Africa there was an assumed lack of government capacity to stretch beyond the centres of power and a long-term expectation about the vital place of missionaries in the colonial project, especially in rural areas. By contrast, 1950s British national health care increasingly detached from church support and the state was expected to assume wide responsibilities. In colonial Africa missions had a far greater say in how the voluntary sector emerged. In the colonial govern-ment in Tanganyika, missions felt threatened during the 1950s by new colonial objectives, and although the government could never have radically reformed health services, missions defended their corner. By 1952 links with certain forms of mission were increas-ingly formalised.[105]

This pattern of state empowering picked up in the 1950s after Burns left; Charles Arden-Clarke, the governor of the Gold Coast from 1949 to 1957, was pro-medical mission and he consciously aimed to further embed a voluntarist culture. In the early 1950s, as a result of many pressures (such as changing international poli-tics, the emergence of NGOs, ecclesiastical devolution, and concerns about communism), missionaries and pro-mission colonial officials actively tried to cultivate a culture of Christian voluntarism through centralised Colonial Service organisations. John Stuart has shown how the first attempt at this was the Oversea Service, which aimed to 'foster a sense of Christian fellowship' amongst new colonial service recruits. Notably, at the opening conference for the Oversea Service in 1953, the Gold Coast governor Arden-Clarke contributed as a speaker.[106] Arden-Clarke's father was a Church Missionary Society (CMS) minister in India into the 1920s, and Arden-Clarke himself had originally considering going into church ministry. He wrote to his parents in 1922 about his younger brother becoming a mission-ary, which he wrote would 'buck you up no end, because I'm sure you were very disappointed in me'.[107] In a letter to his father in 1922, Arden-Clarke argued that twelve male missionaries trained in simple medicine would be far better than twenty erecting a stall in the village market and becoming a 'general nuisance' trying to preach monogamy and the Passion of Christ. That way, 'Christianity will be knocked out by Mahommedanism', he wrote.[108] Under Arden-Clarke, medical mission hospitals were hugely financed and well staffed.[109]

By the eve of decolonisation, missions were opening a plethora of medical institutions with government support and government itself was admitting its inability to set up sustained preventive health care. In 1955, the government stated that as mission medical work continued to expand this was 'encouraged as a policy of Government … in so far as the funds available for financial assistance permit'. In the same report, government contributions were extensively listed: in 1954 the new Presbyterian hospital at Bawku had been completed, the Roman Catholic mission hospital at Navrongo was completed, and progress was being made on their hospital at Jirapa – both 'with funds provided by Government'. In addition, the Maternity Hospital and Midwifery Training Centre at Mampong was opened in May and was being run by the English Church Mission. There were also grants to the Methodist Mission at Wenchi in Ashanti, the Basel Mission staff training at Agogo, the Salvation Army at Begoro, and several Roman Catholic missions in the Western and Eastern regions alongside Jirapa in the North.[110] Finally, further plans were made for a hospital at Worawora run by the Evangelical Presbyterian Church. Extra funds were also given for pupil nurses hostels at the mission hospitals in Navrongo, Jirapa, and Mpraeso (Kwahu).[111] At the same time, the government was building their own hospitals, such as at Koforidua for which £25,000 was earmarked.[112] Alongside these ventures there was the admission that systematic preventative health care across the colony was now extremely difficult and had largely been dismissed: 'during 1953, it was appreciated that the basic necessity of improved environment hygiene and the responsibilities of local authorities in this regard were inadequately recognised … It has to be recognised, however, that many local authorities set up under the recent re-organisations of local government are not yet in a sufficiently strong position to permit the establishment of appropriate health services within a co-ordinated framework of supervision by the Central Government'.[113]

Given the long-term sustained focus on large-scale institutional medical provision, the new local authority structure could not make up the shortfall easily. While campaigns in preventative health care were beneficial, they were not in a position to radically alter the infra-structure and administration already in place. In 1956, £475,075 was granted by government for hospitals, clinics, and dispensaries alone. This was spread across a variety of government and mission projects: for example, £2,000 was given to support the Salvation Army's construction of a clinic at Boso.[114] The rapid growth of mission hospitals and clinics continued.

THE BOUNDARIES AND BENEFICIARIES OF THE VOLUNTARY SECTOR: MEDICAL MISSIONS AT KWAHU AND SANDEMA

Government actual expenditure on medical services increased year on year in the early 1950s; it was £965,020 in 1950, £1,037,795 in 1951, and £1,607,545 in 1952. Missions were building hospitals and dispensaries abundantly. By 1958 the minister of health stated that the government paid the recurrent costs for the Catholic hospitals at Jirapa, Damongo, and Navrongo, the Basel Mission hospital at Bawku, the English Church mission at Mampong, and the Seventh-day Adventist church at Kwahu. The independent Ghanaian government also provided annual grants to the Worldwide Evangelization Crusade's Leper Settlement at Kpandai, the Basel Mission Hospital at Agogo, and the Methodist Hospital at Wenchi. They also provided annual grants to the Salvation Army clinics at Begoro and Boso, and the Catholic clinics at Akim Swedru, Eikwe, Dzodze, and Nandom.[115]

Many new mission actors in the 1950s capitalised on government funding to set up flagship institutions and work in places beyond where state medical services could readily staff. The SDAs set up a hospital for the first time in the Gold Coast at Kwahu in 1955 (and officially opened in 1957).[116] Moreover, the British Salvation Army formed their first clinic at Begoro in 1952, leading later to seven others by 1982, and the Worldwide Evangelization Crusade built a Leper Colony at Kpandai in Northern Togoland in 1952.[117] Old mission actors, by contrast, took the opportunity to expand. For example, in 1953 the Presbyterians at Dunkwa Hospital built a new site with £49,000 of government development funds, with an

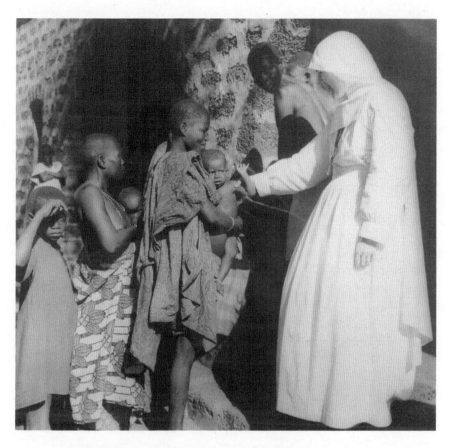

Figure 1.2 | 'The dispensary at Nandom gives an average of 37,000 consultations each year. Here a White Sister chats with a mother who is waiting her turn in the queue with her baby' (c.1950s).

extra £26,000 earmarked for 1955–56.[118] Unlike the government, who struggled to staff large institutions in the far-flung reaches of the colony (especially lacking medical officers and nursing Sisters to meet increased demand), missionary bodies were at a zenith of recruitment from Europe and America.[119] However, there also many that chose not to capitalise on the money and those who were unable to gain any funding. Medical missions in this period were formalising but they remained complex, varied, and independent in many regards.

Given issues with independence and their desire to bypass government interests, many missions also set up their own institutions without consulting the government and actively refused to participate.
The Roman Catholic Medical Mission Sisters Hospital at Berekum
declined government financial aid of around £21,800, which the
government could not 'force' them to accept. In the same Legislative
Assembly debate, the government declined to help Catholics at Foso
set up a clinic and were not setting up their own health centre in
the area.[120] In some cases, missions did not even inform government as to their aims; for example, in 1955 the minister of health
declined to give a government subsidy to the Catholic hospital plan
for Akrokerri because there was 'no information ... received of any
intention on the part of the Catholic Mission to build a hospital at
Akrokerri'; 'if the Mission has this intention it is hoped that it will
first seek Government approval to implement it ... (and state) at the
same time what financial assistance, if any, would be required from
Government'.[121] A similar issue occurred with regards to Roman
Catholic aims to build a maternity hospital at Takyiman, for which no
application for funds was received.[122] In the same year, the Catholic
White Fathers had the Gonja Development Company Hospital at
Damongo purchased for them by the government.[123] The government then debated whether to buy them an ambulance.[124] This was
not simply a denominational issue, but a question of particular congregations or groups who had specific aims and agendas at specific
times. Moreover, some missions changed their minds when circumstances changed: the Catholic hospital at Berekum originally had
been allocated £21,000 (part of which also was sequestered for the
Anglican hospital at Mampong), but when funds were insufficient
they were diverted and reconsidered.[125] At the end of the process,
Berekum turned down the money offered, choosing to promote their
own independence over gaining further financial or national political power. The concept of the 'volunteer' often suggests freedom and
agency, but its implication in emerging statecraft in the Gold Coast
ensured that its practice was bound up with government visions for
health infrastructure and population management. Adopting such
volunteer roles within a state-formalised voluntary sector could have
significant downsides for the restriction of activity and identities, in
which many Catholic missions did not want to engage.

By contrast, in 1955, the Seventh-day Adventists (SDAs) successfully gained funding from the colonial government's voluntary

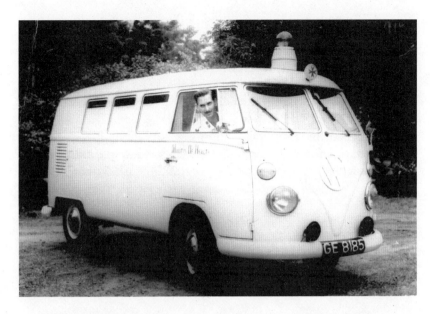

Figure 1.3 | 'Captain Jeffrey Roberts received new Ministry of Health ambulance for Salvation Army clinic' (c.1960s).

provision to build their first hospital in the Gold Coast. Their work was part of a general expansion of SDA medicine across the world: in 1940 SDA health-care assets amounted to $9,687,457.49 with 6,184 employees, but by 1956 they totalled $53,841,675.96 with 10,292 employees. In the Gold Coast the government built the hospital and the SDAs staffed it. As planned under the Maude Commission's voluntary sector suggestions, it was established by a combined committee.[126] Along with money from offerings for foreign mission from the Northern European Division (for Ghana in 1957 alone this totalled $30,802.33), the SDAs also had doctors from their Skodsborg Sanitarium in Copenhagen who could train staff in specific skills such as physiotherapy.[127] In the first few years the SDAs sent two European doctors and three European nurses, as well as employing many 'national' nurses and assistants.[128]

The initial doctors at Kwahu were presented in SDA newspapers as fired up by evangelistic zeal and a pioneering spirit. According to the *British Advent Messenger*, the second SDA doctor at Kwahu

had 'cherished the ambition' of becoming a medical missionary
since being a 'schoolboy'. He had committed to two-and-a-half
years at Kwahu with his wife, and the paper called on all to pray for
them to prosper in this difficult task far from their home in Derby,
England.[129] Little was said about the people Peter was going to help;
the focus was on where he had come from and how big a leap it was
to uproot to Kwahu. The first SDA doctor at Kwahu, Dr J.A. Hyde,
lauded the medical work there in terms of both modernity and effective Christian care. For example, in the SDA newspaper *Northern
Light* in 1956, a column entitled 'Progress in Our Mission Fields'
described how:

> Dr. J. A. Hyde reported on one of West Africa's newest institu-
> tions, the Kwahu Hospital, erected for us by the Gold Coast
> Government. In its first year it treated 28,844 out-patients and
> 557 in-patients. Every available space of the hospital has had
> to be used to try to house these. An indication of the regard
> in which the hospital is held was given by a recent visitor. On
> inquiring whether the institution was a mission hospital, and
> being told that it was, the visitor continued: 'I knew it must be;
> I could tell it by the way you cared for your patients'.[130]

In this account, alongside statistics of patient treatment and struggles at housing them, is an anecdote meant to encapsulate the effect
of Christian care. According to the comment, the hospital both
helped those inside the institution and proclaimed the meaning of
that care to surrounding people.[131]

The SDA's interpretation of the formal voluntary sector fit in colonial government terms, but it was not determined by them. The SDAs
showed off their biomedical effectiveness to the WHO and to the government, and also directed attention toward community evangelism.
According to the same Dr J. A. Hyde in 1958, the governor-general
(who by that point was the Earl of Listowel) and the WHO advisor
to Ghana both commented that the Kwahu hospital was the 'best
equipped and run hospital they had seen in Ghana'. The latter said
this within the Ministry of Health in Ghana, apparently much to
the chagrin of another representative – but Hyde declared that the
Lord had 'caused His name to be glorified in the councils of men'.[132]
For Hyde, SDA success was imagined in terms of God's name being
lifted high in government. This was a specific theology, taken from

passages across the Bible such as Psalm 22, in which God collaborates with His people to proclaim His power in the assemblies of men. As is often the case when analysing volunteer categories, it is the vulnerability and insecurity of those taking up 'volunteer' roles which mean that their identities and tasks become circumscribed to formal structures. By contrast, the SDAs had an international network on which they could rely for imaginative and material support, ensuring they could carve out their own pathways through the government voluntarist edifice. For the SDAs, they were concerned to appear effective in linking to national and international governance networks, but they conceived of these successes as stitched into much larger narratives about creation and their own corporate relationship with God. The SDAs navigated through changes in political context, but this did not mean that they simply received 'voluntarism' unquestioningly. They had agency to push back at the restrictions placed on the concept of the 'volunteer' in state terms by renarrating it in their own.

In all this maneuvering between different categorisations of their medical work, the SDAs were actually not particularly Janus-faced. They proclaimed their aims for their hospital in ways that were not particularly subtle. At both the opening of the hospital in 1957 and the graduation and expansion in 1962, the SDA presented copies of *The Ministry of Healing* (1905) to the ministers of health. The publication details the evangelistic and redemptive motives of their medical mission.[133] The hope was that it would shape the government's work and 'bear testimony to the healing work of the Seventh-day Adventists'.[134] Thus, while they were pleased to be affirmed by government and WHO representatives in biomedical terms and to benefit from the patronage afforded to state voluntarists, the SDAs were up front about their motives. Again, there was much agency for the SDAs to negotiate what voluntarism meant in Kwahu partly because of the strength of their position. They were providing a high-level medical service in a remote place that was difficult to staff for the government and in ways that were emphasising the colony's success internationally. Even more than this, the SDAs had networks beyond the colony and international health, which meant that they were part of something much bigger in their own eyes. This was fed and encouraged by newspapers where they could self-promote but also bolster their own sense of corporate identity by reading the narratives of others.

Beyond giving out pamphlets, the SDAs used their role in the Gold Coast formal voluntary sector to conduct intense evangelism and supernatural ministry within a government-built hospital. Any voluntarist images that the SDAs promoted did not determine the internal culture of the mission hospital, where they prioritised evangelism and spiritual warfare. The real passion of the medical work at Kwahu was certainly not in secular biomedical terms. The idea that missions secularised as they increased their formal relations with government was not the case here. In several SDA newspaper articles this is well illustrated. For example, in the *Northern Light* in 1957 an article was written emerging from a mission service in London where testimonies of God's ministry were shared between Northern European leaders and guests. The writer, J.M. Bucy, an American SDA and the wife of an SDA pastor, describes how 'during the model Sabbath school and mission service conducted by M. E. Lind, the Division Sabbath school secretary everyone actively participated in the review and the lesson study. Then came the gripping story of the deliverance from fetish worship. Miss Amy Horder, a nurse from our Kwahu Hospital in Ghana, told of a woman delivered from heathen worship and a serious physical condition through prayer and loving medical ministry. Truly a remarkable mission story with a happy ending!'[135]

This picture of simultaneous spiritual and physical conversion epitomised the effect at which the hospital aimed. Moreover, this was no minor service – Miss Horder was presenting to the heads of SDA mission. 'Fetish' and 'heathen' worship, which were reported to be healed through prayer, were as much the hallmarks of the hospital agenda as biomedical illnesses. Furthermore, in an article in the same year in *Messenger*, initially quoting Acts, the director of nursing at Kwahu, Lionel Acton-Hubbard, wrote that the hospital's mission was:

'to labour both for the health of the body and for the saving
of the soul ... healing all who are oppressed by Satan' ... 'the
medical missionary work is to bear the same relation to the work
of the third Angel's message that the arm and the hand bear
to the body. Under the direction of the divine head they are to
work unitedly in preparing the war for the coming of Christ'.
The gospel ministry is needed to give permanence and stability to the medical missionary work; and the ministry needs the

medical missionary work to demonstrate the practical working of the gospel – neither part of the work is complete without the other.[136]

The article sets the hospital's ministry in the spiritual battle which 'prepared' the coming of Christ, giving their medical mission eschatological significance. Though this was not completely different from other missions formulating roles within the colonial state, the emphasis on the supernatural within government-funded health care is striking.

The media produced from Kwahu Hospital was about building personal and social identities, as well as beneficial political ones. Isabel Hofmeyr has argued that missions created an international '"archive" of strategies for reading and interpretation' across the world, allowing them to imagine themselves as if addressing a 'vast international Protestant public', whatever the reality.[137] Hofmeyr's thesis rings true for the SDA authors. With a limited readership and an isolated existence in rural Gold Coast, Acton-Hubbard was nonetheless constructing a sense of self on an imagined larger spatial and temporal plane by narrating his place in the hospital. These articles provided a platform for him to individuate and distinguish his role, and a way to try to shape his identities for himself and for others in dialogue with all the competing demands that the mission field placed on him. As Guido Ruggiero puts it in the case of Italian Renaissance self-fashioning, 'family, friends, neighbours, fellow-citizens, and other social solidarities ... each constructed in dialogue with a person a socially recognized personal identity for that individual. Identities based upon "consensus realities" could be quite different for the same person depending on the group that shared them'. The personal narratives that Acton-Hubbard was creating afford perspectives on how he related to colonial discourses, theology, the supernatural, other people, objects and institutions, and his alien position in the Gold Coast. They do not provide an authentic picture of what was really happening in the hospital, but of how subjectivities were fostered within the context of missionary medicine.[138]

An SDA article from 1956 on electricity, prayer, and preaching at Kwahu Hospital shows more detailed aspects of how medical missionaries imagined their roles and experiences. Acton-Hubbard recounts in his article 'The Light Shines at Kwahu' that he imagined one night how impressive the hospital must look to the outside,

illuminated by electricity, and how much the locals must desire the
'light' of Jesus Christ. In consequence he gathered the 'young people'
around the hospital, largely a group of male students, and set out
to organise an event in the town in which they could proclaim the
'Story of Redemption'. Having gained the chief's permission (navigating these local politics was vital to the survival of a medical mission), Acton-Hubbard and his group prayed together and began eight
weeks of preaching to assemblies of 'the chief, the Queen mother ...
the elders ... (and) about 80 nonbelievers'. The male students sang
anthems and people came to hear them, sometimes before going
to the hospital's Sabbath service. Acton-Hubbard and his disciples
were replaying the Acts of the Apostles in the wilderness with even a
make-shift Pharisee from a local mission to battle:

> Yes, Friends, the young people of the hospital are sharing the
> light that has been given to them and the Lord is adding His
> blessing. The students are holding several before and after
> meetings and are gaining interests. In the course of one meeting
> a catechist from another mission in another town intruded and
> asked awkward questions at the end of the meeting. He was
> given a hearing and his questions were answered to the obvious
> satisfaction of the chief, his elders, and the assembled company.
> Yes, a new day is dawning in Atibie, Kwahu. The Holy Spirit is in
> this work and I feel we are right as we reiterate the words of our
> Lord 'Say not ye, there are yet four months and the cometh the
> Harvest? Behold I say unto you, lift up your eyes, and look on
> the fields: for they are white already to harvest'. John 4.35.

Having seen off the challenge of local politics in competing missions and powerful chiefs, Acton-Hubbard declared that the evangelism was charging forward with success. Not one mention of any
actual medicine in the hospital can be found in his account; the point
of the institution was a base for mission and the shining of spiritual (and literal) light. His declaration that the 'Holy Spirit is in this
work', combined with quoting Christ, is a classic trope of Protestant
testimony, in which the feelings and experiences of the believer's
relationship with God are set within the limits of scriptural authority.[139] For his own sense of destiny and with an audience of potential
supporters in prayer and money, Acton-Hubbard was constructing
a 'socially recognized personal identity' of the evangelist, out on the

frontiers of the faith, in dialogue with the movement of the Holy Spirit and the local culture. This was an alternate 'consensus reality' to that of the sanitised medical director which Acton-Hubbard performed at hospital openings and graduations for government officials. The SDA's role within the formal voluntary sector was an identity affirmed publicly to the state and the WHO, but largely separate from Acton-Hubbard's spiritual and evangelistic life personally.

As for their biomedical role, the SDA spiritual agenda was bound up with the desire to administer medicine and produce physical healing. Pamela Klassen has argued that, for many early twentieth-century Canadian doctors, technology was imagined as a way of communicating divine love, power, and prestige. Liberal Protestants were prominent on hospital boards and teams of determining clinical practice, and they perceived the point of the needle as the channel of the Holy Spirit. While sacral texts disseminated ideas, new materials such as electricity, radio, and X-rays were seen 'as both metaphorical and physical channels for healing'.[140] As with Acton-Hubbard's epiphany when realising the powerful effect of the light from the hospital, Klassen argues that many Protestants blended 'scientific and romantic discourses of experience ... proclaim[ing] the salvific and therapeutic benefits of technological and medical progress as tools for staying alert to the workings of the spirit'.

In drawing everyone into medical aid, for Dr Hyde of the SDA mission, general medicine itself expressed the complete work of Christ's ministry in which all become one in Him. Alongside their healing work, Acton-Hubbard was also training what he referred to as 'Lightbearers' – that is, students who were charged with 'going out Sabbath by Sabbath, distributing literature and tracts, holding compound meetings and of course giving Bible studies'. They were equipped with 'visual aids, special tracts, source material, marked Bibles ... [and] the coloured sign "Lightbearer", suitably set off on each side with a flaming torch'. Yet, as well as being a team of roving preachers, the photo with the article shows that these were also nurses and medical auxiliaries, half of them dressed in white medical uniforms and hats.[141] Acton-Hubbard wrote that a group of visiting 'evangelistic students studying health and First Aid at Kwahu' were 'absorbed into the working of the hospital'. The students attended lectures on helping on the wards and outpatient departments, and even attended major operations. On Sabbath morning they prayed, praised, and sang, they also had Bible studies prepared by Dr Hyde.

For example, Dr Hyde would share his thoughts on 'the complete-
ness of the work in God's remnant people', describing 'most vividly
the tragic results of over specialization' as well as counselling the
group 'to look to the Master' as their 'guide in living and working',
reminding them that the 'medical evangelist work has always been
near to the hearts of Seventh Day Adventists'.[142]

Not only was evangelism an outworking of the hospital ministry,
hospital ministry was also used to train evangelists in the meaning
of body and soul healing. Giving them physically demanding tasks
within the hospital was not to teach them how to be doctors alone,
but also to show them how to discipline their work as local evangelists. For example, appealing to the problems with 'over specialisa-
tion' in restricting a doctor's capacity to help lots of people, Dr Hyde
instructed the evangelists on how exactly they should live: looking
to Christ and not narrowing intellectual tracks. In some sense there
was no real split here between physical and metaphorical healing,
because the healing of the body and soul were joined.

While the SDA mission exposes the underlying complexities and
variety of identities at work within the voluntarist sector structures,
not all missions could navigate the tensions so deftly. A contrasting
mission, who struggled to find their place as state volunteers and
who began their medical missionary work in the 1950s, were the
Pentecostals and Scottish Presbyterians at Sandema in the Northern
Territories. Whereas the strength of the SDAs ensured that they
could evangelise locally and even innovate in remaking boundaries between medical authority and spiritual authority, the Scottish
Presbyterians had little of the resourcing, personnel power, or state
links that would make this possible. Notably given their role only
a decade or so previously, by the 1950s the Scottish Presbyterians
found themselves unable to benefit from the resources the voluntarist sector was affording to many medical missions. The category
of the volunteer was not neutral or depoliticised in development,
but bound up with national and international political changes that
informed its shape and determined who it empowered.

The Scottish Presbyterian mission began with two Assemblies
of God Pentecostals who pioneered mission work in the Northern
Territories in the 1930s. In 1951 Reverend William Lloyd Shirer, who
had been at odds with the Gold Coast colonial government for twenty
years, took a job with them as a community development officer.
Shirer and his wife Margaret had toured the hinterlands since 1930

and built an Assemblies of God station among the Dagomba. In 1950, British colonial policy shifted direction and the Northern Territories was included partially in the expansion of mass literacy and health care, reshaping missionary roles within the neglected region. With fluency in two African languages and a wide network of local contacts, Shirer became a prime target for government recruitment. Shrewdly he accepted the new offer to the Department of Social Welfare and Community Development, and Margaret was given a role as director of the Vernacular Literature Bureau.[143] With little evidence of why they made the switch from strictly 'religious literacy' to government education work, it has been suggested that debates over 'social mission' encouraged their move.[144] Perhaps as well, the Shirers exemplify the pure opportunism that mission sometimes required. Abruptly, they had gone from religious mavericks to hot property in the eyes of the state and it seems likely that the couple simply used this to the advantage of Protestant mission. As shown in their work with the Scottish Presbyterians, in addition to the Shirers' new employment they continued to scout out opportunities for missions, using their knowledge and political clout to open the doors wide to incoming teams.[145]

Through their government position, the Shirers facilitated the Scottish Presbyterian medical mission among the Builsa in the Northern Territories which ran from 1955 to 1972. As it was originally designed as a church planting mission and then adapted to suit the large medical needs of the local population, the project was desperately underfunded. It was mostly staffed by volunteers and unpaid Scottish nurses married to clergy. Nevertheless, with the Shirers' advice and contacts, the mission drew in crowds of local people for the church and medicine, forged long-term relations with communities, built several buildings, became a focus for vaccination programmes, and set up an ad hoc but vital ambulance service to the local Catholic hospital. With only an empty government clinic arriving in the 1960s and a couple of Catholic priests in the adjacent area, for almost twenty years the Presbyterian group provided the sole biomedical care to a region of around 70,000 people.[146] As a result of the Shirers and alongside evangelism, ministry, and sustained church growth, the Presbyterians created the first elements of biomedical health infrastructure in the area.

The mix of government administration and church-funded mission work between these adroit Pentecostal ministers and Presbyterian medical workers typifies how fluid the boundaries continued to be between the sacred and the secular in health care on the eve of the Gold Coast's decolonisation. Health care in Sandema was part of a large-scale increase in medical mission in the 1950s which spanned across the Gold Coast, including the North, and was backed by a great deal of government funding. There was a plethora of different forms of medical mission involved in this process, which together had nevertheless transitioned into a formal voluntary sector by the end of the 1940s. As a result of a blend of colonial policy making, government decisions, and missionaries' aims, the expansion was defined by contractual relations to the state. At the same time, informal collaborations remained essential to the sustainability and effectiveness of the missions, especially in local relations with communities, government, chiefs, and other missions. There were limits to formal government control and informal relations remained significant to the growth of mission.

By contrast with the SDA mission, the Scottish Presbyterian medical mission in Sandema in the Northern Territories had a stronger sense of themselves as volunteers, but could not fully benefit financially from the formalisation of the voluntary agency sector. In terms of their own self-identity, a form of voluntarism mattered far more to the Scottish medical mission at Sandema than it generally did to the SDAs. All of the health workers and nurses at Sandema were literally unpaid until 1966 when they employed their first professional member of staff. Before that, the medical mission was informal and unsystematic; it was funded by the Scottish Foreign Mission board but only for the church ministry that it was setting up. It must be noted here that while the Northern Territories were included in the 1950s development agenda, this certainly was not such a radical alteration, since it still remained the neglected region of the colonial state. The medical work, which comprised a huge amount of the mission's actual efforts, did not earn anything. It was supplied by individual nurses and ministers' wives filling their suitcases with medical equipment and drugs on the way to the Gold Coast. They also personally fundraised on furloughs by travelling around Scotland in all weather conditions including thick snow, and at churches' 'bandage Sundays', women's guilds, and Sunday schools. In a letter to the partners of the mission, its leader Colin Forrester-Paton wrote that '30 or 40 ... [come] every morning for treatment ... government had to withdraw the African nurse from the existing Sandema Dispensary ... Mrs Duncan originally planned to do something for mothers and their children but as soon as it became known that she was a nurse, people began flocking to her'.[147]

Louise Duncan was the wife of Robert Duncan, the minister attached to the mission, and had almost no knowledge of the Gold Coast or Africa at all when she arrived in 1956. Unlike the Forrester-Patons who had Oxford degrees, the Duncans were working-class Glaswegians with Robert being the first to attain higher education in his family. Using local networks and connections, Colin Forrester-Paton attempted to get funding from the government under their expansion of medicine in the Northern Territories, but was never successful. He wrote in 1957 that the government offered 'to provide a building, medical supplies and a junior assistant for any missionary nursing sister', but nothing arrived, except an assistant in 1959. Instead, the medical mission was set up on a shoestring, with a Jeep for taking emergency cases to Navrongo Hospital about 18 miles away, catering for around 70,000 Builsa in the region.[148]

The Sandema missionaries struggled with disgust, contracting diseases, and treacherous journeys, and retold these experiences in terms of a volunteer's sacrifice and overcoming. Unlike the settled hospital at Kwahu, the work at Sandema far more obviously exemplified the kind of adventurous 'voluntarism' that was being promoted in the OS, the VSO, and the Peace Corps in the 1950s. Some who staffed the medical mission were not even trained, and had to get used to dealing with sores and wounds. For example, Jean Paton, the wife of Colin Forrester-Paton, writes in her memoirs that when she had to bandage a septic leg in the dry heat of rural Sandema, she wished that she had had medical training. This visceral experience in a makeshift clinic without any real support or financial help pushed these missionaries to the edge. Similarly to how Julie Livingston has described negotiating disgust in Botswana, such experiences were also used in memory to construct a life-narrative of overcoming difficulty with self-sacrifice and by cultivating more dependence on the love of Christ.[149] Like many Peace Corps volunteers who reported not knowing what to do or how to help the places to which they had been sent, the Sandema missionaries were throwing their work together as it came to them.[150] Sometimes this was narrated in terms of impossible struggle, and other times in terms of achievement against the odds. Instead of working solely in the clinic, Jean Paton attempted to produce community health education and teach basic hygiene in order to best use her skills.[151] Robert Duncan wrote to the mission board that 'we are faced with the possibility of closing the clinic if we do not find someone. The great physical strain was seen in the contemplated outstation work, which has never been developed for obvious reasons. If a women's worker were appointed of whom you had doubts about her ability to tackle the trekking, then there is no need for her do it. The clinic, the women's class and the Sunday school in Sandema would offer her enough work without that strain'.[152]

Local politics were a significant concern for the medical mission at Sandema. At the outset of the mission it was building relations with local chieftaincy, via interpreters, that ensured they were able to settle in the area. Across the life of the mission these negotiations continued to be vital. For chiefs the mission was useful: acting as 'gatekeepers' between the medicine, land, and community bolstered their legitimacy as spiritual and political leaders. In order to continually empower themselves, as Justin Willis has shown, chiefs constructed 'elaborate political structures' using different forms of knowledge.[153] Before colonialism most chiefs in the Northern Territories were not custodians of the land, but in the 1920s creating such administrative roles for them allowed 'indirect rule' to function.[154] Navigating these power dynamics was crucial: as Robert Duncan writes, for example, the chief in Doninga was pro-Roman Catholic so they could not go there. However, when a fight occurred between the Chuchiliga and Sandema Nabs the missionaries capitalised by joining in the peace process and making new contacts without having to travel. The result was that they ensured their welcome in Chuchiliga, and the 'Kasem towns of Gbenia, Chiana and Ketiu'. As with many earlier pioneering missions, such as those described in nineteenth-century Uganda by Robert Rothberg in 1964, the Sandema missionaries were dependent on chiefs to make their ambitions grow into reality.[155] This was significant in an everyday sense. For example, Forrester-Paton describes how 'by coming to our service in the Local Council Hall from time to time, with a group of elders and once at least with a large retinue of drummers', the chief pronounced his authority as a Builsa and was able to surveil who was doing what. Forrester-Paton noted that this could be 'awkward for the preacher who might find halfway through his sermon that he was speaking to a very different congregation'. The priority, he notes, was not in 'converting the Chief' but in 'managing him'. The chief was the central authority in an area sidelined by the colonial state; he would invite an imam, he would attend the White Fathers events, and he would aid the Presbyterians because, as he once commented to Forrester-Paton, 'when a girl has several suitors, she gets more gifts'.[156]

In Marianne Gullestad's *Picturing Pity* about a North Cameroon mission, she argues that missionaries fostered one-way relations with local communities because they only gave out aid instead of entering into meaningful, interdependent processes of exchange in which they received gifts too.[157] This has much merit: missions which had stronger and more formal relations with the voluntary sector in the Gold Coast did not need to ask communities for as much, and therefore they did not need to spend as much time considering the community's way of seeing the world.[158] Situations of interpretation and exchange, in which intermediaries such as translators were critical power brokers, were not as common once missions had bureaucratised and formalised.[159]

However, the missions Gullestad describes were still shaped by the cultural encounters into which they entered. As Jamie Scott has noted, even in contexts in which there was a significant imbalance of power, there was still a 'constant commerce' in which missions were changed by the places where they found themselves.[160] What was different about missions like the one in Sandema was that over a long period of living in the area, negotiating with political leaders, conducting clinic work and health care in homes, and eating in local markets, the missionaries became a part of the community. Robert Duncan wrote of one extraordinary moment when he led the community, who came to him for help during a drought, to pray over their crops – he recalled how rain suddenly began to fall.[161]

Though, for all their negotiations, not everyone in the community was enthralled by the Sandema mission – only illiterates, children, and the Sandema chief, according to nearby Catholics. From the local Catholic perspective, the Sandema and Assemblies of God missions were battling for influence amongst the population by negotiating with the chief and giving handouts to the poorest elements of the community (including soap and sweets), but not always successfully. In the White Fathers' annual mission report for 1958 and 1959, the author wrote that the Sandema mission was brokering deals with the Sandema chief to its advantage. The Presbyterians were 'working against the will of the Chief of Chuchiliga', whereas in Sandema the chief seemed to be using 'his influence and authority to more or less

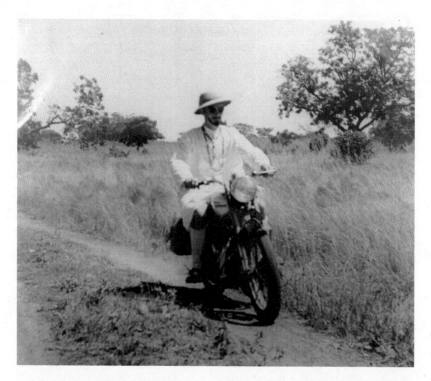

Figure 1.4 | 'White Fathers in the Northern Territories of the Gold Coast.
The White Fathers – are responsible for a great deal of welfare work
among the people of the Northern Territories of the Gold Coast ...
The motor cycle – which can get through narrow tracks which no four-
wheeled vehicle could tackle – is the favourite means of transport among
White Fathers in the North. A large number of remote villages are
regularly visited'.

force some people to follow their catechism-classes'. The chief was
also backing their move to place a Presbyterian teacher in their middle
school by getting him to write to the Education Department at Tamale
saying that there was no Builsa teacher capable of the post. The head
teachers in the district attempted to force the chief to retract his letter
regarding the lack of capacity. 'Needless to say', the White Father concluded, 'the Presbyterians are looked upon with more and more sus-
picion by all the teachers and literate people'. The White Father noted
that the Presbyterian pastor was giving milk to women and selling

pieces of soap 'at a greatly reduced price', which was enabling them to enrol a 'moderate group of illiterates'. By contrast, the literate classes had abandoned the Protestants and, according to the White Father, joined the Catholics. Finally, the report explained that another ploy of local Protestants, this time the Assemblies of God mission, had been to literally hand out 'candies' to children to attract them. This was followed, the report fumed, by a 'violent outburst of shocking insults towards the Catholic Church'[162] – though it claimed, with some satisfaction, that there were those who chose the Catholic Church over the candy.[163]

Overall, the Sandema mission's partial exclusion was part of a wider pattern in the 1950s; a key limit of the voluntary sector was that as the government focused on hospital provision, maternity and child welfare clinic work declined and then stagnated. New government funding was clearly not going into the same types of medicine that it was in the 1920s and 1930s when missions led the way in provision for child and maternal health. In 1952 the Ministry of Health had complained that it was struggling to find a sufficient number of trained health visitors.[164] In 1953 the death of rate of women during childbirth increased from 18.4 per 1,000 total births to 19.0 per 1,000. By 1954, it was at 21 per 1000 total births.[165] That year the medical report declared that 'there appears to have been no real improvement in the Infantile Mortality Rate during the past 20 years'.

Infant and child mortality was generally lower in the 1930s than in the 1940s and 1950s; in the 1930s infant mortality was even reduced to 100 per 1,000 related births in one year. Obviously, the incorporation of greater amounts of people, population rises, and the extension of state surveillance will affect these statistics, but the general impression is of mixed success in the 1930s and serious issues in the 1950s. The infant mortality problem in particular was hotly debated in the Legislative Assembly, where the ministerial secretary for the Ministry of Health, J.K. Donkoh, blamed pregnant women for failing to attend hospitals regularly. At this some honourable members replied 'Oh no! No!' and Dr Ansah Koi argued that it was the lack of sufficient oxygen in hospitals. Another minister, Mr Boakye, blamed the problem on the lack of maternity clinics across the country.[166] Given how difficult a long journey to a hospital might be for a pregnant woman, and the general reduction in clinics and lack of local care, in a sense all these arguments had merit. As the

Table 1.3 Gold Coast child and maternal health providers in 1945
(This was a considerable change from the dominance of the Red Cross in
the earlier 1940s.)

	Red Cross	Government	Missions
Children attending in 1945	42,819	52,738	97,126
Expectant mothers attending in 1945	36,893	30,990	6238

Source: *Gold Coast Colony Report on the Medical Department for the Year
1945* (Accra: Government Printing Department, 1946), 13, Liverpool School
of Tropical Medicine (Liverpool, UK).

Table 1.4 Gold Coast child health providers in 1950

	Government	Missions
Children attending in 1950	84,520	93,856

Source: 'Infantile Mortality Rate', *Report on the Medical Department for
the Year 1950* (Accra: Government Printing Department, 1952), 8, Liverpool
School of Tropical Medicine (Liverpool, UK).

Table 1.5 Gold Coast child health providers in 1952

	Government	Missions
Children attending in 1952	59,725	67,664

Source: *Gold Coast Government Report on the Medical Department For the
Year 1952* (Accra: Government Printing Department, 1952), 10, Liverpool
School of Tropical Medicine (Liverpool, UK).

Table 1.6 Gold Coast maternal mortality between 1934 and 1949
(Both rates reduced further slightly in the subsequent two years.)

	Maternal mortality (per 1,000 live births)	Maternal mortality (total)
1934	48	
1949	18.3	310

Source: *Gold Coast Colony Report on the Medical Department for the Year 1951* (Accra: Government Printing Office, 1952), 3, Balme Library, University of Ghana (Accra).

Table 1.7 Infant and child mortality in the Gold Coast between 1934 and 1954
(It must be noted that for 1950–54 there was no accurate survey of the whole colony given the difficulty of gaining full government registration – for maternal morality, the figures were based on thirty-six registration areas.)

Year	1934	1945	1949	1950	1951	1952	1953	1954
Infant mortality per 1,000 related births	115	119	125	122	117	125	113	119

Sources: 'Infantile Mortality Rate', *Report on the Medical Department for the Year 1950* (Accra: Government Printing Department, 1952), 8, Liverpool School of Tropical Medicine (Liverpool, UK); 'Infant and Child Mortality', *Report of the Ministry of Health for the Year 1954* (Accra: Government Printer, 1959), 21, 97, Wellcome Trust Library (London, UK); *Gold Coast Colony Report on the Medical Department for the Year 1951* (Accra: Government Printing Office, 1952), 3, Balme Library, University of Ghana (Accra).

American political scientist and sociologist David Apter wrote in 1955 from a field study with Gold Coast University on the Akuse dispensary, in the colony 'the death rate is high, how high no one knows in precise terms. Dispensaries are few and far between. Health facilities are overcrowded. In some areas people are afraid to go to a hospital because so many people die there after having traveled many miles on foot, by canoe, or by lorry, arriving too late for effective treatment'.[167]

Hospitals might provide a high level of care, but to even access one came with a high level of risk for most people. At the same time, it must be noted that when an antenatal care mobile clinic was run in HuHunya, it was 'very poorly attended'.[168] At an antenatal care at Sandema some women were discouraged by their husbands from leaving the house to visit clinics. Therefore, house visits were required, which in turn required relationships of trust to be fostered over a long time so that decent care would be possible.[169] Skimming the surface of the problem could be just as ineffective as sporadically setting up white elephants. Though not everything had changed, in 1947 rising child and maternal health attendances had been assessed by the medical department as due to their becoming a 'pleasant social event', similarly to the Kumasi health weeks in the 1930s.[170] Overall, in spite of the issues, hospital construction continued apace.

CONCLUSION

The aim of the late colonial state was to create a large system paid for by government and staffed by Christian missions within a formal voluntary sector. Following the decline of the Scottish Presbyterians after 1927, the makeup of this sector was diverse, and the results of these various trajectories was complex, not uniform or unilinear. Mission culture was not simply determined by voluntarist political agendas, financial aid, or softly shaped voluntarist norms within the colonial state. Missionary responses and culture were determined by denomination, specific congregation, theology, location, timing, and generation – as much as by other forces. The concept of 'voluntary' was ambiguous and was deployed in contested ways across this period. The mission clinic at Sandema much more clearly shows the relevance of volunteering and the voluntarist lifestyle; however, unlike the SDA mission at Kwahu, the Presbyterians could not fully benefit from the formal voluntary sector. The path was set for interventions which were scattergun and largely top-down, with much of state financing propping up hospital care that the majority of citizens were unable to access. A wholesale system based on sanitary policies driven by African voices was ignored. Instead, mission hospitals became the backbone of Ghanaian health care for the ensuing decades. This is the foundation on which later global health was based.

Religion and Africanising Health:
Ghana, 1957–68

The vast horizons of expectation for African postcolonialism often are judged to have been a mirage. As contemporary Chinese invest- ment creates new power dynamics on the continent, local African leaders can still look like gatekeepers whose political cultures are shaped ultimately by external resources rather than internal tra- ditions, cultures, and beliefs. For postcolonial nation-states like Ghana, the early years of independence were heady and optimistic. The triumph of self-governance quickly turned into the opportunity for modernisation and the realignment of international politics. The kernel of hope in this critical period seemed to have been destroyed by the 1970s, after coups and devastating economic crises appeared to show that the visions of 'Africanisation' were chimeras. How- ever, the power of the African nationalists in this period to lay claim and shape development and health should not be dismissed. Their choices and how they operated within their constraints had long- term ramifications. The pattern of colonial voluntary sector provi- sion was not broken, but it was reshaped and empowered in new ways by nationalists. Throughout the late 1950s and 1960s, tensions over religion, regional divisions, and conceptions of medical mission were key features of making 'modern' health.

To address unjust health access and to empower continued Africanisation requires close attention to how national health has been formed. Civil society, national infrastructure, the voluntary sector, religion organisations, and communities have been sites in which Africanisation and capacity building have occurred. Though Africanisation should not be conceived in the restricted terms that European missions often conceived of the process (with their attendant concerns for maintaining their role), global health still needs to recognise the significance of what those missions produced and how they were managed by nationalists. A deeper history of Africanisation in global health requires exploring the rivalries and local leadership battles whose unique political dynamics had complex outcomes. As long as the understanding of the early years of independence is oversimplified, the 'extraverted' continent will be at the whim of dominating global historical narratives, rather than charting a course which, amidst immense internal diversity, is distinct. Africanisation in independent Ghana changed the landscape of medical mission and development without uprooting the infrastructure built in the 1940s and 1950s.

Africanisation can be defined as simply the process of installing Africans in roles previously held by Europeans and Americas. This institutional form is the most obvious to assess and the easiest to chart. This chapter will track the Africanisation process emerging within the national Ghanaian churches, within European perspectives on the meanings of development, and within Kwame Nkrumah's government. It will compare the differences in Catholic and Protestant responses to 'Africanisation', analysing how local, regional, and transnational politics could shape this process as much as national political change.[1] Yet, there was a significant detachment between high-level concerns for modernity and sovereignty in the Ghanaian Parliament, and medical missions' own experiences and perspectives on decolonisation.[2] This chapter will argue that Catholic medical mission 'Africanised' in the sense of training many Ghanaians as nurses. However, because expatriate missionaries kept control of many of the higher positions in health care, 'Africanisation' in the sense of responding to ideas, structures, or perceptions of 'Africanness' was more limited. To keep clarifying this term is a continual and important process in mapping how global health has been changed by Africans and by uniquely 'African' perspectives, and how this relates to the legacies and networks of medical missionaries.

Africanisation was also conceived within a more specific conceptual and temporal framework that cast back to J.E.K. Aggrey and the development context of the 1920s. Aggrey's legacy for African leadership and elite education shaped how Africanisation was understood by Ghanaians nationally and globally. Aggrey's legacies, particularly the enduring achievement of Achimota College, were the subject of contests and battles, largely because of their symbolic place in the meaning of 'Africanisation'. Aggrey and Achimota could be seen as pillars in the restoration of Ghanaian traditional ritual in modernised postcolonial leadership, or they could be seen as lasting examples of accommodationist Christ-centred missionary internationalism. The definitions of the Africanisation process were unstable and at times fluid. Nevertheless, through commemorations and rituals, as well as through organising global health campaigns, Aggrey and Achimota's symbolic meanings were the focus of attempts to secure and fix the meanings of Africanisation.

This chapter will first explore Nkrumah's relationship with medical missionaries and the need and desire to fund them. Second, it will explore the other voices within the Ghanaian government supporting medical missions and Christianity more widely. It will examine a moment in 1958 when a high-ranking Muslim politician, Alhaji Mumuni Bawumia, argued in the Parliamentary Assembly that all Ghanaian health care should be given over to missions.[3] It will contrast this with the invocations on behalf of missions of Joseph Emmanuel Appiah. Appiah wished to be seen empowering high-level technical medical missions such as the Basel Mission at Agogo, in order to distance himself from his former 'tribalism' in the early 1950s. Not all political actors in Nkrumah's Ghana knew how to navigate the tensions between missions and development to their advantage. On their own initiative, 'leftists' in the Northern Territories took control of all the Catholic hospitals in Navrongo. This was shortly followed by Nkrumah returning all the hospitals to the missionaries and funding them even more extensively. By contrast, as the final section will conclude, one medical missionary touched a raw nerve by remaining in a key role at Achimota after independence, and was hounded out in the early 1960s. Nkrumah's developmentalism could seem inconsistent, it changed across his tenure, it homed in on specific symbolic battles, and in various contexts it could be confusing – even for his adherents.

THE AFRICANISATION OF MEDICAL MISSION
IN DECOLONISING GHANA

In Kwame Nkrumah's years as president of Ghana (1957–66), expatriate medical missionaries could be cast as necessary experts and health care workers because of the consolidation of their power in late colonialism. At the same time, because of their place in colonialism and their long-term linkages to its structures, they also could be attacked as vestiges of imperial rule. Missions thus could be seen both as representatives of scientific modernity or as stooges of colonial anti-modernity. Ultimately, how this contested role played out in the development narrative depended on the political utility that Ghanaian nationalists found in identifying themselves with either missionary modernity or their colonial roots. Simultaneously, missions could be identified as important supporters of technocratic development and as detractors from postcolonial independence, when it suited Ghanaian political actors. Yet, throughout these battles, missions continued to expand their coverage and funding from government. It is perhaps missions' reticence to challenge the status quo, in contrast to the bombast of political actors at the state level, which has contributed to their invisibility and perceived early decline. By 1967 there were thirty-four mission hospitals in Ghana staffed by a wide variety of congregations and denominations, only a handful fewer than the thirty-nine government hospitals.[4] Local hospitals carried on their work, often regardless of government changes.

Often detached from these high-level battles over modernity and colonialism, in local and regional contexts, missionaries continued to reformulate development in their own ways and by processes and localities that mattered to them. While Nkrumah was able to create a political context of which missionaries had to be aware, medical missionaries generally cast the major changes within decolonisation in terms of Africanisation rather than in terms of modernisation or separation from colonialism. Concerns for Africanisation arrived with decolonisation, but they did not exactly match up with the perspectives of nationalists on development or mission. Nkrumah could not be ignored, but his efforts could be challenged out of the public view, away from the symbolic centres of power such as Achimota College. Africanisation was divided by denominational changes, national churches' power, missionaries' awareness of their need to adapt, and the choices of local chiefs. These processes did not directly parallel Nkrumah's rise and fall; instead, they evolved in relation to changes in the national church and local chieftaincies. In general, the Protestant missions handed their hospitals over to Ghanaian church boards by 1967, which empowered them to challenge the state. By contrast, Catholic missions incorporated many Ghanaian nurses and health workers but kept many of their hierarchies dominated by expatriate missionaries into the 1980s, which limited some of the hopes of African autonomy.

There is an intense debate within the history of mission over how quickly and how extensively the historic mission church 'decolonised' and Africanised its hierarchies. David Maxwell argues that, often slightly in advance of political changes, ecclesiastical hierarchies were Africanised through the decolonisation era, with the Catholic Church making twenty African bishops in the 1950s. This proceeded apace with the Vatican II in the mid-1960s, and gained a 'critical mass' with the second of wave nationalism in the 1970s.[5] By contrast, Elizabeth Isichei has emphasised how much missions were desperate to retain control of their health institutions. She also noted their slow transition generally: in Sub-Saharan Africa there were 5,502 expatriate Catholic priests in 1949 and 8,703 in 1959, and by 1980 in Sub-Saharan Africa there were still 30 to 40 thousand Christian missionaries.[6]

However, Africanisation can be defined more broadly than just in terms of incorporating Africans into the running of churches and hospitals. It can also be considered in terms of changing methods, structures, and ideas in response to perceptions of 'African-ness'. As Ogbu Kalu has argued, the 'theological state' had imploded and the mission's 'passive revolution' failed to respond to African-initiated churches (AICs) and African indigenous Christianity. Kalu has argued that between 1965 and 1975 'people increasingly found the missionary version of indigenization to be unsatisfactory and restrictive'.[7] Simultaneously, medical missions could both retain power over their structures, methods, and ideas, but also be seen to Africanise by incorporating more Ghanaians into hospital work. The Catholics did this by training up many Ghanaians in low-level health care and holding onto the major positions of control within hospitals and clinics. The Presbyterian shifts were more profound, as they had to transfer power to an Africanised ecclesiastical hierarchy – though, as with the Catholics, they were limited by a lack of Ghanaian doctors.

Alongside personnel changes, battles around notions of Africanness were elaborated by key Ghanaian individuals within national and international health (sometimes, as with Nkrumah, these laid claim to the legacy of Aggrey – described further in the next section). Africanisation as a process of identity formation beyond an institutional personnel change figured significantly in how global health was shaped by Africans in in the 1960s, 1970s and 1980s.

For Ghana, where there were fewer histories of oceanic immigration into the country, much of Africanisation therefore related to how the continent was perceived as a modernising force. Nkrumah's Pan-Africanism linked to wider socialist networks and to the non-aligned movement, and though it may have been a largely failed project, its efforts at emphasising a particular racial role globally continued in different forms. This global slant to Africanisation is perhaps partly because much of the oceanic history of Ghana was in slave labour leaving the country, rather than, as in eastern and southern Africa, the imposition of systems of indentured labour or the colonial stratification of older trade routes being codified and increased. It also may be the result of the role of US and European University-educated elites occupying many of the leading roles in the first decades of postcolonial Ghana. Medical advocacy intersected with a conception of African racial difference and the challenge to the racial traditions in certain kinds of medical policy making. As for ethnic differences locally in Ghana and issues of autochthony, the way in which Africanisation of health shaped these is yet to be explored by historians, and funding such work would make extraordinary inroads into understanding postcolonial identities. This would build on the work already done on the 1920s and 1930s on the ethnic rivalries on the coast as well as their intersection with conceptions of development (explored in the introduction). Currently, the conception of Africanisation in this section remains partly narrowed to specific church and government institutional policies. However, a specific conceptualisation of Africanisation in its relation to the emergence of development and Aggrey was fought over by later Ghanaian leaders. This will be expanded in the next section on Nkrumah and further in chapter 4 with larger imaginaries of the unique African identities in global health.

Focused on its institutional roles, the Presbyterian Church of Ghana (PCG) announced in 1967 that it had Africanised all its hierarchies and taken national control over the Presbyterian missionary health infrastructure. This sat in awkward conjunction with the continued presence of expatriate missionaries.[8] By the early 1960s, new medical missionaries were being paid for by the PCG, such as the Scottish Presbyterian nurse Doris Hodds who was employed to move to Sandema to run the clinic. The Ghanaian Presbyterian synod clerk recorded that 'her salary is to be paid by the PCG which will also be responsible for her accommodations at Sandema'. Moreover, this was described in Afro-centric language: instead of 'missionary', Hodds was described as being 'engaged primarily as a "fraternal worker"'. Writing to the permanent secretary of health, A.L. Kwansa declared that 'the Church of Scotland ... is fully integrated in the Presbyterian Church of Ghana'.[9] In 1967 and 1968 the PCG produced a report to assess their health-care system in which their control over the medical system was emphasised: 'For the first time in the history of the Presbyterian Church of Ghana, members were asked to sponsor the medical work of the church which is done in six places in Ghana'.[10] For the large, symbolic Basel Mission Hospital at Bawku, the PCG proclaimed the 'considerable change ... made in replacing expatriates with Ghanaians, as part of the Africanisation'. Though most of the main medical positions were occupied by expatriates, the report proudly explained that 'the following posts held by fraternal workers were taken over by qualified Ghanaian personnel: Pharmacist, Nursing-Tutor, Laboratory Technician and Ward Masters'.[11]

In terms of perspectives on theologies of medicine, there was little that the PCG explicitly defined as a uniquely 'African' perspective, but the PCG did ensure that their own standards for evangelism were consistently being met. The 1967–68 report shows how there was inspections of standards of moral education through health care. These were detached from government perspectives on mission and modernity at the time and detailed how Christian mission was being extended. For example, at Agogo Hospital, one chaplain fiercely denounced the leadership for dropping 'Bible studies' and instead was encouraged by 'the branch of the Scripture Union which is gaining grounds among the Pupil Nurses'. An inspector wrote of the daily morning services and intercessional prayers on 'Saturdays for our patients and sick-friends', which were ensuring that the hospital's true mission was being practiced. Furthermore, the inspector wrote of nurses' evening services in the wards, in which there were 'guest preachers' and in-patients were 'given bibles and tracts to read'.[12] Yet the PCG were not looking to extend their independence to the point of financial self-reliance. On the report on the Bawku hospital, the account began by registering the 20,000 national cedis (NC) provided by the Ghanaian government and the 14,000 NC given by the Basel Mission to underwrite the hospital. In the analysis of Agogo, the Presbyterian contribution of 20,000 NC was printed alongside the government contribution of 50,000 NC and the Basel Mission's donation of 30,000 NC.

Scottish Presbyterians, who by this point had not been close to the government for more than two decades, generally found the PCG's authority an important safeguard against perceived nationalist excesses. Some expatriate Presbyterian missions saw the Ghanaian leadership as a bulwark against the kind of overreaching of state power as they had experienced under Nkrumah. Colin Forrester-Paton wrote in his penultimate letter to his partners in January 1970 that the PCG were an important ally in the need to be vigilant and 'to prevent the abuse of power'. This was especially the case as 'the problems of unemployment and the drift of people into towns, and of course the old evil of corruption, remain as daunting obstacles'.[13] On the other hand, Forrester-Paton could find the PCG difficult and inefficient himself. In the mid-1960s the PCG wrote to one of the Sandema missionary leaders explaining the necessity of training the nurse, Doris Hodds, at Navrongo or Bawku because of her 'lack of experience'. Forrester-Paton noted in the margin of the document, 'I am not clear how Dr. Warmann deduced this', adding that he could not see why she could not be moved straight to the mission when they were so desperate for help. This was a part of the PCG attempting to systematise health-care practice under their control. For example, in 1968 'Sister Lewis Fraser ... [had been] taught for five months at the Nurses Training School at Agogo and was transferred to Sandema in February 1968 to replace Sister D. Hodds for another period'.[14] Given the freedom with which Forrester-Paton had been able to run the Sandema mission in the previous thirteen years, at times he resented PCG oversight, especially when they set up bureaucracies which left the mission understaffed in the short term.[15]

Another aspect of Africanisation was the changing role of chiefs, who became more intimately involved with the local running of medical missions. At the Sandema Presbyterian medical mission, the first Builsa presbyter was Johnson Akobrika. Akobrika was a member of the Sandema Nab family and took over the mission work at Chuchiliga in the late 1950s.[16] From early on Akobrika had become indispensable to the Presbyterians' ability to settle in the area, but his involvement went further than a standard intermediary role. With his leadership as Chuchiga, Akobrika also became a supervisor to the Presbyterian clinic, chapel, and health centre.[17] The effect was wider than just for the mission itself. Akobrika's role in taking over some of the key supplies of health care in the area and co-opting the Presbyterian mission led to him being able to unite the Sandema chieftaincy with the

Chuchiliga chieftaincy. The chiefs had tied themselves to the medical mission and in doing so resolved a power battle at the centre of Builsa regional politics. At the local as well national levels, Ghanaians were able to drive institutional change in medical missions to fit their own agendas and according to their own priorities.

For missions, local chiefs could be relied upon to ensure their continued expatriate control and independence from the government. As Richard Rathbone has argued, Nkrumah's government embarked upon wholesale legal and administrative changes in order to eradicate the traditional constituents of Ghanaian social and political life.[18] The chiefs in the late 1950s began to infiltrate the church, as well as to co-opt it from the outside. The strategy for the chieftaincy from the late 1950s was to draw foreign interests into local political structures, with the chief as sort of head manager. Moreover, as Justin Willis has argued, chiefs detached themselves from state failings by continually reinventing their traditionalism.[19]

By contrast, with the Presbyterians, foreign funding allowed some Catholic missions' independence from political changes. The Holy Family Hospital at Berekum and their sister dispensary at Techiman consistently turned down government funding. In 1956 the hospital had turned down a £21,000 grant from the government.[20] Again in 1957, C.S. Takyi asked the minister of health if he would provide funds for the expansion of the dispensary at Techiman, but he was told that all of the £143,000 in the annually recurrent estimates for 1957–58 were committed because 'the Roman Catholic Mission that operates hospitals in Techiman and Berekum are not eager to have financial help from the government'.[21]

In another debate mentioned in the previous chapter, it was noted that the government could not force missions to take the money. It was not only Catholics who could sidestep government power: in 1961, Takyi asked which mission hospitals were rejecting government funding, and was informed that the Baptist mission hospital at Nalerigu had turned grants down as well.[22] Government development perspectives and narratives sometimes had little to do with how missions viewed themselves or their work. The Medical Mission Sisters (MMS) were keen to maintain their independence and, unlike other missions described in previous chapters, they could afford to do so. As will be explored in chapter 3, part of the reason was that they were receiving large amounts in donations from Dutch and West German Catholics.

Catholic medical missions in Ghana produced nurses' training and by the 1980s the majority of health workers in Catholic hospitals were Ghanaian; yet, it was often still expatriates who were the doctors and senior staff. Some hospitals, such as at Apam, had no expatriate personnel at all by this point, but Catholic health institutions were mostly a mix of Ghanaian and expatriate. Generally, where expatriates were available, they occupied higher-ranking positions such as doctors, senior nurses, and medical officers; Ghanaians generally did not find themselves in such positions. As is noted in the statistics on Holy Family Hospital at Nkawkaw, 'All the senior nursing sisters are expatriate personnel with considerable nursing experience'.[23]

Catholic medical missionaries were more concerned with Africanisation in response to decolonisation than they were with modernisation. It was through the construction of difference in terms of race that the missionary development narrative was given definition and identity. From 1953, the hospital at Berekum had also been beginning to develop a facility for training nurses, which struggled in the first four years with many candidates unable to pass state examinations and others leaving the hospital discouraged. In 1957 the programme was rearranged and by 1958 'nine students received their caps'; a further three passed preliminary examinations in 1960.[24] Training of locals as nurses was a key part of the way in which the MMS imagined the distinctions between themselves and Ghanaians: creating nurses both facilitated their work's sustainability and showed clear separation between Ghanaians who were educated and developed and those who were not. In material terms, with their MMS-style uniforms, trained nurses embodied racial and human development within Berekum. By 1982, only thirteen of the 193 staff members at Berekum were expatriate missionaries, and only another eight were MMS. Forty-seven of the Ghanaians working at Berekum were enrolled nurses.[25] In terms of hierarchy little had changed, though the nursing work had hugely expanded. Racial difference mattered for how medical mission was imagined and practised.

While the Catholic historic mission church was empowering African bishops, its health-care institutions were continuing to ensure some dominance of European and American Catholic doctors – both laity and in religious congregations. Catholic medical mission in Ghana maintained the control of expatriates partly because of, and

Table 2.1 Breakdown of Catholic health care between European and
Ghanaian staff in 1982

Function	Ghanaians (1982)	Expatriates (1982)	Total (1982)
Enrolled nurse/midwife	605	0	605
State-registered nurse/ midwife	99	66	165
Chaplain	7	6	13
Doctor	7	26	33
Laboratory personnel and X-ray technicians	80	0	80
Ward assistant/auxiliary	621	0	621
Matron	9	7	16
Administrator/clerk	79	4	83
Labourers/domestic auxiliary	569	2	571
Medical officer	0	4	4
Pharmacist	1	3	4
Senior nursing Sister	0	20	20
Village/community health workers	41	1	42
Tutor	8	5	13
Qualified registered nurse/midwife	15	0	15

Source: Compiled using statistics from the surveys contained in Patrick A.
Twumasi, *Survey Report Health Services in Ghana: National Catholic
Secretariat January–April 1982 (April 1982*, Department of Health, National
Catholic Secretariat, Accra), private archives of the National Catholic
Secretariat (Accra, Ghana).

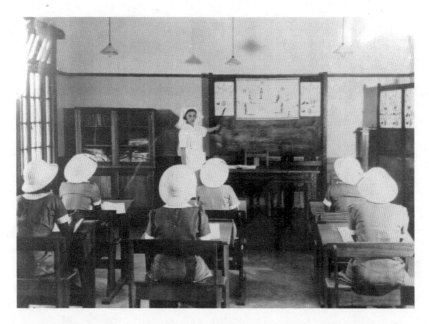

Figure 2.1 | 'Princess Marie Louise Hospital, Gold Coast: Miss Pittock, Health Nursing Sister giving a lecture in the Lecture Rooms' (c.1950s).

not in spite of, Vatican II. Expatriate medical mission Sisters, such as the Holy Family Hospital at Berekum, were affected by Vatican II, but in ways that actually contributed to their control. Vatican II not only encouraged the making of African bishops, it also relieved nuns of having to always wear habits in public. For the MMS at Berekum, this meant they could do work in ecumenical and secular settings more easily.

Continued expatriate power was also partly an issue of training and immigration more generally. From the 1950s, Catholics had been training Ghanaians to become nurses, but not in higher level qualifications. At Berekum where there was a nursing training college, there were sixty-seven enrolled Ghanaian nurses and midwives but only one Ghanaian doctor out of a total of five. This was generally the case across Ghana. The cadre of Ghanaian doctors was limited, and missions did little to help this process. As will be explored in chapter 4, Nkrumah's attempt to create a medical school faltered and, as will be described in chapter 5, half of Ghana's doctors and nurses left the

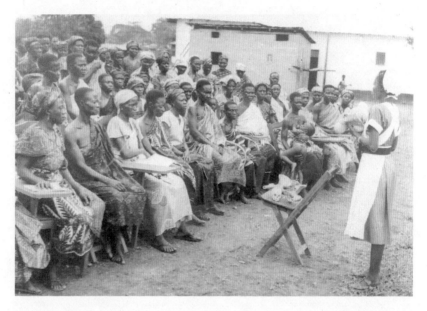

Figure 2.2 | 'A course was recently held at Kwaso, in Ashanti, for tradi-
tional village midwives, and proved of immense value. This picture shows
Miss Agnes Ofori, the midwife in charge of the course, lecturing village
women on child welfare' (c.1950s).

country during the economic and political crises of the late 1970s
and early 1980s, resulting in further expatriate control.[26] In Catholic
health in Ghana by 1982, expatriate doctors still predominated,
whereas Ghanaians held the majority of administrative and auxiliary
roles. Though one significant shift was that, by this point, there was a
third more Ghanaian nurses than European ones.

CHRISTIANITY, MISSION, AND KWAME NKRUMAH

In contrast with the medical missions, Nkrumah's Africanisation
came with far more intellectual energy and with the drive to reformulate the previous meanings of development, as well as to recapture the symbolic meanings of its earlier African creators like Aggrey.
These changes took place in the context of Nkrumah's increasing
consolidation of political power. Nkrumah formed how Ghanaian

politicians and medical missions imagined the process of development and independence in the 1950s and 1960s. He dominated structures and culture, though in complex and contested ways. Nkrumah was concerned to re-sacralise the Ghanaian state when he took over as president in 1957. He began a process of redefining Christian development in his own terms, in relation to pre-colonial pasts and traditional African religion. Amidst his challenges to missionary tradition, he promoted Christian beliefs. Moreover, alongside his attacks on medical missionaries Nkrumah needed the formal voluntary sector and historic forms of mission medicine to run health care. Given the consolidation of medical mission across the colony in the 1950s, Nkrumah focused on culture wars in visible places in the capital that symbolized African achievement – such as Achimota College – where Nkrumah has been a pupil and a teacher, as well as being mentored by Aggrey.[27] Concurrently, mission health care in Ghana grew across the country. Nkrumah constructed a narrative of modernity free from imperial and religious bonds by focusing on key points of significance that would be seen by specific audiences, not wholesale or systematic change. Nkrumah did not wholly reject the religious past, but modified older economies of the sacred. Sacraments were reconceptualised, traditional rituals were retained and developed in new ways, and in cultural exchanges and negotiations old and new beliefs were mixed.[28]

Nkrumah's relationship with religion, development, and Africanisation were complicated to say the least. He had trained as a Presbyterian minister in the United States and yet allowed a cult to form around him as a messiah while he was president. He advocated a type of civil religion and noted that because religion was an 'instrument of bourgeois social reaction ... the state must be secular', and ejected clergy he did not like, planted party officials in churches, and carried a walking stick and white handkerchief like a 'priest of African religion'.[29] This was a state that wished to influence religion, while not wanting the church to influence it in return. Notoriously, Nkrumah infuriated the church and missions when he put up a statue of himself outside Parliament House with a sign saying 'Seek ye first the political kingdom' (an authoritarian twist of Christ's invocation to 'Seek ye first the kingdom of God'); yet alongside this avowed secularism, he also drew on all forms of spiritual authority, from animism to the freemasons.[30] What can be said is that Nkrumah shifted from a relationship with God, which he described as 'very personal ... [and] direct', to a focus on the aggressive pursuit of pan-African cultural and political independence as his primary concern when he assumed power.[31] As much as was practically feasible, secularisation and attacking missionaries were important tools in Nkrumah's arsenal – but as rhetorical and symbolic strategies, rather than literal policy. In spite of his image as an ideologue, Nkrumah did not let any animosity toward the colonial government-mission nexus interfere with his paramount aim of African independence, and for the moment that meant the success of his brand of Ghanaian nationalism at all costs.[32]

In general, Christianity was also incredibly useful to Nkrumah. As John Pobee puts it, Nkrumah's party, the CPP (Convention People's Party), realised that 'homo ghanaiensisis is homo radicaliter religiosus and could, therefore, be reached through religion'. As Rupe Simms has shown, the party newspapers used biblical language, comparing taking up CPP principles to being filled with 'new wine'. Moreover, several times in the early 1960s the *Evening News* described Nkrumah as the Second Coming of the transfigured messiah. From 1963 the Newspaper Licensing Act had meant that only party newspapers could exist and the evening news had become one of the foremost mediums of state propaganda. Yet, as early as 1950, the same newspaper had rewritten the beatitudes in Matthew in terms of self-government and activism: 'Blessed are ye, when men shall vilify you and persecute you, and say all kinds of things against you for Convention People's Party's Sake'. In another instance the party changed the Lord's Prayer to read: 'Give us this day our full self-government/And forget about the infringement of charges'. Moses's exodus from Egypt, Ethiopianism, and the challenge of the early Christians to Rome were all recast in terms of the fight for freedom from empire. Christianity was also useful because it acted as a unifying system, language, and set of practices for a nation riven by ethnic and political differences. Nkrumah cast himself not only as a messiah but also as a 'non-denominational Christian'.[33] In this period, the heterogeneity of missions and Christianity was constructed according to its significance in building the nation. Resacralising the state was part of reconstructing Ghanaian citizenship and consolidating political power. This was particularly important given that Nkrumah's main supporters were school leavers whose limited literacy was mostly from mission schools, which meant that they would have known many of the most common phrases of the Bible.[34]

Nkrumah's relationships with missions were also complicated. In 1951 Nkrumah was given the title 'leader of government business', winning a democratic election which was a colonial concession to trade unions and nationalist organisations demanding 'self-governance'. Shortly after, in 1952, Nkrumah was given the title of prime minister.[35] At this point, when Nkrumah was first successful in national politics and no longer in a prison cell, he denounced general poor health care and missionary education for their places in colonial injustices: 'There were slums and squalor in our towns ... All over the country great tracts of open land lay untilled and uninhabited, while nutritional diseases were rife among our people ... our existing schools were fed on imperialistic pap, completely unrelated to our background and needs'.[36]

By 1957, after violence, constitutional impasse, and political turmoil, Nkrumah had capitalised on the economic success of the Gold Coast and on his status amongst school leavers to win victory for the CPP and establish himself as president without a formal opposition.[37] This laid the groundwork for his dictatorship. Across this period Nkrumah developed one of his conceptions of missionaries (in tandem with his changing ideologies) as harbingers of colonial oppression and as roadblocks to socialist modernity. In 1963, Nkrumah wrote that missionaries had participated in colonial theft and slavery: 'While missionaries implored the colonial subject to lay up his treasure in Heaven, where neither moth nor rust doth corrupt, the traders and administrators acquired his minerals and land ... Assuming the Christian responsibility of redeeming Africa from the benightedness of barbarism the ravages of the European slave trade were forgotten; the enormities of the European conquest ignored'.[38] In the same year, Nkrumah's minister for foreign affairs and the president of the UN General Assembly agreed in his own book that, 'in short, the personality of the African individual was systematically being debased and eventually denied, if not obliterated, by the support missionary activity gave to colonial rule'.[39]

Another of Nkrumah's foreign ministers and one of Ghana's 'founding fathers', Emmanuel Ako-Adjei, described mission as 'spiritual aggression' and 'spiritual imperialism' – in spite of being a devout Christian himself who was educated in a Basel Mission school.[40] Yet, Nkrumah still funded the medical work of missionaries extensively because the experts and staff were necessary to ensure a stable health-care system across the emergent Ghanaian state. As with his notions of religion and resacralisation more widely, Nkrumah saw missions as a relative problem compared to his absolute focus on the success of Ghanian nationalism and pan-African independence. Where and when he drew the line on his ideological commitments was not simple.

In terms of ideology, Nkrumah's form of socialist transformation was not focused on changing property relations, eradicating religion, poverty, or economic slavery, or really on 'class' at all, but rather on economic productivity and modernisation. Socialist mass welfare was his long-term version, but a mixed economy was its short-term, evolutionary means.[41] Nkrumah had argued in his earliest speeches that he wanted to cut a diplomatic path through East and West and to continue the technocratic developmentalism of his colonial predecessors. He funded European and American missions at the same time as building relations with the Eastern Bloc. This positioning was complex – as well as supporting foreign missions, Nkrumah's socialism meant mobilising youth for self-discipline and self-reliance, in ways that were tied to aviation and modernity.[42] Yet, by 1960, and perhaps even by 1958, his concerns for retaining power, his fear that he was being spied on by American intelligence, and an attempt on his life forced him into choosing a single course publicly.[43] Once president, Nkrumah was quick about ensuring his hold on power and silencing dissent: the Preventative Detention Act in 1958 consolidated his grip on the state, regional and sectional politics were stopped by 1959, and in 1964 the One-Party Act finalised this process.[44]

Nkrumah's visions of modernity were widely disseminated, but he could not control their interpretation or actual effect. Nkrumah claimed that the Ghanaian state needed to go through a process of resacralisation because historic colonial-mission relations had harmed society. Nkrumah argued that he did not want to create a 'political war on religion' when insisting on the 'secular nature of the state', but he did have very strong ideas about the African path to modernity which cast 'colonial' religion as backward.[45] However, Nkrumah's attempts at encouraging resacralisation faltered outside of state newspapers and state monuments. During his time studying for the ministry in the US, Nkrumah had attempted to remake the identity of J.E.K. Aggrey by performing Aggrey's funeral with libations and traditional ritual – much to the chagrin of his college. The aim was to recast Aggrey as a bridge between African ancestry and African modernity. Yet, this did not automatically mean that Ghanaians reimagined who Aggrey had been. Aggrey's legacy was seen by many as bound up with the historic mission church, with Cape Coast elitism, with the Fantes, and with the Guggisberg vision for Christian human development. Aggrey had preached continually in these terms without rejecting foreigners. Aggrey's most famous invocation – for the 'black and white keys' to work together – was not immediately thrown asunder when Nkrumah mourned him in a different way.[46]

Nkrumah's attacks on the historical role of mission also did not discourage their medical work in Ghana or stop him from funding them. In some decolonising areas, such as Sudan and Indonesia, state unification problems were blamed on missionaries; they were held responsible for disruptions because their faith was contrary to the process of promoting national Islam. In other areas, authoritarianism and civil war led missionaries to flee.[47] In Ghana, many medical missions were not only unharmed, they continued to receive government funding. The first ten-year development plan based on the recommendations of the Maude Commission did not stop in 1957, but continued until at least 1960.[48] In 1957 the ministerial secretary to the Ministry of Health, F.K.D. Goka, responded to a question as to whether the recommendations of the Maude Commission would be dropped by averring that there would be 'no deviation from the programme' – to which the Assembly responded with cheers of 'Hear, hear'.[49] Many hospitals run by missions, which were constructed and equipped by government in the 1940s and early 1950s, still had their recurrent costs covered by the government after independence.

The effect of the Burns Hospital agenda, the Maude Commission, and Arden-Clarke's missionary zeal was long lasting, and was compounded by Nkrumah's development plans. As B.A. Konu put to F.K.D. Goka in May 1957 in a debate over whether Ada would get a hospital: 'Does the Minister not appreciate the fact that it is more in the interest of the country as a whole to build at last one health centre in each of the 104 constituencies than to build central hospital in two or three towns where patients wait for hours on end to be attended?'[50]

The minister prevaricated and was a little riled when another question asked: 'Is it not a fact that the Government care very little for the health of the people in the rural areas?' Goka responded: 'That is not a fact, Sir'.[51] The predominance of mission hospitals continued well beyond Nkrumah's rise to power and actually increased. Though there was certainly some opposition to the lack of government interest in hospitals, it did not steer them from the course set out by the mission-government relations which began in the 1940s – none of Nkrumah's hostile public rhetoric was even registered in the Assembly. Nkrumah's five-year and seven-year development plans included significant provision for health-care and medical education. In the second development plan commencing in 1959, of the total £350 million requirement presented to the National Assembly, £200,000 was proposed for endemic diseases and health education, and £1,130,000 was made for the new regional hospital at Tamale and new hospitals at Walewale, Wiawso, and the first phase at Tarkwa. It also included mission hospitals at Mampong and Nsawam. £705,000 was provided for the extension of existing hospitals and £800,000 for health centres in non-cocoa-producing areas.[52]

In spite of Nkrumah's support, some Protestant missions struggled with funding and staffing from the later 1950s. In June 1957 there was a debate in the National Assembly over the Presbyterian hospital at Worawora which was having difficulty getting nurses, running an ambulance service, and housing its staff.[53] F.K.D. Goka, at the time the parliamentary secretary to the Ministry of Health, declined to add to the funds for the hospital: 'The Voluntary Agency which manages this hospital was given a capital grant for £80,000 for the buildings. When this arrangement was made it was clearly understood that the Voluntary Agency would be responsible for equipping the hospital and for paying all recurrent costs other than those involved in training nurses ... The management of the hospital is in the hands of the Voluntary Agency and it is its obligation and not that of my Ministry to take any steps that are necessary to provide an ambulance and staff quarters'.[54]

Unlike Goka, the challengers Mr Kodzo and Mr Kusi were demanding more money from the government because 'the hospital is now in dire need of nurses', 'the buildings in the hospital were put up by the Government without the quarters', and the £80,000 grant was not sufficient 'to buy an ambulance besides meeting other expenses'.[55] Goka replied that 'nurses are in short supply all over the world' and that 'it was clearly stipulated that the Agency will provide quarters for the nurses'.[56] He added that '£80,000 was used in building the hospital' which had been running for some time (it was built in 1952).[57] Nowhere during this debate was the question of the validity of funding missions raised; the problem was that Goka did not want to extend the original 1952 contract. That both Kodzo and Kusi were repeatedly challenging him shows how much the mission hospital mattered to the region. In spite of the failure of the mission to honour their agreement to provide nurses' quarters, two Ghanaian representatives were promoting them in a nationalist assembly.

The mission's problem was not with government but with their financial circumstances. This was not an anomaly. As David Hardiman has shown, six out of eleven Protestant mission hospitals were shut down between 1956 and 1965 in Gujarat by Indian churches because of a lack of finances.[58] It is possible that the Presbyterians' efforts to staff another hospital at Adidome was straining their health-care resources, given their reduced power over education. The 1950s were the high point of world mission and many missions expected to keep growing – whatever happened with decolonisation and the Cold War. According to Adrian Hastings, the amount of expatriate missionaries in Africa increased until 1966 and subsequently declined.[59] As David Maxwell has shown, because of their loss of education to postcolonial states, many mission churches started working more in health care, female self-sufficiency, and environment and sanitation.[60] However, for some missions this may have been logistically too difficult, whatever the political context.

MEDICAL MISSION AND EARLY POSTCOLONIAL GHANAIAN HIGH POLITICS

Within the political culture of development, Africanisation, and Christianity that Nkrumah was trying to construct, Ghanaian politicians used different strategies to consolidate their own power. One of the tactics was to identify with certain aspects of medical mission but not others. At the various levels of Ghanaian politics, creating links with and defending aspects of medical mission could be vital to retaining a foothold in the government of the postcolonial nation-state.

It was not only because of old commitments to colonial recommendations that the independent government funded medical mission: some Ghanaian ministers wanted to spread medical mission right across the new nation. David Maxwell has emphasised that the

'mission-educated leadership of nationalist movements was distinc-
tively lukewarm towards the Church'.[61] While this argument holds
true for most at the very top of nationalist movements, many of
those who were one rung down from the presidencies, without such
a great public-facing role, were proud of their mission roots and
keen to see mission control expanded into other services. This is
more in line with revisionist historiography that has differentiated
between the views of the rank-and-file and the leadership within
African nationalist parties; but here it is extended to more subtle levels within government leadership itself.[62] Crucially, it was not only
ministers who liked mission itself that advocated for medical missionaries, it was also politicians who knew that supporting it could
be used to their own political advantage.

    One of the most striking examples of a senior government socialist
supporting medical missions was Alhaji Mumuni Bawumia. Around
the same time that Nkrumah was strengthening his grip on power
by ending sectional and regional politics – and in the same week that
Bawumia 'crossed the carpet to join with CPP' to a chorus of cheers
from CPP members – Bawumia advocated for all of health care to
be transferred to missionaries. All of it, that is, except the central
hospitals. He asked on 20 June 1958 in the National Assembly: 'In
view of the shortage of doctors and the difficulty experienced by
the Government in recruiting doctors, will the Government consider
handing over all hospitals, with the exception of central hospitals to
the Missionaries'?[63]

    This statement was made only three days after Bawumia had joined
the CPP. At one of the most pivotal and controversial moments of
Bawumia's career, he claimed that missions should take over the entirety
of Ghanaian health care. Two months later Nkrumah attempted to
give Bawumia a ministerial post but was persuaded against it because
of internal issues in the CPP. Bawumia's statements had clearly not
antagonised Nkrumah. If anything, it may have been that, given
Nkrumah's own private attitude to missions, Nkrumah had considered Bawumia's comments as a serious potential policy direction. In
1962 Bawumia was made minister of state and northern regional
commissioner, and was given 'all … the support and cooperation he
needed' by 'Chiefs, [and] old and new CPP members'. Though it must
be noted that relations were not always so easy, given Nkrumah's
increasing volatility and paranoia; for example, in September 1962
Nkrumah accused Bawumia of attempting to assassinate him.[64]

For Bawumia, supporting medical missions was a ploy for other political means – and one he was experienced in making. In 1955 Bawumia had used the building of a Baptist mission hospital to consolidate regional political power for Mamprugu. Bawumia helped to ensure the building of the Nalerigu Baptist Mission Hospital when he worked for the Mamprusi Native Authority. In his memoirs Bawumia explains that the district commissioner had been hoping in January 1955 that a US Baptist mission tour might settle in Mamprugu. The aim was, according to Bawumia, 'to ensure the development and expansion of Nalerigu to befit its state as capital and seat of the King of Mamprugu'. This was not about Christian evangelism but about regional geographies of power. Bawumia knew that the government was not going to support the area and had not included Nalerigu 'in its development programme for either a health centre or hospital'. Regardless of national government interests or those of the CPP, Bawumia said that he would go to 'any length to get the hospital established' – this to ensure that Nalerigu retained and enhanced its regional status.[65]

In order to make this support of the Baptist hospital possible Bawumia then worked with Naa Sheriga (the paramount chief, king of Mamprugu – the Nayiri), to purchase 'a big ram, eggs and yams to welcome them', and then when they arrived, he 'assembled all sick people in and around Nalerigu ... includ[ing] the blind, lepers and chronic chest pains ... and pregnant women'. He mobilised the Elders to show support and marshal the sick to show need. The Nayiri aimed to convince the missionaries by arguing that the people and chiefs in Upper Volta (Burkina Faso) and Northern Togo still paid 'allegiance to him' and so would be patients for the hospital too. Moreover, Bawumia produced a map to prove that, apart from Gambaga and Walewale which were Muslim dominated, the rest of the area had no particular religion. As expected, the Baptists agreed to build a hospital on the land that the Naa offered.[66] Bawumia knew how to play missionaries to his own advantage, partly because he knew what they wanted and how they worked. This was not because he desired Christian evangelism; Bawumia was a Muslim. It seems far more likely that it was a ploy to create local political power and garner foreign investment.

While Bawumia's experience was of CPP opposition to the mission at Nalerigu, it was actually with Nkrumah's help that the Baptist hospital was built; this Bawumia may have taken as a general principle for political operation in national government. After the mission decided to settle at Nalerigu and applied to reside there, the CPP minister of health (J.H. Alhassani) blocked the process because the Nayiri did not support the CPP. However, Bawumia outmanoeuvred him using his relationship with Richard Akwei, who had lived in Gambaga in the medical field units as principal secretary. Akwei was unsuccessful at first, but Bawumia went to Accra to force Akwei into pleading to Nkrumah for the hospital. Awkei did, and was successful in convincing Nkrumah, going over the minister of health's head, who was extremely dismayed again because of the Naa's opposition to the CPP. In response Nkrumah argued that 'if the people were not CPP today they could be CPP tomorrow'.[67] Three years later, and three days after joining Nkrumah's party (at which time Bawumia clearly advocated for medical mission), he may have been utilising his experience with Nkrumah during the conflict over the mission at Nalerigu.[68] Bawumia was probably aware of how he could sideline other CPP members and ingratiate himself to Nkrumah. Nkrumah's rhetoric about missions might have fooled some, but according to his autobiographical reflections on Nkrumah's intervention at Mamprugu, Bawumia knew better. Bawumia consistently managed the role of missions for political advantage in specific contexts, here interpreting correctly that Nkrumah's socialism was necessarily limited by the needs of development.[69]

Buwumia was not alone in supporting missions from within Nkrumah's party. Associating missions with modernity could be a useful political tool for other Ghanaian nationalists. Joseph Emmanuel Appiah, the United Party (opposition party under the one-party state) member for Atwima Amansie, proclaimed in a major speech to the National Assembly that medical mission should provide for a huge proportion of Ghanaian health care, just as mission education had produced 'ninety per cent of those of us who sit in this House':

> We know that in the far North, in Agogo, in Brong-Ahafo, all over the country, these missions have tried to satisfy the health needs of our people by setting up hospitals. I know that in some places it is the misery of the people that has compelled them to set up these emergency hospitals, as I call them. I have always felt that whenever and wherever a missionary body has done a thing like that the Government of the day should be ready to help

them in all ways without their crying for it. Look at the hospital at Wenchi, for example; it is satisfying a growing need in a very large area and yet building facilities, accommodation and so on are very poor because it is the work of the Methodist Mission. I know that they have not got much funds and they could only do what their purse would allow them to do. The accommodation of the doctor in that hospital, not to take even of that of the nurses, cries to high heaven to deliverance.

Another example is the Agogo Hospital. The number of people who stream into that hospital from all over the country, makes one feel that here is a job that has been well done again by a mission. I happen to know that if they have the wherewithal they will expand the hospital to meet the growing needs of the people who come from far and wide. It is always a source of pity to go to Agogo Hospital and see people standing outside the gates because all the beds are full ... [there is] terrible congestion in this place and I am almost constrained to say that I beg the Ministry to do something about this missionary hospital.[70]

Appiah went on to argue that not only should mission hospitals be far better funded, the government should do more to restrict 'herbalists' and 'witch-doctors'. As he put it, 'we cannot mix up science with superstition'.[71] Given the historic animosity between medical missions and the 'juju' of their African counterparts, Appiah was not only promoting their hospitals, he was also repeating one of the traditional tropes of their struggle.[72] In this he was showing himself to be a defender of Agogo, a mission hospital in Asante which represented the heights of modern biomedical achievement with its ophthalmology unit funded by the German Blinden mission. It seems likely that Appiah was trying to associate himself and the region with the drive for national modernity.

This type of missionary modernity was in contrast to the 'tribalism' of the Asante chiefs and Asante politicians such as Appiah, who were under fierce attack within Nkrumah's Ghana.[73] Particularly significant to Appiah was that Nkrumah's charge of anti-modernity and colonialism had been levelled at the National Liberation Movement (the previous opposition party to the CPP) earlier in the 1950s because of its association with Ashanti. In 1951, during an escalation of violence in Ashanti, the CPP had proposed to break up the region into two administrative regions, capitalising on divisions between the Kumasi chiefs and those in the Brong region. At this point Appiah, an Asante himself, left the CPP to join the NLM. This was a big blow to Nkrumah as Appiah had been one of his close companions and a delegate at the 1945 Pan-African conference. However, what was crucial was that Appiah with the NLM could now turn the charge of 'tribalism' back on the CPP, claiming that they wanted power over Asante instead of national unity. However, by the 1956 election, the CPP had been able to regain ground; they propagated the message that the NLM would cause an Asante invasion of the South, they decreased internal CPP rivalries, and they allied with the chiefs in the North. Continuing support from school leavers who had moved the South, the CPP won in 1956 and the NLM were forced into appealing to the United Nations and to the British Colonial Office for an independent Asante. In 1957, the secretary of state Lennox-Boyd did promise safeguards in the constitution to the NLM leadership protecting the region's autonomy and chieftaincies. Yet when Nkrumah consolidated power in the late 1950s he destooled pro-NLM chiefs, empowered pro-CPP chiefs, ended chiefly power within local councils, and divided the Asante region.[74] By contrast, the chiefs in the Northern Territories were largely untouched and continued to form the basis of the Northern People's Party (NPP), a vital political bloc following the downfall of Nkrumah in 1966.[75] As for Appiah and the NLM Asantes, they were left with the burden of their earlier attempt to sidestep Nkrumah and were now easily labelled as 'tribalists' who did not support modernisation. Thus, given the political culture that Nkrumah had set up, associating with national 'modernity' rather than Asante 'tribalism' was vital to retain a political footing within the one-party state.[76]

Nkrumah and CPP members like Appiah valued associating with missions because they could be used to bolster claims to scientific advancement, biomedicine, and technology. Far from being backward stooges of tradition, Appiah's comments show how missionaries could also be viewed as the key players in a postwar developmentalism, as Joseph Hodge describes in the case of the Swynnerton Plan in Kenya, and Sabine Clarke argues for in the case of the Colonial Office.[77] As Clarke argues, there was technocratic turn in official Colonial Office thinking between the 1940s and 1960s, when development solutions were rationalised based in a faith in science and influenced by the large-scale research projects of E.B. Worthington and Lord Hailey's African Survey. Nkrumah and Appiah may have been influenced by these as well, perhaps through development economists brought into Ghana such as William Arthur Lewis.[78] Yet, going beyond Clarke's argument, this thinking occurred alongside the longer-term missionary traditions of challenging 'superstition' and indigenous practices perceived as demonic.[79]

However, visions of missions as development surrogates coexisted with Nkrumah's links between missions and colonial legacies of inequality, and this coexistence demonstrates the complexity of Nkrumah's development vision. Modernity was related to national unity and the sidelining of the Asante chiefs. It was not modernity at all costs; modernisation was specifically intended to defeat regional political opposition. Depending on its utility to national political control, for Nkrumah and others, missions could either be cast as colonial manipulators or as modern medical scientists. In postcolonial Ghana, development could reduce the significance of missionary proselytism and divides. As shown across various National Assembly debates in the late 1950s and 1960s, missions could be cast as neutral drivers of necessary development projects to help the Ghanaian people. In some ways this corroborates James Ferguson's famous thesis that development can function as an anti-politics machine in which the performance of 'extremely sensitive political operations involving the entrenchment and expansion of institutional state power' can be undertaken invisibly through 'neutral, technical mission'.[80]

In Nkrumah's socialist CPP the response to the promotion of mission medicine was generally positive. C.S. Takyi (CPP Wenchi East) directly agreed with Appiah in the same debate in 1960: 'We have Mission hospitals at Berekum, Techiman, and Wenchi but these hospitals do not get subsidies from the Government; they operate on their own. I am suggesting that the Government should give them sufficient grants'.[81]

That said, it must be noted that in another debate the following year Takyi was furious that government officials were not being allowed to use mission hospitals free of charge and therefore had to travel 40 to 50 miles elsewhere. He also criticised mission hospitals that 'were not giving their best' and should be taken over by government. For Takyi as for Nkrumah, promoting mission hospitals was pragmatic on the basis of what the government could get out of their facilities or how the government could control them through funding contracts.[82] On the other hand, some CPP members were more concerned about how the government was failing the voluntary sector. For example, Daniel Buadi from Asim argued in 1960 that 'the hospital at Fosu is being run by the Roman Catholic Mission. Originally, it was decided that a Health Centre would be built at Fosu but because of the Roman Catholic Church hospital the plan has been suspended. I am asking the Minister to see to it that whatever the Government have provided for the putting up of a Health Centre at Fosu, must be given at once for the work to be put in hand'.[83]

Not all of the attempts to finance missions would be affected; at no point was 90 per cent of Ghana's health care run by missionaries as Appiah had hoped, but much was added. Already in 1959 the Ministry of Health set out its plans to provide a 'new 24 bedded ward ... for isolation and Tuberculosis cases' at the Basel Mission Hospital at Bawku.[84] In addition, they 'proposed to erect an X-Ray Department at Bawku' with necessary equipment in the same year.[85] By 1960 there were plans to double the number of hospitals beds, which, by that point, were at one for every 1,750 citizens (including government, mission, and mining hospitals). Part of the plan began with adding additional wards of thirty-two beds to the mission hospitals at Axim and Mampong.[86] In 1960 a second female ward was provided at Bawku for £14,000.[87] In May 1961, missions provided a quarter of the total national bed strength.[88] Overall, between 1960 and 1961 mission hospitals £290,000 was earmarked by government.[89]

Other major politicians under Nkrumah advocated for the expansion of medicine on the grounds that doctors were performing the miracles of Christ – not those of modern science. J.A. Owusu-Ansah, the United Party representative for Offinsu Kwabre, made a long statement in a debate on hospital staff in 1958 in which he argued that doctors were the 'most important people in this country' because they 'perform miracles in the same way as Jesus Christ did when He was on earth'. Therefore, their working conditions should be 'fitting and proper ... in order encourage them' because they are 'our saviours'.[90] The connection between Christian ministry and surgery particularly was emphasised, but in a further statement he argued that because doctors are miracle-makers they 'should not be confined to the municipal towns alone; rather, they should be given every encouragement to help the rural areas too'. Owusu-Ansah continued to extend his vision for Christ's healing on earth through medicine when in 1965 he advocated that 'the health needs of the people will continue to receive urgent attention of the government and party. Our aim is to provide free health facilities for the entire people of Ghana by the end of the Seven-Year Development Plan period'.[91] Not all Ghanaian politicians chose to claim medicine for modernity, however; others chose to use it to bolster their claims to promote Christianity.

In other cases, medical mission was supported for its commitment to Ghana in direct attacks on unpatriotic Ghanaian doctors who were leaving the country. In the National Assembly in 1965, Jambaidu Awuni (Kumasi Central) argued that a medical mission in the North was a model for Ghanaians. In saying this he girded it with attacks on colonial limitations on African potential:

> In one of the mission hospitals in the North, there are about five doctors attending to patients and they do not have time for closing. Sometimes they even sleep in the hospital ... In spite of the volume of work they always say their prayers each morning before they commence their daily work. These people do not complain that they have left their homes thousands and thousands of miles away to come and serve here in the North. These doctors have not come from Germany to serve their fellow white men but they are here to serve us the black. It is high time that our doctors follow the example set by these white doctors. Even some of our people who are qualified abroad do not want to come back ... It is unfortunate that I am not a doctor but it is not my fault. If the imperialists had allowed me, I would have become a doctor.[92]

Given Awuni's constituency, he was not trying to gain money for a local mission hospital out of pragmatic reasons, but was actually making a larger argument about the brain drain of Ghanaian doctors training abroad. In doing this he spent a considerable portion of his speech proclaiming the diligence, self-sacrifice, and faith of the Basel Mission Hospital at Bawku. Awuni contrasted the failure of Ghanaian doctors with the heroism of German doctors. It was not simply modernity that made missionaries useful to Ghanaian politicians, it was also their role in arguments about character and national identity. The model of missions could be used as a political weapon in arguing for increased dedication to the cause of Ghanaian postcolonial success on the behalf of Ghanaians themselves. For

Awuni this was clearly linked to his own patriotism: he notes in conclusion that he would have committed so sacrificially if the imperialists had allowed him. Perhaps in the intense political battles in the final stages of Nkrumah's regime, Awuni's claim of loyalty to his country and his challenge to the loyalty of the doctors was an important performance to secure his government position.

Crucially, in spite of all these advocates for medical mission in government there were socialists who were confused by Nkrumah's mixed messages on mission, development, and modernity. In the Northern Territories in 1961 'leftists' took over the Catholic hospitals near Navrongo and had to be stopped by Nkrumah. Given the slippages and contradictions between Nkrumah's rhetoric, development needs, and structural legacies of the Ghanaian state, some socialists misunderstood – perhaps wilfully but also understandably – the attitude of CPP to medical missions. In 1961, the White Father and regional superior J. Alfred Richard wrote to the Reverend Richard Walsh in the central Padri Bianchi (White Father) offices in Rome that socialists had stolen the mission hospitals in response to news put out by 'leftists' and 'pressure groups': 'Hospitals run by the Missions were to be taken over this year according to the T.U.C. the big Trade Union here'.[93]

In response Nkrumah officially denied any involvement and enacted countermeasures. The missions had their hospitals returned 'indefinitely' and even more money was given to the missions. As Richard explained, in the aftermath of the conflict, 'more grants than ever are available for our hospitals' and the missions were urged by Nkrumah to 'open more school and especially staff schools for the government'.[94] Unfortunately there is no evidence as to exactly how the leftist usurpers responded to this stamping-out by a government to whom they were allied. What this does show is either how confusing socialism in Ghana could be at the time or how trade unionists and socialists locally could act for their own concerns without national legitimacy. Whatever the case, Nkrumah was able to enforce the mission hospitals' return, demonstrating the extent to which he was able to control the Northern Territories in spite of not eradicating chiefs in the area. It also represents Nkrumah's concern to encourage missionary health care even at the expense of alienating his own leftist foot soldiers.

After 1961 medical missions were in more conflict with Nkrumah's increasingly paranoid and authoritarian regime, but in general mission grew and was supported by pro-mission African Christians, some of whom held considerable power. Around 1961, particularly after an assassination attempt, Nkrumah clamped down on civil liberties and threw out foreigners he suspected of being spies. For example, Colin Forrester-Paton wrote back to the Scottish mission board of 'a drive by the governing and almost all-embracing Convention People's Party to form branches within the congregations of the Churches'. However, Forrester-Paton also wrote of how this was 'quietly and successfully resisted by the authorities of all the Churches in the Christian Council; and even more important, there has been no spontaneous move by the many C.P.P. members within the Churches to form such branches, despite a propaganda campaign directed to this end'.[95]

As Forrester-Paton wrote, there was considerable church resistance to Nkrumah's reaching out to claim power and his rhetorical claims about planting CPP members in churches. Much of this was 'quiet' and did not hit the headlines. Brian Stanley has argued in his edited book on missions and nationalism at the end of empire that African churches could act as a hindrance to African nationalism and often stubbornly held their ground.[96] As Maxwell has argued, for postcolonial states, the body of the church was greatly desired in part because it was a critical mobilising unit.[97] With Nkrumah, even propaganda and infiltrating party branches could not co-opt the Christian Council. Though perhaps deals were cut behind closed doors, in public resistance was effective, according to Forrester-Paton. For example, at the Ridge Church in Accra which Forrester-Paton helped to set up, alliances outside the state were formed.

In 1962 the medical missionary David Murray returned to his home at Achimota College to find it burned down. He had worked there since 1956 as a doctor for the school and unofficial medical officer for the Scottish Presbyterian Church before taking a long furlough of three years back in Scotland in 1959. When his family first arrived, on the eve of independence in 1957, they had been warmly welcomed into Ghana. The Murrays' first years mostly went without a hitch and they were given a grand house on Achimota land. However, when they returned, Nkrumah's regime had hardened its attitude towards specific groups. Seated at Achimota, which was Nkrumah's alma mater and a beacon of Ghanaian development, Murray was a prime target for a symbolic attack on the aspects of Africa yet to be decolonised. Burning down the Murrays' house was only the beginning. In public, locals turned on the family, the press denounced them, and the local chemist hindered their access to pharmaceuticals. Around them expatriates were being expelled. On one occasion, the brother of Sister Vicky Teye of Achimota Hospital demanded that they remove and burn his name out of their visitor's book.[98] The Murrays managed to leave Achimota and David took a job at the nearby 37 Military Hospital, but there too he was resented by other staff and bullied out as an imperial remnant. In 1968, after Nkrumah had gone, still the Murrays found that it would be better to leave Ghana for Uganda, where they set up a private practice. Eventually David Murray ended up as a bagpiper for Idi Amin and would go on to influence some of the films and books about Scottish remnants under Amin's reign.[99] This snapshot of the Murrays' fluctuating fortunes captures an important aspect of missionary lives in postcolonial Africa, and nuances the argument about closeness in relations – but it is not the whole picture. While this account might be evocative of the sort of challenges missions could face, under Nkrumah such conflicts were largely confined to the centres of state power and key symbolic sites of Africanisation. Far more significantly, missions were utilised rather than rejected in the creation of Nkrumah's modernity and after he had fallen.

In spite of all the pressure, one Ghanaian friend from Ridge Church remained loyal to David Murray: the medical administrator for Korle Bu Hospital and senior officer in the Ministry of Health (and eventually director of the medical services), Michael Baddoo. He would visit the Murrays regularly, helping them out and tipping them off when there was trouble. Baddoo's wife was a white Englishwoman and both had attended Cambridge. Building this relationship at the Accra Ridge was vital for the Murrays maintaining their life in Ghana until the late 1960s.

However, the wider context of Nkrumah's state was one in which mission flourished. By 1966, the year of Nkrumah's downfall at the hands of a coup, medical mission in Ghana had already grown considerably. In 1963 there were fifty-one registered medical practitioners; this grew to eighty-four in 1964, 101 in 1965, and 106 in 1966 – over double what it had been three years earlier. 106 doctors was just under a third of the amount of registered medical practitioners in the Ghana, which totalled 320 and had only grown by nine since 1963 (though there were heights of 337 in 1964 and 159 in 1965). Moreover, there were 149 non-Ghanaian medical practitioners in government service, though this had dropped from 192 in 1964 and 190 in 1963. By contrast, the amount of non-Ghanaians in non-government service as medical practitioners was 220, up from 134 in 1963, peaking in this period at 232 in 1964.[100] Child welfare clinic distribution had regrown by this point, however, climbing to 242.[101] There were 160,690 new antenatal cases, 362,511 old ones, and 47,059 postnatal cases.[102] Furthermore, out of 70,000 leprosy patients, 21,500 were receiving treatment.[103] Notably, two out of the four leprosariums were run by missions.[104] Moreover, mission hospitals were 'fully subsidised by the Government', according to a National Assembly debate in 1965.[105]

CONCLUSION

Two core narratives of medical missions supporting or corrupting postcolonial development and Africanisation have been consistently in tension since independence. Navigating these competing identities was one of the critical aspects for Ghanaian nationalists such as Bawumia and Appiah in retaining their foothold within the one-party state. The analysis of both shows how concerns about missionary modernity could be bound up with long-term political battles over regional independence, religion, local political power, and tribalism. Battles over who controlled development, as Frederick Cooper has shown, were central to claims to independent African rule. In this, missions more commonly figured as an asset to Ghanaian nationalists, but they could be perceived also as a challenge to government sovereignty over development, disrupting the connection between state and citizens. Generally, for Nkrumah the historic mission church might obstruct some of his grand visions, but it was a vital part of his state. It offered the sorts of biomedical, scientific technologies of modernity that he wanted for his development policies. Medical missionaries' association with colonialism and British rule was only a major issue in the symbolic centres of power and development like Achimota College. However, these complex layers could confuse even loyal socialists who in 1961 took over the mission hospitals around Navrongo, only to be thrown out again by Nkrumah himself. Not everyone could navigate the tensions in missionary identities for political gain.

Within these contests over the possible identities of medical mission, medical mission grew. By 1966 thirty-four mission hospitals had been built, as well as many dispensaries, clinics, and mobile stations. Medical missions' experiences and perspectives were generally separate high-level debates in the Assembly. Medical missions reformed their development practices and their hierarchies in response to decolonisation in terms of 'Africanisation' – not in terms of the modernisation or detachment from colonialism that mattered to nationalists. From the 1960s onwards, both Catholic and Protestant medical mission did 'Africanise', but in different ways. These differences were shaped by local and regional actors, and by changes in the national and transnational churches, as much as by government politics. Both Africanised institutionally a great deal from the 1960s, but expatriate Catholics retained much control over the hierarchies of their health care. This was in contrast to the Presbyterian Church of Ghana, which took power over all the former Scottish and Basel missions, yet faced significant limits to their ability to Africanise. For all missions, the lack of Ghanaian doctors, especially in the late 1970s and 1980s, meant long-term expatriate control.

In the bigger picture of the meanings of Africanisation for development and its attendant identities, Nkrumah attempted to align himself within the reconstructed symbol of African internationalism, modernity, and religion – J.E.K. Aggrey and his key institution, Achimota. This process of commemoration and ritual was not stable. In subsequent memorials across the century, Ghanaians challenged Nkrumah's transnational imaginary, forming their own set of global, accommodationist, and missional frameworks around the same figure. As Europeans also tried to make sense of the postcolonial and postwar world, they attempted to redefine the meanings of health and development in order to form new national narratives. All this was bound up with global health and being increasingly shaped by processes of Africanisation as well, but in ways that disseminated different visions of what development could mean and who it helped. How such transnational networks were funded, how they were interpreted by patients, practitioners, donors, and governments, and how they facilitated multilateral health campaigns will be the subject of the next chapters.

3

Reframing Postcolonial International Health: Ghana, the Netherlands, and West Germany, 1957–90

Beyond the early years of postcolonialism, religion remained vital in formulating the meanings and practice of health development in Ghana, and in global health more widely. During the remaking of modern Germany, through aid tied to Catholic medical mission and financing, global health was articulated in postcolonial states. Historians and practitioners have traditionally framed postcolonial international health in two broad ways: the US and the Soviets in a global Cold War battle to control the 'third world', or the former colonial powers trying to retain their control over the new nationalist rule of their old colonies.[1] In addition, recent work in development studies has also examined 'South-South' international health. Finally, Erez Manela in his work on the Smallpox Eradication Programme (SEP) has, following Akira Iriye, emphasised that US involvement was not determined by the Cold War or imperial expansion. Instead, the US place in SEP centred on 'the growth and articulation of a global community'; this was through NGOs which were an expression of an older international idealism within 'technical' health fields.[2]

However, this chapter will argue that there is another, significant, framing that has been largely absent from the historical literature on international health: old colonial powers establishing health development through medical mission in areas that they had never ruled or had almost no relation with since before the 1880s imperial 'scramble'. From the late 1950s, West Germany and the Netherlands conducted international health work in Ghana – an area to which they had, in recent times, almost no connection. This was elaborated without the 'global community' of the WHO and UNICEF. It was a process not simply determined by Cold War agendas, old colonial patterns, or the emerging global community; it was truly fresh development work in a decolonised setting. These arguments challenge Iris Borowy's categorisations of East German international health and development aid to Nicaragua in terms of 'Cold War logic', North-South relations, and international health models. Instead, this chapter will show how West German and Dutch Catholic medical mission transcended these categories.[3] Mission and development were cast in wider narratives of suffering, the rebuilding of the German state, and the dreams of reunifying German national identity which emerged after the Second World War.

This chapter will first explore how and why Dutch and West German Catholics funded such a great deal of medical mission in Ghana, and what this meant for reconfiguring European identities. The second section will examine German Catholic missions and especially the German Catholic development organisation: Misereor. This section will assess what could be achieved on the ground and how this was experienced by missions. It will show the limits of Catholic transnational networks in tying together a global citizenry by the bonds of shared human endeavour and sacrifice.

The chapter's last section will demonstrate that Dutch and West German Catholic postwar medical mission was a global phenomenon including Asia, Africa, and Latin America. Yet, it also will emphasise that Ghana *was* a country of focus for Dutch Catholic mission, and there was an influx of Dutch Catholic medical missionaries to Ghana in the 1960s and 1970s. This was supported by the Dutch government and the Catholic aid organisation Memisa (Medische Missie Actie). Memisa was established in 1925 (becoming Memisa Mediscus Mundi from 1984 following a merger with Medicus Mundi Nederland), but, like Misereor, gained extensive financial support from campaigns in the 1960s and 1970s. In Ghana, Memisa funded staff accommodation, medical supplies, and even salaries for this stream of new recruits.

Finally, for additional detail, the appendix at the end of the book evidences the sheer range of Catholic medical missions in Ghana to which Misereor and Memisa made contributions. These processes created an infrastructure which made possible and shaped how global health was outworked in postcolonial Ghana, as will be explored in chapter 4. Chapter 5 will then detail how this specific framework and style of missionary health care worked in coordination and competition with shifting visions of global health.

FASTENAKTION AND EUROPEAN POSTWAR RENEWAL: WEST GERMAN AND DUTCH MEDICAL MISSION IN GHANA

West Germany and the Netherlands funded Catholic health care in Ghana from the late 1950s into the 1990s to a huge extent. This was an entirely new process and represented a major change in medical mission, development, and international health. Between the 1950s and 1980s both the Netherlands and West Germany, supplying millions of deutsche marks and guilders, established many Catholic medical missions in independent Ghana. In spite of their lack of colonial heritage in Ghana, there was a massive growth of Catholic medical mission in Ghana after the 1950s from West Germany and the Netherlands. The two countries not only financed their own new institutions, they also funded European and American Catholic missions such as the Medical Mission Sisters (MMS, based in Philadelphia) with a million deutsche marks and guilders at a time. Furthermore, when Indonesian nationalist-led revolution ended Dutch rule in the mid-to-late 1940s, and then again when the republic became an authoritarian dictatorship in the 1960s, Dutch Catholic missions fled – not home – but to Ghana. There they came in droves, setting up new hospitals and supporting old ones.

Neither the Netherlands nor Germany had had a significant national colonial presence in the Gold Coast since 1871. Before the British ruled the Gold Coast, it was named the Dutch Gold Coast or Dutch Guinea and had been controlled by a Netherlands colonial government since 1598. Nonetheless, without a large settler population, when the Gold Coast was ceded to the United Kingdom in 1870–71, the Dutch role in the colony almost completely disappeared. The transition to British rule was well documented in Douglas Coombs's history in 1963; however, in national Ghanaian history, other than notable fortress landmarks, the Dutch are almost as forgotten as the Portuguese who preceded them.[4] The Swiss and German Protestant presence through the Basel and Bremen missions has had more of a mark on Ghanaian national life. Their flagship hospitals at Agogo and Bawku forged international reputations for high-level service, such as in ophthalmology. The Basel Mission workers were involved in planting the first cocoa crops on which independent Ghana's economy was based. However, there was little national German power in the country and these missionaries were swiftly ejected by the British government in the two world wars. The Gold Coast was strategically vital as the base for the American air force and the British RAF to launch campaigns in Europe and North Africa.[5] Overall, Germany and the Netherlands' role in colonial Gold Coast was, by the beginning of the 1950s, a feature of either the distant past or restricted to a specific Protestant group.

However, by the end of the 1950s West German Catholics chose to identify with a denazified, Catholic internationalist and democratically liberal narrative which emphasised shared humanity with other Europeans and shared suffering at the hands of the Nazis. This was physically embodied in the Misereor Lent collection campaigns in which West German Catholics fasted and thus suffered to help the world's hungry and the poor. For West Germany and the Netherlands, international Catholic mission networks provided an alternative route to lay claim to a development narrative that was different from old colonial connections, new US-led Cold War strategies, or the emerging international community. As Nils Brimnes shows for the Danish, tuberculosis aid was used to separate themselves from claims of Nazi collaboration. In the late 1940s and 1950s initiatives began as an 'effort to create good-will in war ravaged Europe' before UNICEF funding turned into a large-scale international health campaign.[6] Moreover, the Danish worked in India where they too had had no previous colonial role. For West German and Dutch Catholics, development in Ghana offered a way of joining in the postwar reconstruction efforts of the Europeans and the US who were presenting an internationalist vision of a reborn humanity after suffering the violence of war. Moreover, instead of simply trailing the old colonial paths or aiding the emerging global community, West Germans could build upon an older, traditional Catholic development. Again, it was one which could be linked to a different Catholic war narrative of suffering and resistance, rather than collaboration or acquiescence.

Through Konrad Adenauer's tax policy and huge donations from West German Catholics, Misereor was extremely well funded in the 1950s. From 1949 to 1963, Adenauer was the chancellor of the Federal Republic of Germany (FRG) and chair of the foremost political party in West Germany, the Christian Democratic Union (CDU). In West German politics Catholics dominated; though the CDU included both Protestants and Catholics, Adenauer himself was a devout Catholic. As Tony Judt has described, Dutch and West

German Catholic communities became far more integrated within the wider political culture after the war, and Adenauer emphasised ecumenism in order to gain national support and reduce church-state conflict.[7] The CDU had cross-denominational support even in Bavaria.[8] Continuing older German policies, Adenauer apportioned tax money to churches depending on their members, which benefitted Misereor particularly.[9] Yet, at the same time, Catholic and Protestant aid programmes were separated, with Catholic bishops gaining especially massive amounts of donations from West German churches.[10] Misereor emerged out of the World Union of Catholic Women's Association and the West German branch of the Pax Christi movement, which in the mid-1950s campaigned against starvation and leprosy overseas. Out of this the German bishops began fasting in 1958 to protest against worldwide hunger under the banner of 'misereor super turbam' (pity for the crowd), raising money for poverty relief. In 1959, Misereor collected over 34 million deutsche marks (DM) in donations from West German Catholics; this would reach hundreds of millions by the early 1960s.[11]

Misereor's work was mostly confined to work amongst West German Catholic churches because of historic regional affiliations. The smaller German Protestant relief organisation 'Bread for the World' also began in 1959, focusing on the famine in India and gaining tens of millions of deutsche marks. Combined, the total was over 50 million DM, which exceeded the West German parliament's international aid budget.[12] Unlike Misereor, which could rely on West Germany alone, Bread for the World also collected 11.8 million DM from East Germany in the first three years of its operation. By contrast, East German Catholic Bishops did not collect in East Germany until 1968 when their efforts were organised as 'Need in the World' – separate from Misereor and mainly funded by non-aligned or communist former colonies.[13] As Dora Vargha has shown for Hungary, in some cases international health was shaped by Cold War rhetorics and in others threats such as polio offered a safe place for 'unprecedented, open cooperation among governments on the two sides of the Iron Curtain'.[14] Catholic development aid from Germany, where collaboration crossed the Iron Curtain or not, depended as much on deep historic regional loyalties as it did on more recent Cold War divisions. For example, as will be further elaborated below, places in Bavaria provided a great deal of Misereor funding, ensuring that they did not need East German help.

The scale of aid from West Germany and Misereor to key postcolonial states was large. In 1962, West Germany was the first member of the Development Assistance Committee to start co-financing.[15] In one instance in 1967, the West German government gave $200,000 to the Medical Mission Sisters' (MMS) nursing programme in Berekum, Ghana, alongside a grant of $58,000 from Misereor and 25 per cent of the costs from the MMS itself.[16] In 1965, for a project that ran from 1966 into the 1970s, the West German government gave 7,783,000 DM to a plan between the Vatican, Misereor, and the Indonesian bishop. A further 65,000,000 rupees was to be paid by the Indonesian bishops, jointly funded with Misereor.[17] Simultaneously, the Ghanaian government was being given massive loans by KFW (Kreditanstalt für Wiederaufbau), the German development bank. Between 1966 and 1969, 10 million DM was lent to the Ghanaian government, which was around 12 million new cedis, for the first phase of a national electrification project. The second phase after 1968 was funded by the World Bank. This was crucial for wider Ghanaian development aims such as the aluminium smelter. KFW funded Ghana again in 1989, extending electrification to the North for the first time.[18]

In the Netherlands too, Catholic medical mission was given massive funds from the early 1960s. In the Netherlands co-financing programmes, in which matching grants were distributed to development agencies, had a similar consequence for both Catholic and Protestant aid, and secular organisations were given a far smaller share. As C.H. Biekart put it, the 'German and Dutch aid agencies that were founded in response to official co-financing programmes would later become the largest private aid agencies in Europe'.[19] As Karel Steenbrink has shown, modelled on Misereor, the Dutch Catholics set up 'Lenten Campaign' (Vastenactie) in 1961, and in 1963 they partnered with Protestant development organisations and gained government funding. In 1965, the Dutch government co-financed both Catholic and Protestant development agencies with 5 million guilders. In 1946 the newly formed Catholic People's Party (KVP) went into coalition government with the social democratic Labour Party until 1956. Between 1958 and 1965, the KVP dominated Dutch politics, supplying every single prime minister in the period. According to Steenbrink, from then on it became 'common policy that the government supplemented up to 75% for development programmes ignited by Christian churches with their overseas partners'.[20] Steenbrink further shows how in 1971 the Dutch Catholic medical organisation Memisa gained 20 million guilders in its first television campaign event; its second in 1975 gained 8 million guilders. Alongside the Protestants the 1972 television event KOB I collected 58 million guilders in the campaign.[21] As will be discussed further in the final section of this chapter, one Memisa member recalled that Ghana was a focus country and that (very) roughly 500,000 guilders were being given annually to Catholic aid for ambulances, medicines, hospitals, and doctors in the 1970s.[22] The Medical Mission Sisters at Berekum were given millions of guilders from Memisa.[23]

There have already been studies of Dutch and German (both East and West) development aid being poured into their old colonial territories, but their role in previously disconnected nations has not been studied. Carola Rensch and Walter Bruchhausen have explored how West German relations with Africa were fostered through development aid given to Togo, an old German model colony, and to Gabon, where the notable mission doctor Albert Schweitzer had been based. West Germany also financed international cooperative efforts through the WHO. For Togo, much of their reasoning is similar to the work of Manela, namely that the benefits to technical expertise and longer-term capacity building for research were the drive behind funding: '"development aid" claimed to bring and the promises of science' and modernity.[24] Furthermore, implications for German aid to Africa in the Cold War have also been discussed; most notably, like with Cuban medical internationalism, the ideological affinity East Germany held with Nyerere's socialism in Tanzania resulted in development aid to bolster their shared endeavour. For example, John Iliffe has noted this with regard to East German doctors staffing hospitals in East Africa, though Iliffe particularly emphasises the long-term colonial connections with the area.[25] There were also disjunctures in German relations with their former colonies. With the UN taking trusteeship over Namibian territories and handing control to South Africa, as soon as independence occurred for Namibia in 1990 Germany began giving development aid – before which relations were restricted.[26] However, there was far more that was new and independent with regard to German aid than this. It must be noted at this point that Matthias Egg in his doctoral dissertation at Universität Bonn has, in German, detailed some elements of German Catholic mission work across the colonial/postcolonial divide for Zimbabwe, Cameroon, the Congo, Namibia, and Ghana.[27]

Identifying with a denazified, liberal political culture was vital to the reconstruction of West German and Dutch politics in the postwar period. As Christoph Müller has argued, many West Germans in the late 1940s, 1950s, and 1960s were hostile to the modernisation and globalisation of their country, and as a defence against this, 'West-German anti-Americanism could be found in all social strata'. In an attempt to articulate a resurgent German nationalism, there was a desire to find a place for Germany between the East and West blocs.[28] Moreover, Barbara Marshall argues that antipathy toward the denazification process actually stopped a resurgent Nazism by ensuring that the occupation forces soaked up animosity which could have been directed at German political parties.[29] Lutz Niethammer famously argued that denazification's greatest effect was to produce a 'mitläuferfabrik' or a 'follower factory'. This was distinct from restricting the definition of denazification to the official American programme which was abandoned by the West German government in 1951. The initial American programme had had practical issues with too many Germans with Nazi pasts needed for necessary work such as in the civil service, difficulty with enforcement and recording, and Cold War expediency requiring the rapid restoration of West Germany. Instead, by only convicting a small section of the population and releasing the majority of them, the denazification process after 1951 provided most Germans with clean pasts. Combined with the consistent effort of the West German government and the Catholic Church not to address the Nazi past, the most obvious result of denazification was that it swept the horrors under the carpet and it was not until at least the 1970s that liberal culture would consider them properly again. As Ian Turner and Barbara Marshall have suggested, denazification helped stop any political resurgence of Nazism by eliminating Nazis for long enough that a new political culture could develop.[30] This political culture was heavily dominated by a quietist Catholicism which washed over national guilt.

Like Germany, the Netherlands also had an intense denazification process that resulted in the internment of around 100,000 collaborators.[31] The Netherlands, too, had to re-establish a fresh political culture while being unable to root out everyone with pro-Nazi allegiances, and they also chose to base their state on Catholic democratic politics. The KVP became incredibly powerful in the 1950s and 1960s, only waning in the 1970s. Moreover, much of the Catholic development efforts, as Steenbrink noted, were directly copying initiatives like Misereor in West Germany. Catholicism, as in West Germany, offered a set of older moral and domestic norms, perhaps bolstering the restoration of protected private realms, all of which were felt to have been overturned or destroyed during the violence and dislocations of war. Moreover, it may have been that the scriptures, communal rituals, and causes of Catholicism held spaces and narratives in which 'strong but restrained' masculinities could develop, as the boundaries between men and women were questioned at work and at home by changing employment patterns.[32] Crucially, Catholicism provided a version of the national past that could ignore the horrors of nationalism and recall an international order around the Holy Roman Empire and the Vatican. Via Christian democracy there could be a different and Catholicised political fit that neither subjected itself to Cold War blocs or to the older colonial traditions. Even if the latter did not have the bad odour of the former, given the annexation of many old colonial territories for Germany at least, another route was required.

Dutch and West German Catholics identified with a common European political culture based on older missional traditions, empire, and development. For both the Netherlands and the West Germans the liberal international order, the global community forged largely by the Allies and including new nationalist states, may not actually have been that popular (though more study would need to be done here). By contrast, missional Roman Catholicism, considering the amount given in donations and through the government, clearly was a very popular alternate kingdom and form of international belonging. Crucially, these development efforts were not simply a response to war guilt. They were about identifying with a narrative of shared suffering with other nations, distinguishing themselves from collaboration and Nazism. Colonial administration and European integration could go hand in hand: postwar commonalities could be expressed through empire, rather than it being a field of competition. In the case of West Germany and the Netherlands, development in a colony administered by the British offered an opportunity to enter into the commonalities of a shared imperial past as well as shared hardship. Development in Ghana offered a seat at the table in European reconstruction. Just as Brussels laid claim to the European machinery, West Germany had to attain a role in the reconstruction of Europe and European empire, but was shut out from gaining too much institutional power. Therefore, it forged its own path in the emergence of the international order within a flourishing Catholic internationalism, which in the early 1960s was spreading across the United States and Latin America. In the latter, liberation theology was encouraging priests and nuns to the front line of social justice issues from the 1950s.[33] Moreover, perhaps if we consider Ghana as a British context even in the 1960s, West Germany could also have been showing its ability to be effective in development work, in ways better than perfidious Albion who were being pushed further out.

As Frederick Cooper has shown with African nationalists, so too with West Germany: showing leadership in a form of development that served national interests legitimised rule in government and democracy.[34] This was significant given that West Germany was blocked from developing its former colonies in southern Africa. Instead, it could join in with a Catholic internationalism that was widely resurgent in the 1960s, during Vatican II, the attendant social justice movements, and the pioneers of the 'preferential option for the poor'. While some Dutch Catholics fell out of favour at Vatican II, there was still a significant movement here, amidst decolonisation, in which development leadership and European commonality narratives could be proved in Catholic medical mission.

Developmentalism through Catholic mission was a form of civil society-state coordination which distinguished West Germany from the tyranny of Nazism. In the aftermath of the fall of the Nazis the German evangelical churches collectively apologised in the 'Stuttgart Declaration' for 'not loving more ardently'. By contrast, Pope Pius XII's postwar radio broadcast eschewed the collective guilt narrative in favour of emphasising Catholics as themselves victims at the hands of the Nazis.[35] The German postwar state was underpinned with the 'Persilshein' attitude in many areas of national life in which those who previously had worked in key positions regained them without reproach. Though not nearly to the same extent, the Netherlands also had issues with Nazi pasts that had political consequences such as the empowerment of Catholics. Vital to the maintenance of the denazified narrative, given the contrary realities, was that civil society was shown to have an active role in keeping the government accountable, putting checks on the overuse of power and showing the healthiness of state institutions which were not closed to associational life. These features of liberal democracy, especially in the American setting, were important to perform to the world. In the case of development – driven by the Catholic bishops, funded by citizens themselves and then supported by the state – it showed aspects of German liberal governance and was crucial to the denazification process.

These ways of understanding the meaning and purpose of Misereor's development work were articulated most notably by the federal president, Heinrich Lübke, at a large rally in Cologne in 1964. Alongside the CDU chancellor Ludwig Erhard and the famous Nazi resister who helped to start Misereor, Cardinal Frings, Lübke lauded the work of Misereor to more than a thousand guests in early 1964. Key parts of the speech were recorded and further disseminated in national and regional presses. The most significant aspect of the speech repeated in newspapers was the connection between Misereor's work in development in its rebounding effect for German unity and restoration. In *Der Spiegel*, Lübke was quoted as having said that 'the unselfish works' of Misereor would 'reverberate' back upon Germany and thus 'all who serve sacrificially and cooperatively' and who contribute to aid for the needy would be also be working 'simultaneously to restore German unity'.[36] This added to links between national unity and Misereor's development work being forged with everyday items such as national stamps which depicted the charity branding alongside ears of corn. Moreover, in the Bavarian newspaper *Passauer Neue Presse*, who also reported on the Cologne speech, this quote was extended to include the relationship with the Nazi past. They described how Lübke had explained that 'the German people must earn peace, freedom, and unity, as a result of what was done in the last 30 years' and that 'they (the German people) will be shown through development aid a way in which they can effectively help others'. Lübke particularly encouraged the German youth to join in this development aid in order to gain the adventure that they sought in places that were 'waiting' for them.[37]

In tying the funding of Misereor's development aid to the traditional fasting period of Lent, there was a sense in which Germans were choosing suffering in order to alleviate the suffering of others. *Passauer Neue Presse* commented on this major event and Lübke's speech, and regularly featured articles and adverts about Misereor between 1961 and 1964, perhaps because of the large Catholic contingent in Bavaria. There were articles on how much the Bistums Passau diocese had raised their giving from year to year (such as in 1963, which was said to be up 33 per cent on 1962), and from a local bishop encouraging even more donations because of the scale of global need.[38] These articles were featured along with pieces on developing countries such as Ghana. For example, in one article Kojo Botsio, the minister for Foreign Affairs in Ghana between 1961 and 1965, welcomed young doctors from overseas because Ghanaian health care urgently needed them.[39] Overtures about need, hunger, and the desire for help from 'developing countries' were tied with fasting, a cause and performance captured by the term 'Fastenaktion'. Donating to Misereor was a collective Catholic act during Lent in which churches would give up food, money, or habits in order to provide for the hungry in poorer countries. Such a physical embodiment of purposeful suffering had restorative aspects, both in terms of participating in the redemptive suffering of Christ and in the narrative of European suffering during the Second World War. In 1958, Cardinal Frings had made similar points at the outset of Misereor, arguing that misery had entered the German consciousness and they had become aware that most of the world was hungry.[40] In 'Fastenaktion' Catholics were invited to physically participate in the pain of the world in order to help it recover.[41] As many articles in *Passauer Neuer Presse* showed, they did so in their droves.[42] In 1963 alone the Bistum Passau diocese donated 552,584 DM. In 1964, the Passauer Pfarrelen gave 70,416 DM to Misereor, slightly less than the 72,577 DM the year before. Almost like competition results, printed figures in the press were even broken down by individual church donation, for example, Pfarrel St Nicola in 1964 donated 13,553 DM.[43] It was these kinds of contributions across Germany that ensured Misereor gained hundreds of millions of DM annually in the 1960s. In 1961 Frings's Adventiat campaign had gained 170 million DM.[44]

The effects of these development narratives and denazification processes were not paltry: medical mission in Ghana gained millions of deutsche marks as a result. One of the old international Catholic networks that benefitted most from this process was doing medical mission in Ghana, which gained substantial grants from Dutch and West German governments and Catholic development agencies between the 1950s and 1980s. From its beginning in 1959 to 1990, Misereor gave around 40 million DM to Catholic health care in Ghana. This began at a time when the deutsche mark was one of the strongest currencies in the world. The breakdown of the financing can be viewed in the appendix, converted into euros. According to this table, in the 1960s around 7 million DM were given to Catholic medical mission. However, taking into account the tendency for loans to be converted into grants because hospitals could not repay the money, the figures may have been even higher than suggested. It must be noted that, given the array of different denominations in which donations were made and the difficulty of comparing across decades of changing exchange rates, the appendix table represents the most consistent information on how much Misereor was giving. For a simple breakdown, it shows that between 1950 and 1990 Misereor spent over 40 million DM on Catholic medical mission in Ghana (around 18.3 million euros).[45] David Maxwell has showed that in Katanga, European issues such as Irish conflict were being replayed in the mission field between Catholics and Protestants.[46] In Ghana, from the 1960s, issues over German reconstruction were being outworked in the mission field with large-scale consequences.

Partly as a result, Catholic growth in health care outpaced Protestant mission across the period, and it also was much larger than the Islamic revival of the Ahmadiyya movement. In 1967 there were thirty-nine hospitals, fifty health centres, and eleven health posts under the Ministry of Health. By 1972 this had grown to forty-nine hospitals, fifty-four health centres, and fifty-eight health posts. In 1975 this had reached fifty-four hospitals, fifty-nine health centres and seventy-eight health posts. Government health expenditure as a percentage of GDP had grown steadily from 1.11 per cent in 1966–67, to 1.48 per cent in 1973–74, and 2.21 per cent in 1975–76.[47] Unfortunately consistent statistics across these decades are not available for mission beds or expenditure. By 1971 missions had only increased by one hospital to thirty-five from thirty-four in 1966 (however, this may have been the result of greater focus on health centres or health posts); this then rose to thirty-six in 1972.[48] The Islamic Ahmayidda movement did establish a hospital at Agona Swedru in 1971 in order to 'regain the lost heritage and glory of Islam'. This was certainly key to the revival of Islam in an area which had previously been a Christian town and, according to the chairman, 'now had a considerable population of Muslims'.[49] While deserving much more attention in scholarship and future research, the medical mission of the Ahmaydiyya movement did not have the national scale of Catholic mission. As for government institutions, by 1971 there were 5,218 hospital beds (the largest amount of these, 1,761, were in Greater Accra) and only 2,950 mission hospital beds. The largest amount of mission beds, 800, were in the Eastern region, showing the continued division between government priorities in the South and missionary priorities further north and in the East.[50] By contrast, there were 511 mines hospital total beds and 200 private hospital total beds. The total across all the institutions meant that there was one bed to every 830 Ghanaians in 1971.[51] By 1985 the Christian Health Association of Ghana (CHAG), including the majority of Catholic hospitals and health institutions, had thirty hospitals, thirty-three clinics, and four Primary Health Care (PHC) projects, resulting in a bed capacity of 4,400. In 1982, 2.5 million outpatients were seen in CHAG institutions with 1 million being children. Crucially, 69 per cent of CHAG was made up of Catholic health institutions. Only 17 per cent were Presbyterian, 7 per cent Salvation Army, 2 per cent Evangelical Presbyterian, 2 per cent Methodist, 1 per cent Baptist, 1 per cent Anglican, 0.5 per cent Pentecostal, and 0.5 per cent Church of God. By the 1980s, Catholic growth had outstripped Protestant growth, making Catholics the main actor within CHAG.[52]

The new funding streams from Misereor and Memisa fit into a continued large-scale funding of medical mission by the national Ghanaian government on top of local contributions from patient fees. A large proportion of mission hospital funding came from the government in the 1960s and 1970s, consistent with earlier patterns. This continued until at least the mid-1970s, after which statistics of government expenditure on mission are unfortunately unavailable. However, in the table in the appendix, Catholic hospitals' data shows that they were gaining a lot of government funding as well as patient fees in 1982. For example, Jirapa Hospital in the Northern Territories had 95.5 per cent of its total income derived from the national government. In 1975–75, the government estimated that they would give around 15 million cedis to mission hospitals out of a total 200 million cedis on health generally and compared with 128.5 million cedis given to the Ministry of Health. As government expenditure fluctuated in the 1970s, Protestant growth slowed but Catholic mission was still benefitting from both national and international sources.[53]

CHAG, dominated by Catholic health institutions by the early 1980s, was also largely funded by Memisa, Misereor, and the Dutch government. As will be discussed further in chapter 5, the organisation CHAG (which coordinated missions in Ghana, ensuring they could lobby as a group from 1967), was funded by Memisa and

Table 3.1 Episcopal Aid Agency Misereor e.V.: Ghana – number and grant amount of the approved project of the DAC-Group 1, in euros, in the period from 1959 to 1990

DAC	No.	Grant Amount €	No.	Grant Amount €	No.	Grant Amount €	No.	Grant Amount €
100	0	0.00	0	0.00	5	116,574.55	5	116,574.55
103	4	53,039.35	17	1,258,755.05	43	3,447,084.21	64	4,758,898.61
111	33	3,302,383.14	26	1,511,455.50	69	6,921,533.72	128	11,735,372.36
112	1	43,255.29	7	426,417.42	15	1,089,051.72	23	1,558,724.43
113	0	0.00	1	14,316.17	0	0.00	1	14,316.17
114	0	0.00	0	0.00	4	123,732.64	4	123,732.64
116	0	0.00	3	8,819.78	0	0,00	3	8,819.78
Total	38	3,398,677.78	54	3,219,783.92	136	11,697,976.84	228	18,316,438.54

Source: Compiled using statistics from the surveys contained in Patrick A. Twumasi, *Survey Report Health Services in Ghana: National Catholic Secretariat January–April 1982 (April 1982*, Department of Health, National Catholic Secretariat, Accra), private archives of the National Catholic Secretariat (Accra, Ghana).

Misereor. While CHAG was set up by the CMC (Christian Medical Commision) to which Misereor also donated, Dutch and West German aid actually facilitated its work.[54] Given the large percentage of Catholic health institutions within CHAG this is hardly surprising, as it gave them a stronger voice in voluntary sector negotiations with the government and trade unions. This further allowed Catholic medical mission in Ghana to expand and dominate the health landscape from the late 1960s onwards. Vitally for CHAG and for PHC, Memisa and various other Dutch organisation also supplied drugs in 1981. The donations totalled 300,000 DFL. Furthermore, in the 1983 refugee crisis in Ghana, when over a million Ghanaians entered the country from Nigeria, emergency donations were given by the Dutch government (260,000 DFL), Misereor (750,000 DFL), the Christoffel Blind Mission (500,000 DFL), ECHO, and the Christian Council of Ghana. This was combined with a further Dutch government grant of 2,000,000 DFL. These were recorded as having covered 'all the needs of the CHAG units for at least 1 to 2 years'. In addition to all this, in 1985 EZE (German Protestant Association for Cooperation in Development) gave a further 2,000,000 DM for the drug supply programme and ICCO (Interkerkelijke coödinatie commission ontwikkelingsprojekten/interchurch coordination committee for development projects) gave 750,000 DFL.[55] Memisa contributed 200,000 Nfl, Brot für die Welt gave 250,000 DM, Cebemo gave 300,000, Eén voor Afrika Relief gave 150,00 Nfl., Christian Aid gave £40,000, and CIDA gave $50,000.[56] As chapter 4 will show, combining with Canadian aid was not unusual. What was incredibly striking about these numbers, as will be seen in chapter 5, is that they aimed to bolster CHAG and Catholic medical missions' ability to continue building PHC even against international trends away from the movement.

MISEREOR AND GHANAIAN DEVELOPMENT: EXPERIENCES, IDENTITIES, AND NEGOTIATIONS IN MISSION

Through Misereor a wide range of Catholic medical mission in Ghana was extensively funded, but this did not mean that it could impose its development narrative on medical missions. Grand visions of German restoration and humanitarianism were detached from the lived experiences and priorities of medical missionaries themselves. Moreover, local circumstances and national changes shaped what was possible for mission. Missions relied on Misereor but they also continued to need patient fees and government grants. Crucially, development narratives in West Germany were detached from the ground-level realities and concerns of medical missionaries. They were also detached from the ways in which Ghanaians themselves experienced health as patients or created health care as practitioners. The ways in which Germans embodied their aid in 'Fastenaktion' suffering did not create direct bonds of fellowship with Ghanaians, and there were ultimately disconnects in the lived experience of Roman Catholic transnational networks.

, By contrast, the medical missions on the ground who were actually interacting with Ghanaians directly – and who were embodying their sacrifices in the hospital and in ways that were visible to the Ghanaian state – did manage to construct some sense of international brotherhood, whether Catholic or not. They also seemed to have separated themselves from the 'imperialists' and the national traitors who did not return to the homeland. As discussed in the previous chapter, the narrative of sacrifice and dislocation was repeated and recast by Jambaidu Awuni. Awuni contrasted it in the National Assembly in 1965 with Ghanaians who did not seem to feel the same call:

> In one of the mission hospitals in the North, there are about five doctors attending to patients and they do not have time for closing. Sometimes they even sleep in the hospital … In spite of the volume of work they always say their prayers each morning before they commence their daily work. These people do not complain that they have left their homes thousands and thousands of miles away to come and serve here in the North. These doctors have not come from Germany to serve their fellow white men but they are here to serve us the black. It is high time that our doctors follow the example set by these white doctors. Even some of our people who are qualified abroad do not want to come back.[57]

In that sense, German transnational identity was fostered, but not in ways that aid agencies may have imagined it or that European states conceived of its potential to tie together donors and recipients. The many layers of international health, national identity, and religious motivation were complex, varied, and divided between local, regional, national, and international contexts. How racial unity, transnational networks, and a context like Ghana were perceived was dependent on a plethora of interlocking demands, encounters, and concerns. Significantly, it appears that direct physical encounters in medical settings could create transnational unity, but these were seldom related to the wider picture of how they were financed, even in government debate.

Misereor's ability to create developmental transnational identities again was shaped more by medical encounters on the ground than it was by the imaginaries of European development campaigns. Misereor was involved in financing a wide set of Catholic medical missions in Ghana from the early 1960s onward and it was in these specific settings that development was made sense of and reconstructed: in its practice. As Barbra Mann Wall has shown, Family Hospital at Berekum received a considerable amount, including $200,000 in 1967 from the German government.[58] In the 1970s (beginning in 1971 with an initial grant of around 5,000 cedis and ending in the early 1980s) the Holy Family Hospital was granted over 1,037,000 DM for a hospital extension.[59] Misereor also had an array of other projects. In 1961, the committee gave 134,400 DM as an aid loan to help complete the St Martin's Hospital at Agroyesum.[60] In 1963, the hospital at Kpandu received 286,000 DM and a nurses' training centre received 214,000 DM. 300,000 DM of this total was in donation and 200,000 DM was in loans, with the majority of the loan being borne by the nurses' centre which only received a 14,000 DM donation.[61] In 1971, the hospital at Kpandu received 72,910 cedis for drainage. In 1974 the hospital at Assin Foso received 90,000 DM for X-ray apparatus.[62] In 1980, Misereor built staff accommodation costing a combined total of 240,000 DM at St John's Clinic and Maternity at Akim Ofoase, Holy Family Hospital at Nkawkaw, and St Michael's Maternity Clinic at Ntronang.[63] These huge sums of money shaped how hospitals could create a culture of development and transnational connection. Finding out how Ghanaians themselves interpreted this development encounter and how they perceived this scale of investment is beyond the scope of this study but would be hugely worthwhile further work. Nevertheless, Ghanaians at an elite level did figure in the combinations of how the money was used and what it created.

These large amounts of money from Misereor were combined with local Catholic initiatives and financing, which Misereor managed to exert some control over but which were in a dialogue of exchange with local Catholic institutions. In 1979 Misereor worked with the National Catholic Health Council, Diocesan health committees, and the Catholic Bishops Conference in Ghana to produce an 'Essential Improvements Fund for the Preparation of Church

Health Institutions in Ghana for Basic Health Care Work' – that is, a fund to equip hospitals, clinics, and mobile clinics to support Primary Health Care. The fund was to improve water supplies, sewage systems, electricity, and minor auxiliary buildings, but not new wards, staff buildings, or running expenses such as salaries or drug supplies. On average the financial split was around 25 per cent local and 75 per cent Misereor. This amounted to a local contribution of 340,000 DM and a fund contribution of up to 1,000,000 DM.[64] By 1986, the local Catholic diocese and archdiocese had contributed 2,032,085.05 cedis.[65] Monitoring and evaluation would be done by independent agencies and the Ministry of Health. In another case in 1982, 60,000 cedis were collected from the National Catholic Secretariat in Ghana for the Papase Hospital, Dzodze Hospital, and Weme-Abor Clinic. This was transferred to the Procure in Oosterbeek, Holland on the account of the bishop – rather than being kept in Ghana.[66] Well after formal Ghanaian independence, by working with local Catholic networks Misereor significantly extended their financial power in a range of projects and even could gain direct control over local Catholic fundraising. While they tended not to be the weaker player in coordinating development projects, they did work with local stakeholders and the government (which in the 1950s, the Holy Family Hospital had shut out).

Misereor funding was divided up in a range of amounts between a variety of projects and could draw in other financial actors such as the government and the local church. In 1981 Misereor set up a mobile eye clinic out of Nandom Hospital for 7,023 cedis.[67] Smaller amounts of funding, as in this case, may not have been able to ensure that a hospital functioned without support, but they provided leverage to gain funding from other areas too. Continuing the long stream of government funding for mission hospitals, in 1981 the hospital at Nandom also received 397,500 cedis from the government, 350 in ambulance fees, 86,817 in patient fees, and 15,215 in other fees. As in the original set-up of Nandom, built by the government in an area of long-term Catholic medical mission and staffed by the Catholic Church in 1965, the effective application of even small grants could have wide-ranging effects.[68] The small eye clinic out of Nandom Hospital may have been at the lower end of Misereor funding, but it was part of a network of income streams which had to be combined to make the institution function. Moreover, because the government-mission relationship had been established over the long term, each of Misereor's grants could encourage more spending from the state in certain areas by pooling resources. At St Anthony's Hospital at Dzodze, Misereor consistently contributed 11.36 per cent of funding, which amounted to around 40,000 DM a year between 1979 and 1981, combining with local contributions and project revenue of 30,000 DM to ensure that the hospitals continued functioning.[69] The sheer range of Misereor involvement, with the West German government, Memisa, and the Dutch government, is shown in the appendix. In a wide variety of Catholic medical missions across Ghana they were cooperating with local authorities and smaller-scale non-governmental agencies to produce a range of projects and health-care institutions.[70]

Misereor also worked alongside a variety of international health organisations and could use these to ensure their independence from the Ghanaian national government. In 1961, in a project to construct a hospital at Papase, the Germans worked with both Dutch and Northern Irish Catholics. Memisa contributed 70,000 florins, Father Smith in Northern Ireland collected 50,000 florins, and Misereor only needed to add 55,000. In combination they were able to put forward 185,000 DM to the bishop of Keta to begin construction. However, as will be explained later on, given the lack of government funding to help repay the loan, the bishop of Keta had to decline the money.[71] By contrast, at Berekum, Misereor spent even more in grants-in-aid (though it must be said, given the general pattern of combining resources, that the Holy Family Hospital at Berekum may have been something of an anomaly). By dividing up funding between different projects at different levels and in different ways, alongside other Catholic international health organisations, Misereor could manage the level of involvement of local governance. Again, as can be seen in the appendix, Misereor and Memisa fit into a patchwork of funding for Catholic medical mission for which they were two of the most common donors.

Misereor did not have a free hand in every area, but they were incredibly powerful and resourced Catholic mission across the length and breadth of Ghana. They used a variety of different projects, cooperating and collaborating with other international health organisations, local churches, national governments, medical missions, and communities. In some cases their attempts at certain plans, health innovations, or theologies were obstructed by opposing institutional interests, hostile nationalists, difficult circumstances, and long-term infrastructural patterns such as with hospital care. Nevertheless, by using intermediaries and building networks of trust, they hugely financed Catholic medical mission and ensured that even in the 1980s, when health care in Ghana all but collapsed, mission hospitals still had resources, staff, and funding. The scale of their aid work in Ghana shows the significance of West German Catholic aid. They fit within older networks and also with other new actors, while making certain that Catholic missions negotiated from a position of financial strength.

All these new initiatives were shaped by political instability and economic decline in Ghana. Rural decolonising Ghana was in some ways a traditional mission field and in other ways a completely new landscape: a rapidly decolonising nation which by 1972 entered a period of successive political coups, economic failure, and racial tension. While West German development narratives mattered in Germany, in Ghana development work itself was reformulated by specific contexts, circumstances, and groups. In the 1970s Ghana underwent the disastrous military dictatorship of Ignatius Katu Acheampong (1972–78), who in his own terms wanted to make 'war' on the economy. This was followed by further labour repression, protests, and violence by the state under the first regime of Flight Lieutenant Jerry Rawlings. Between 1957 and 1971 economic growth had been slow and fluctuating, but from 1975 it went into massive decline, culminating in total collapse by 1983. Between 1975 and 1978 cocoa income plummeted, and between 1975 and 1983 real output per head fell by 40 per cent to a quarter below the level it had been at independence. By 1983 the currency was valued at 5 per cent of the official exchange rate and GDP had been declining by 5 per cent each year (it would increase 5 per cent annually in the decades after structural adjustment in 1983).[72] Thus, around Berekum, and in the Ashanti region which had been historically strong in capitalist development and the creation of a cash-economy based on cocoa, the 1970s and 1980s were extraordinarily impoverished times. Resources were extremely limited and the black market was rampant with producers attempting to sell outside the price controls and heavy taxation of the state.

The West German development narrative of suffering, restoration, and international commonality may have been performed and constructed within Ghana, but it was not generally experienced or perceived as such by missionaries themselves. The German development narrative had to be constructed within this context, but it could not simply be deployed exactly as its European interests would have liked. Given the negotiations with Nkrumah and struggles with economic decline, there were far more pressing concerns than the reverberations on German society of missions' medical work in rural Ghana. Mission had greater issues with adapting to new circumstances, negotiating with locals, growing the local mission, and ultimately evangelising. Misereor's grander visions were detached from missionary realities. In an impoverished landscape, the physical realities of poverty and emigration gave physical shape to what the postcolonial medical mission meant.

Mission stations could act as hubs within their wider, more fluid networks; in these hubs biomedicine was created in ways that cut against the bigger narratives that the network as a whole tried to present. Alice Street has shown that in analysing the place of biomedical encounters, the competing orderings of the world that create 'the hospital' can be more visible. In places where there is 'institutional instability and medical uncertainty', where people are forced to make biomedicine work as best as possible, focusing on 'peripheral' biomedical institutions can show how these doctors and nurses have to take control of alternative orderings (such as kinship relationships) in order to secure authority.[73] Following Hokannen's idea of mission stations as hubs with networks, it is possible to tease out how biomedicine was created using various orderings of the world. Mission networks may have been funded and empowered by German nationalism, but in specific places, hubs in the network, those grand narratives were made into ground-level biomedical relationships in nuanced ways.[74] Moreover, missionaries themselves often lived by older 'master narratives' of missionary self-sacrifice and dedication, which in biomedical hubs could have varied meanings and performances based on need, local culture, and patient and staff orderings of the world that competed with their own. Finally, MMS missionaries who were not German themselves but often American and African (a general shift in mission makeup from European to American and African which Adrian Hastings has mapped) differed from their funders about why they were doing medicine.[75]

Catholic medical missionaries were focused often on the theological intent of their medical aid. Unlike in broader international histories, it is often assumed within historical literatures on international health that in the 1960s at the latest, organisations had secularised and that medical missions had left behind evangelistic priorities in favour of biomedical ones. However, Misereor in the early 1980s were still theological in their motives, at least insofar as they were directly collaborating with those who were, such as the National Catholic Secretariat. This evangelism was more subtle and more about the defence of the faith and the expression of the faith's values in bodily care than it was about direct proselytism. For example, at the outset of the National Catholic Health Council meeting in 1980, Bishop J. Owusu's address asked that the groups continue in their discussions 'the Church's tradition of dedicated service based on Gospel values'. He preached that 'in the world today, confronting us lie many challenges to our values and beliefs along with numerous risks … The temptations are many'.[76] In another meeting with two more Misereor delegates, Owusu encouraged freedom from reliance on foreigners and also urged Christians to give back to health care as they had received from God through Misereor. He explained that rural health care, the sort Misereor had financed with capital grants, was that which Ghanaian Christians should take on themselves: 'Let the love of Christ be deepened in us through prayer and expressed by the giving of ourselves, our time, our talent in the spirit of self emptying for the sake of our people in the rural areas … in bearing our trials with fortitude … following Christ in the Gospels each in his own work as a committed Christian'.[77]

In the following talk from Professor A. Foli and then from Sister Ancilla, Misereor was praised as offering help to the Catholic Secretariat medical missions, without which they would be in a 'bad way'.[78] The aim of Owusu's talks was not to attack foreign aid, though independence was a high priority, but to walk in the footsteps of Misereor Christian mission. Misereor's medicine was to them an expression of faith which they wanted to produce too. How the Misereor delegates felt about these convictions and interpretations of their work is not clear, but the continued funding and close relationship with the Secretariat suggests that their Catholic theological priorities were in some accord.

Misereor's German developmentalist concerns were not considered very much in Catholic medical mission in Ghana itself. As shown in chapters 1 and 2, whether evangelism or a particular development narrative was expressed on the ground and how it unfolded depended on the mission station itself, the particular missionaries, and the timing of an encounter. However, to some extent, there were

Catholic-specific trends and theologies, as can be seen in the MMS at Berekum. At Berekum in 1961 the MMS produced a film document-ing their hospital and nurse training, in which they concluded that their work achieved the unification of the care of the body and the care of the soul: 'We are all of one kind, alike in body everywhere in God's creation, each of us alike in his immortal soul. The soul the end. The care of the body the means. End and means made one through the medical mission apostolate'.[79]

The film also emphasised the commitment to science against the 'juju' of the 'fetish priest'.[80] Their version of proselytism was expressed through the boundaries they put on their scientific work: what was acceptable and what was not. Moreover, the wearing of the habit – a striking white feature amidst a local Ghanaian market – performed the purity and holiness of the medical mission. This was not explicit gospel preaching as Seventh-day Adventists and Scottish Presbyterians did in other areas of Ghana; it was performing a set-apart, modern community of belonging through disciplines such as the sacrifice of caring for the sick, scientific practice, and donning the white habit. Belief was not displayed in spiritual performance but through exemplars of virtue and building relationships based on care.

Though Misereor managed to retain a great degree of control over local actors and their funding, Ghanaians also had agency to manip-ulate Misereor to support their own agendas – they may even have helped to change the whole course of Misereor away from an early preoccupation with hunger. In 1959, Joseph O. Bowers, the bishop of Accra, managed to gain 66,000 DM of funding for a 'Hospital for Crippled Children' from Misereor. He did this through a variety of persuasion tactics. First, he made an emotional appeal that had almost no relevance to his actual bid but that emphasised the scale of health need and the lack of interest of the government when it came to the care of children. He attached a newspaper clipping about sev-enty-one babies dying in a period of only four months in Agona Abodom, with no apparent cause and no medical officer going to examine the epidemic. Perhaps another reason that Bowers used the article was that it described how health officers that tried to get mothers to send their children for medical treatment by having the Abdomhene beat gongs found that some mothers 'expressed reluc-tance' sending their children to doctors 'because of religious faith'.[81] He may have been trying to show the dangers of not allowing the historical mission church to continue its authority over health, as those mothers 'would continue to prefer spiritual healing at open air church services where the sick are subjected to all forms of blessing which ultimately end with presentation of a holy crucifix'.[82]

Given the challenge the ecstatic Pentecostal congregations could pose to traditional medical mission, Bowers may have been looking to foster the image of a shared enemy of the true church. Second, Bowers added to this newspaper clipping his own vicious attack on the government, aligning himself with the Catholic Church rather than the evils of the secular state:

> We are in the process of establishing the ONLY HOSPITAL
> FOR CRIPPLED CHILDREN in Ghana. The Brothers of St.
> John of the God are despite their many obligations bearing the
> major part of the financial burden for this urgent work of mercy.
> Unfortunately, the government seems to pursue the pagan policy
> of leaving such works for the deaf, dumb, lame etc. almost
> entirely to Voluntary Agencies, and despite assurances given in
> Parliament cannot be moved to give timely assistance to this
> project for which also we have been making appeals to various
> sources without adequate success.[83]

Finally, adding to his critique of the 'pagan' and deceitful government, Bowers emphasised his ties of concern to the foreign Catholic missions already attempting to do this work. Not only was he arguing that it was incumbent on Christians to do such an 'urgent work of mercy', he argued that other Catholics have already heeded the call but were not being supported. Later in the letter, Bowers spoke a language of universal brotherhood in Christ, attempting to build trust and a kinship of passion in order that his specific aims might be met: 'I wish to conclude by thanking our numerous benefactors in Germany who under the direction of their Shepherds in Christ are contributing so efficaciously to the spread of the faith in Africa and the Diocese of Accra, and by assuring them of my prayers for a double portion of the rewards that Christ has promised to those who assist even the humblest of His little ones'.[84]

Drawing on both biblical invocation to help children and also on a tradition of mission work in which Africans (particularly African children) were viewed as a lower, needy group of humanity requiring Christian charity, Bowers hammered his message home.[85] The

Misereor response from G. Dossing in May 1959 encouraged Bowers to go through the official process of five separate petitions and also to consider agricultural projects, given the starvation and hunger about which Misereor were particularly interested.[86] Nevertheless, by November, Bowers had been given his 66,000 DM for a 'Hospital for Crippled Children' in Koforidua.[87] While Misereor may have already been considering widening their approach by this point, it is clear that local agents like Bowers were also shaping the change in policy and gaining from it.

The development narratives that were prevalent in West Germany and that fuelled Misereor were detached from the realities and concerns of medical mission in Ghana itself. Misereor policy could also be shifted by local agents by not repaying loans. In 1975 A. Konings, the bishop of Keta, informed Misereor that they would not be able to repay the loan for the completion of the Kpandu Hospital and construction of the nurses' training centre (this had been financed with government money too). The 140,000 DM loan would not even be met in part. This was due partly to the collapse of the Ghanaian economy in the mid-70s, following several coups and the slump of cocoa prices worldwide in the 1960s. Konings offered a four-point explanation:

1. On account of the devaluation of Ghana Cedi by approximately 30% I could no more be held accountable for refund of 140,000 DM but only for the 25,200 Ghana Cedis at whatever the rate of foreign exchange that might be.

2. Since that time two more devaluations of the Ghana Cedi took place with the result that now the foreign exchange value of 25,200 Ghana Cedis is just over 50,000 DM.

3. I kept the loan of 25,200 Cedis up to last year, 1974, but due to the sharp increase in prices of medicines, drugs and hospital salaries I was forced to put all financial resources at my disposal, including the loan of 25,2000 Cedis into the hospital to keep it running, the alternative being having to close down the hospital completely.

4. I was hoping that the situation would improve, but instead of this it is still deteriorating, because we cannot increase the hospital

fees from the patients, as the people are relatively poor and the Government in its hospitals also charges no fees at all, or very small ones, it any.[88]

Furthermore, 'world inflation' had destroyed any possibility of repayment, Konings wrote.[89] Given the relative strength of the deutsche mark to many other currencies, it is strange that this eventuality was not planned for in the initial loan or the funding kept in deutsche marks until it was needed. Perhaps it was not expected that the cedi would collapse so considerably. In 1961, Ann Van den Ende had written to Father Odam at the medical administration in the Bishops' House: what would happen if private hospitals were taken over – would loans be repaid by government instead?[90] Nevertheless, questions of what would happen if the economy collapsed seemed to take a back seat to concerns about political turmoil. Perhaps without having another obvious option, or out of mercy or long-term trust, the Prälat G. Dossing wrote back to Bishop Konings saying that the full 140,000 DM 'has been converted from a loan to a grant on a decision by the Episcopal Commission of Misereor'.[91] While Misereor had considerable control as they held the purse strings, once money had been distributed it was hard to get back and power could be diffuse throughout the medical mission network, with Ghanaians having many strategies they could employ from below.

Government could also hinder what Ghanaian Catholics and Misereor wanted to do. Extra international health aid and shrewd negotiation were needed. The same bishop of Keta, A. Konings, wrote to Misereor in 1961 that he would have to retract a request for aid even though the desired amount of 185,000 DM had already been offered by Misereor, Memisa, and a Northern Irish cleric. This was for the hospital at Papase, mentioned above. Konings wrote that, since the offer had been made,

the situation has changed completely. The Government no longer allows me to build a hospital at Papase, but only a so-called Health Centre, which comprises an outpatients department, maternity and a maximum of 15 beds for inpatients. It would be impossible to refund a heavy loan from the small income which such a Health Centre produces because the running expenses are proportionately identical to those of a hospital. I do not at the moment know what to do in the matter, but you will appreciate that I cannot at this juncture undertake commitments and responsibilities which I would later on not be able to honour.[92]

This statement suggests why Misereor may have forgiven the other debt at Kpandu in 1975. It was not mismanagement on the bishops' part, as he was careful not to ask for many loans he could not repay. Instead the issue at Kpandu was genuine unforeseen change, and Misereor had a long-term relationship of trust with the bishop so they were not going to coerce a repayment. As Hanaan Marwah has shown with the electrification development project in Ghana, it was not managerial failure but economic crisis following the 1971 devaluation which caused rising costs and the burden of foreign debt. By 1975 the government of Ghana was maintaining the existing exchange rate but the cedi was collapsing on parallel markets, and by 1982 the cedi was valued at one-twentieth of what it was worth officially. This was followed by debt restructuring, structural adjustment, and other crises such as the West African drought between 1982 and 1984. However, between 1961 and 1966, the cedi was worth almost as much as the dollar, and was relatively healthy.[93] It was clear that Misereor were happy to take risks in this period on both local Catholic leaders and on the continued funding of mission hospitals by the Ghanaian government. Given the Ghanaian government track record of funding mission hospitals and given that they often tried to force money into the hands of the Sisters at Berekum, without the benefit of hindsight this probably was not considered a particularly dangerous gamble.

Even though Misereor could not directly impose its narrative of development, missions relied on it to ensure the survival of their own work. As with bishop of Keta in the mid-1970s, Ghana's economic collapse meant that mission hospitals would have had to stop growing or even running at all without large-scale funding from abroad. By this point, the Ghanaian government could not financially guarantee that any shared policies would be possible. Misereor had to finance mission hospitals with conversions of loans into grants and resolve urgent issues in institutions that they already supported. On the other side, Misereor needed trusted intermediaries like the bishop at Keta to help them navigate the changing economic situation. Otherwise they were offering money that they would never see returned. Crucially, this dialogue also shows how much missions still depended on government well after formal political independence from the British Empire. Offers of funding were not simply convenient for mission projects: without the backing of Nkrumah in 1961, the hospital at Papase could not be built at all. As mentioned in the previous chapter, 1961 was a turning point for Nkrumah, when he became incredibly suspicious of foreign actors and the church. In most cases funding continued, but in 1961 something occurred that meant the bishop of Keta fell out of favour or Misereor could not navigate Nkrumah's increasing authoritarianism and socialism. Nevertheless, by 1963, Konings was able to construct a health centre at Papase with other sources of money that did not need to be refunded.[94] Misereor did not stop there: the St Mary Theresa Hospital at Dodi-Papase was also built in this year.[95] According to the 1982 Catholic report, its income was made up of government grants (41 per cent), patient fees (46 per cent), and private subsidies (15 per cent). Donations were also being received from Misereor, Memisa, KOOK (Holland), Wor and Wand (USA), and Areon.[96] Perhaps by adding in further actors, or by converting the loan to a grant or by negotiating with the Ghanaian government, they were able to negotiate past the roadblock and construct using different means.

Misereor was not totally empowering: missions still needed government funding and patient fees, which left them subject to local and national changes. The majority of Catholic missions in Ghana largely were funded by patient fees and they were vulnerable to local and national disputes, such as with trade unions. This again shaped the kind of development narrative being created. In general, the table in the appendix shows the extent of the dependence on patient fees across the Catholic medical missions in Ghana in 1982. In the Holy Family Hospital, Barbra Mann Wall has shown how in the 1979 nationwide strike of the Ghana Registered Nurses Association over salaries, 'nurses and midwives did not come to work for five days at a time'. Instead, the missionaries had to use 'Traditional Birth Attendants'. These Ghanaians were probably unqualified in biomedical practice but 'left their families and farms to staff sixteen shifts at Holy Family Hospital'. When the strike continued the MMS had to use the local chief to negotiate with the employees to return to work.[97] While there is little evidence of missions actively stopping the nationalisation of health care (often they were politically quiescent, except in trade union disputes already raised), missions relied on patient fees for their continuation and would not have promoted any government attempts at more radical redistribution.[98]

Overall, all these challenges and constraints shaped the terms in which Catholics in Ghanaian health work narrated their position in the larger tradition of historic mission, its adaptation, and its survival, rather than in the terms laid out by Lübke in Cologne. Catholic transnationalism was difficult to maintain across diverse conceptions of the meaning and performance of development. Without physical and visible contact, the notions of sacrifice and suffering that motivated donors was disconnected from recipients. Nevertheless, the embodiment of their help in the form of medical missionaries themselves did create a medical encounter that in some cases served to foster notions of shared humanity beyond race and organizational links, and the dialogues between donors and institutions also created some shared endeavour. German Catholic transnationalism, therefore, did register on the ground in Ghana, but in terms and narratives that were unstable and multiply. The dissemination of the ideas about German restoration through Catholic unity was difficult to sustain, and controlling the reception and interpretation was difficult to manage. Most significantly, it was in the picture of the sacrificial missionaries themselves that something of that effort found a performance. How Ghanaians generally received it is difficult to analyse beyond key leadership, but would be worth further study, especially in the wider frame of Catholic transnational aid in the postcolonial world.

By 1982 Catholic medical mission, funded by government, Dutch and West German Catholic mission organisations, local fees and churches, and a variety of other international health organisations, had proliferated and settled across Ghana. There were at least fifty-four Catholic mission health institutions, including hospitals, clinics, maternity centres, and PHC centres spread all over the country. Combined, they catered for hundreds of thousands, if not millions, of patients. The list of donors is extensive and a surprising variety were present. The pattern and frequency of Dutch and West German aid is clear: they were involved in the vast majority of Catholic mission institutions, which is highlighted in bold in the appendix. Out of the forty-four Catholic mission institutions with reliable and detailed information on funding, at least twenty-four had Dutch and German aid involvement, and two others were indirectly supported through Jirapa Hospital and the Holy Family Hospital at Berekum (funded by Dutch and West German aid). This bald statistic is just the minimum amount, as it seems likely that many more were also gaining funding from them. Holland and Germany were the most consistent and widespread donors, in the form of embassy aid, government donations, international organisation, and mission funding.[99]

GLOBAL DEVELOPMENT NETWORKS AND THE DUTCH FOCUS ON GHANA

Given the scale and significance of West German and Dutch Catholic medical mission in Ghana, the question is: was this an exception or was it happening elsewhere too? Walter Bruchhausen and Carola Rensch have explored German postwar aid to Togo, in which public health and academic research were combined from the 1960s.[100] Bruchhausen has also shown that from 1961 West Germany was using Marshall Plan funding for development aid, and church projects were around 50 per cent financed by this. Medicus Mundi Internationalis was created to organise European Catholic efforts in West Germany and Austria, Belgium, Ireland, and the Netherlands (though Bruchhausen notes in this regard that Calvinists in the Dutch government did restrict the activities of the large Catholic minority). Financed by lent donations, International Cooperation for Socio-Economic Development (CIDSE) was begun by one of the founders of Misereor bringing together eight bishops from Catholic development organisations to build on the secular-church collaboration work allowed after Vatican II.[101]

There is a paucity of research on Catholic medical mission, but in general it appears that in Africa, Asia, and South America there was significant funding from West Germany. Between 16 October 1959 and 31 December 1959 alone, there were requests to Misereor for almost 20 million DM from all over the world. The largest was from South America which in total requested 3,671,155 DM. Africa was at 3,152,412 DM, Asia at 668,070 DM, Oceania at 753,500 DM, and Europe at 335,000 DM.[102] It is not clearly stated which of these requests were met, but the requests themselves show that Misereor was seen to be a donor across the world, and that world extended well beyond Ghana alone. As Gonzalo Navarro Sanz has shown, the West German government began development work in Latin America in 1952, giving funds to the UN programme for technical assistance; then, in 1961, the Economic and Development Cooperation Ministry (BMZ) was formed. While there were German immigrants to Chile, it was a Spanish colony – again, this was a completely new form of colonialism. Crucially, Sanz also shows that West German Catholic foundations Misereor, Adventiat, and the Konrad Adenauer Foundation (KAF) began even before the BMZ was established. In 1961 the Christmas Eve collection for Misereor was purposefully for aid to Latin America and collected 23 million DM, which then became an annual initiative for aid to Latin America.[103]

Streams of funding and staff from West Germany and the Netherlands lasted at least into the late 1990s. In 1992, Memisa had 130 doctors working in eighty programs (mostly in 'English-speaking Third World countries').[104] By 1998, according to P.W. Kok, Memisa accounted for 'about half the annual number of Dutch health care workers in third world countries', and in 1996 received 1,820 requests for assistance with 82 per cent support-ing structural programs and 18 per cent disaster relief.[105] As for Misereor, by 1994, it was active in 101 developing countries in the Caribbean, Africa, Asia, and Central as well as South America. Their budget total was $258,100,000, half of this from private sources and half from public ones.[106]

There were many other Catholic medical missions in this global network extending across the second half of the twentieth cen-tury who were connected to Misereor and Memisa. Mattias Egg has shown how between 1952 and 1994, the Medical Missionary Society GMH (Gemeinschaft der Missionshelferinnen), the Medical Missionary Union (Missionsärztlicher Bund), and the Würzburg Medical Missionary Institute (Missionsärztliches Institut Würzburg) funded and staffed Catholic medical mission across Asia and Africa. Egg shows that there were twenty-six projects over eight coun-tries and that 109 sisters of the GMH were employed as health workers. These were in Pakistan at Sargodha and around India: in Shrirampur (West Bengal), Jhansi (Uttar Pradesh), Shevgaon (Maharashtra), Chetput (Chennai), Thellakom (Kerala), Allahabad (Uttar Pradesh), and Bangalore (Karnataka). They were also found across Africa in the Congo, Namibia, South Africa, Zimbabwe, and Cameroon (as well as Ghana, for which Egg analyses the work at Tumu, Navrongo, and Eikwe). Egg argues that these organisations were vital to other West German missions' success: 'Due to their permanent mission the sisters of the GMH were able to act as medi-ators between the health policies and strategies of German institu-tions like MI and Misereor and the State and Church authorities in the missionary countries'.[107]

Thus, a network of West German and Dutch aid was significant across large areas of Asia and Africa. Contrasting sizes, timing, duration, and forms were linked up by common denomination, interest, and nationality, creating very effective health infrastructures that in many cases could weather the storms of decolonisation. For example, in the case of GMH, they acted as 'mediators' for Misereor and MI because their 'permanent mission' created stronger local bonds.

At the same time, amidst all this global funding Ghana *was* a particular focus for Memisa and the Netherlands, resulting in many young Dutch doctors staffing Catholic hospitals, especially where there were not local alternatives. When the former Dutch colony of Indonesia became independent and authoritarian, Dutch missionaries hot-footed to Ghana instead. Some worked for the Basel Mission while others went to Catholic missions, and many were progressive idealists hoping to establish their own stations – including followers of the Catholic medical approaches of E.F. Schumacher and liberation theology.[108] With the general stream of Dutch mission, others followed. As the 1969 annual report for St Michael's Hospital in Pramso, Ghana, stated: 'Most of the mission hospitals are run by young, often Dutch doctors'. With its own doctor set to leave in the following September, the report noted the concern that although the young Dutch doctors 'are fully qualified according to the Dutch standards, they generally do not have the obligatory 3 years experience required by the Ghanaian medical and dental board'. Nevertheless, the report explained, without 'sufficient Ghanaian doctors ... available to run these hospitals, a compromise solution must be found', because for St Michael's there could not be 'a sound financial basis' without a doctor.[109] Moreover, it noted that both expatriate nurses were set to leave by 1970, meaning that 'Ghanaisation' was 'obligatory' as well as 'desirable'. However, a shortage of Ghanaian nurses was, as with doctors, 'threatening' for St Michael's.

Dutch and West German missionaries arrived in swaths as a diverse cohort with differing views but all part of the same stream over several decades. Dutch doctors were common across many areas of Ghanaian missionary health care. From its opening in 1958, St Elisabeth's Hospital in the Brong Ahafo region was, according to the 1983 annual report, mainly staff by Dutch nurses and expatriate doctors. This group operated on a consistent turnover, with each doctor and nurse residing around two to three years in Ghana.[110] In many other cases Dutch doctors had little Catholic practice or theology but applied themselves to the missionary work of Catholic hospitals.[111] Dutch and German Catholic medical mission was a complex and even conflicting group. Theological, medical, and reproductive health issues were contested and even viciously disagreed over. One Dutch 'liminal missionary' (as he put it) who came to Ghana in this period was the anthropologist Sjaak Van Der Geest, who stayed from 1971 and, after his PhD, continued to work on sexual relationships and birth control in the town of Kwahu-Tafo.[112] By contrast, the more conservative Catholic Margaret Marquart (discussed further in chapter 5) worked closely with the Ghanaian Catholic archbishop Peter Sarpong.

Along with the growing number of Dutch doctors, making sure that staff were funded and housed was a further feature of Misereor and Memisa aid across several decades. St Michael's Pramso received funding from Misereor to build a senior staff bungalow in 1981 and 1982, and Memisa provided medical supplies and drugs to the hospital.[113] In the 1980s St Anthony's Hospital in Dzodze had successive Dutch Sisters-in-Charge and Dutch physicians as medical officers.[114] At St Anthony's, in the late 1970s Misereor had funded building improvements, and in 1981 Memisa funded the construction of new accommodation for nurses as well as further medical aid.[115] From 1980 until at least 1986 there was also a tradition of medical students from the Catholic University in Nijmegen, training at St Anthony's for 'practical exposure'. In 1986 there were four Dutch students, one researching the incidence of schistosomiasis in the Ketu district.[116] Finally, some doctors in Ghana were specifically funded by Memisa and there may have been many more across this period, though such details tended not to be recorded in the annual reports.[117] One example is the Dutch 'Memisa-nurses' who staffed the hospital at Assin Foso in the early 1960s. Another example, around two decades later in April 1983, is the physician Ineke Bosman who arrived in Ghana and studied Twi at Abetifi until October, then took up a contract as a 'Memisa-doctor' for four years at Nkoranzaman Catholic Hospital.[118]

Yet, it was not Memisa grants and missionary doctors alone that constituted the Dutch relationship with Ghana: private individuals and the Dutch government also funded Catholic mission in the 1970s and 1980s. In their 1983 report the Nkoranzaman Catholic

Hospital thanked the Dutch government for donations, along with Misereor and Memisa.[119] In 1983, St Elisabeth's Hospital in Brong Ahafo thanked the Dutch government for donations of drugs (and thanked Dutch colleges, schools, and Catholic communities as well).[120] There was a Dutch primary school and 'School for the Blind' that supported St Elisabeth's, alongside a series of Dutch private donors who paid for gutters and pipes, and a foundation from Almelo who gave money and donated equipment.[121] At St Antony's, Orion in Delft improved the orthopedic workshop and helped with shipping, and CEBEMO from Holland paid for a water project.

Into the later 1980s and 1990s there were still strong connections between Dutch donors and medical staff and Catholic mission hospitals in Ghana. In July 1987, St Theresa's Hospital and Health Services in Nkoranza noted that, along with other Dutch visitors, Daan Verboom from Orion in Holland had managed to install a solar energy fridge at the clinic in Akuma. This followed Orion's donations of beds, an X-ray machine, and additional solar energy systems for vaccine storage.[122] The Apam Catholic Hospital in their 1989–90 annual report noted that Misereor had recently donated Nissan petrol and a duplicating machine, Memisa had provided funding, Horizon Holland had given bedsheets, a water pump, and an electric typewriter, and the Catholic Mission Board had provided drugs.[123] Staff, too, were continuing to remain in Ghanaian hospitals, such as the physician Jos de Maat who was still stationed alone at St Elizabeth's by the end of the decade – though the report noted that they were blessed to be given locum relief by a Ghanaian doctor in 1989 which was offsetting some of the pressure.[124]

As will be analysed further in chapter 5, one of the notable consequences of this steady stream of supplies and staff was the support of Primary Health Care. At St Anthony's in Dzodze, Misereor funded a Primary Health Care and maternal-child health scheme between 1977 and 1983. The aim was that this would be taken over by the Ghanaian government in 1980, which eventually did happen in 1983 but only for the cost of the salaries. The government could not extend to funding the equipment improvements that the scheme needed, though Memisa did donate a new Land Rover in 1984. This PHC scheme was not alone but limitations were significant. St Anthony's offered the only mobile clinic for the 25,000 people in Ketu district, and covered only 8 per cent of the population under five years old.[125]

CONCLUSION

Ghana was so significant for Dutch and West German Catholic medical mission because of a combination of factors, in which old colonial ties were not important and the Cold War was only one in a range of concerns. This chapter has argued that postcolonial international health requires reframing in order to incorporate post-war Dutch and German mission which does not fit into the current frames that emphasise Cold War causes, old colonial concerns in decolonised settings, and the growth and articulation of the international community. The drive behind West German and Catholic medical mission may, of course, have incorporated some of these – West Germany's political shape was very influenced by the US and the formation of opposing East-West blocs, and Catholic international health organisations were part of a growing international development community. However, the prime causes were identifying with a development narrative that emphasised Catholic internationalism, liberal democratic credentials with strong civil society leadership, and shared suffering under the Nazis.

Focusing on the postcolonial nation of Ghana without a German or (for a long time) Dutch colonial past, and a nation with a strong Catholic heritage and network of missions, gave Dutch and West German mission a very effective focal point for projects to create a new liberal humanitarianism. Moreover, given the lack of patterns of medical mission generally in Ghana and its reliance of mission, there was not the hostility that was encountered in other postcolonial nations such as Indonesia. This did not mean that West German and Dutch Catholic medical mission operated with a free hand; they were constrained by Ghanaian national politics, local circumstances, economic fluctuations, and the long-term priority of mission hospitals in Ghana. It also did not mean that missionaries imagined their development work in the same terms. Missionaries' lived experiences, their perspectives, and their organisational dynamics were frequently detached from abstract debates about development, voluntarism, and nationality. As Emma Hunter puts it in her work on ideas of freedom in Tanzania: 'apparent uniformity at the level of words and concepts can hide the multiple and contested meanings developed in local contexts'.[126]

Nevertheless, because of the scale of funding available, their relations with trusted intermediaries on the ground, the availability of staff from Europe and America, and the combination of a variety of institutional forms in a network of Catholic international health organisations, missions were able to grow considerably. The appendix shows the sheer range of Catholic medical missions to which Memisa and Misereor had contributed in Ghana by 1982. It was here that the performance of a suffering and rehabilitating West Germany and Netherlands found its stage. The result was a well-resourced and well-staffed network of Catholic health institutions in Ghana that became a vital network for international health organisations and national programmes.

4

International Health Campaigns
and Christian Mission: Ghana, Europe,
and North America, 1950–94

A huge variety of actors and voices make up 'international health' and 'global health'. Yet, as historical concepts, the terms are often reduced to only meaning the workings of elite policy makers in the centres of global organisations in Geneva, New York, and Washington, DC.[1] As Sanjoy Bhattacharya has shown, in Frank Fenner's history of smallpox eradication (SEP), the wide array of participants involved in the programme was silenced and national involvement – especially that of smaller nations – was particularly circumscribed.[2] This chapter considers a variety of scales and networks, and argues that in the negotiations between them, medical missionaries and Ghanaian Christians figured as negotiators, intermediaries, and advocates. This chapter will tie USAID (United States Agency for International Development) and the WHO (World Health Organization) together with national health planning in the Ghana measles and smallpox programme, and with health care more widely. It will analyse how Catholic medical missions facilitated USAID's PL-480 food aid programme across Ghana. In both cases, missionaries enabled far greater capacity than otherwise would have obtained.[3] The key claim of this chapter is that understanding global health requires keen attention to the infrastructure and historical networks in a given country – it doesn't happen in a void, and, in the case of Ghana, the role of religious health is absolutely vital.[4]

This chapter will first explore the involvement of Ghanaians, the US, international health organisations, and missionaries in the 'Ghana Smallpox Eradication and Measles Control Programme'. International health was hugely shaped by these Ghanaian actors who had long-term linkages to mission. Ghanaian Christians could straddle both mission and international health, and use both to their own ends. This argument challenges the boundaries of the concept of 'medical mission', showing how, as institutional Africanisation of medical science and medical mission proceeded, there were continuities with older traditions of historic mission. Ghanaian Christians could function as medical missionaries within the hinterlands of the state and away from the urban centres in which they were born and educated. This was through mission hospitals and clinics, but also within international health. International health campaigns could be imagined in similar terms to that of roving colonial evangelists and preachers travelling to remote communities to share the gospel. Ghanaians also challenged older models; while international health actors may have imagined their inventions and use of missionaries as secular and technical, for Ghanaians themselves this work could be seen as a truer expression of their faith than historic forms of medical mission. This first section will detail the driving role of Frank Grant in measles and smallpox control in Ghana. Grant was a Christian Ghanaian, son of the eponymous president of the Methodist conference, medical field unit leader, and nicknamed by his USAID colleagues as a 'Ghanaian Abraham Lincoln'.[5] This part of the chapter will further the exploration of the coordination of Ghanaians, missions, and US aid work by examining the creation of a medical school. In these developments, long-term continuities in both the Africanisation of Ghanaian medicine and mission culture can be highlighted; yet, added to this, USAID also wished to co-opt the Africanisation process to meet their own concerns for state stabilisation and modernization.[6]

The second section will explore the USAID nutrition programmes in the context of severe economic decline in Ghana in the 1970s. It will analyse the role of the US Catholic Relief Services (CRS) in distributing food in the USAID programme PL-480. It was not only Ghanaian doctors but also expatriate missionaries who were working with and shaping international health in ways that linked to new streams of mission funding and personnel in the 1960s, and in a context of long-term continuities in the structure of Ghanaian health care. WHO and US medical aid in Ghana were shaped by powerful and well-resourced Christian networks as well as by America's religious priorities and international health agendas during the Cold War. This will further the analysis of chapter 3 by exploring the postwar expansion of Catholic mission in Ghana. Crucially, the CRS's

links to the global network of Catholic mission, to Misereor, and to
Ghanaian Catholic missions logistically and imaginatively extended
how USAID conceived of their food aid.

'A GHANAIAN ABRAHAM LINCOLN': SMALLPOX, MEASLES, AND THE MEDICAL SCHOOL

International health organisations offered Ghanaian Christian
doctors and medical mission networks a new way to exert influence and control; this had wider repercussions for the international
health campaigns of the 1960s and 1970s. Medical missionaries
adapted to the new international health contexts and were incredibly useful to international health organisations, while constructing
programmes in ways which were useful to them. In doing so, they
challenged the traditional structures and identities of historical
medical mission (such as needing to be part of a specific denominational organisation), but also gave mission new outlets, functions,
and postcolonial roles.

International health programmes often require validation at the
national level and are constructed in ways that are politically useful to local actors. In her recent article on Portuguese India's relations with the WHO's SEARO (World Health Organization's South
East Asia Regional Office) in the 1950s, Monica Saavedra considered international health politics from a national perspective. In this
she challenged common historical accounts, such as that of Nitsan
Chorev, which focus on the institutional agency of the WHO, the
import of its universal visions, the effect of its global agendas, and
its adaptations to political difficulties. By contrast, Saavedra looked
at how SEARO was a 'product and locus of regional politics', how it
served a national political agenda, and how it was one of the forces
which reshaped global health programmes. Saavedra builds on the
work of Sanjoy Bhattacharya, who, in his work on smallpox control
and eradication (SEP) in India between 1947 and 1977, argued that
the WHO's programme was formed and made possible in negotiations with the complex national interests of Indian ministers and
bureaucrats.[7] This point is made even more strongly in his work on
SEP in Bhutan, where the WHO submitted to and had to negotiate
with the demands of Indian authorities.[8] Moreover, in the work of
Sarah Cook Runcie, the medical field units (MFUs) in Cameroon
are shown to have been necessary to SEP being possible – again

national structures and politics needed to be marshalled for international health programmes to function.[9] With Portuguese Goa
and India, global medical programmes were imagined in terms of
the national concerns which they legitimised on the international
level. As Saavedra puts it, it is important to consider 'multiple scales
and actors when analysing the politics of international, and indeed,
global health'.[10]

While the smallpox eradication programme had international
traction, it was actually controlling measles that made it useful locally. The young Ghanaian epidemiologist Francis (Frank)
Chapman Grant became the deputy director of the MFUs in Ghana
in the early 1960s. Already by this point they had much contact
with USAID through the malaria eradication programme in the mid-
1950s, which had ground to a halt because of a change in the direction of international health. Grant was named the head of the Ghana
Smallpox Eradication and Measles Control Programme when it
began in 1965.[11] How this programme was strengthened and formed
by the international health community was not a unilinear process.
It was neither a case of decisions from on high in Geneva controlling
Grant and the MFUs, or Grant freely creating programmes based
solely on need. It was a mixture. Grant was particularly interested
in measles because of the extremely high incidence of the disease in
Ghana at the time, especially for children under five. Around 5 to 15
per cent of children infected before eighteen months were likely to
die. One contemporary report asserted that Ghana had 25 per cent
of all measles cases in Africa – which led to a CDC team of doctors
using USAID funds to commence a measles identification project at
a national hospital and clinic in Ghana.[12] Grant combined the two
in order to create a national immunisation campaign. Once Grant
had the backing of the CDC and also the WHO, he wanted to bring
in USAID. The USAID programme officer in the mid-1960s, Fred
Gilbert, recalls how Grant forced his hand in getting the programme
started:

> One of my first Ghana memories was that Gordon Evans handed
> me an airgram about the idea of a smallpox-measles program.
> He said, in effect, 'I don't know what this is, but figure out
> what to do with it'. When I finally found time to flip through
> it, my reaction was that it was an unrealistic, lobby-driven
> initiative from left field. It certainly hadn't followed a normal

path through the AID programming process (not that there was much definition of that). CDC ... and WHO were the instigators, and there had surely been some communications from either Washington or Atlanta with the Ghanaians because one day a wonderful man named Dr. Frank Grant (a Ghanaian) from the Ministry of Health came by and wanted to talk about smallpox and measles ... He also had a message and said, 'Maybe we should talk about this'. That was a pain in the neck – it meant that I REALLY had to read the damn thing. It was clear that this wasn't something that would go away if we scoffed. It was coming at us a hundred miles an hour, and we really had to get moving even though we already had too much on our plates. And nobody else on either his side or mine could focus on the matter. So the two of us sat down and 'whomped up' an agreement for an activity financed by AID, sponsored by WHO and implemented by CDC – thus fitting no model or guidance available in the Manual Orders – and got it signed with precious little fanfare – or, at least, none that I recall. And that exercise turned out ultimately to be a good, even fun, experience since Frank Grant was such a good guy. And then, lo and behold, all kinds of crazy things started happening. People started arriving. Soon CDC people were working out of a local office in close collaboration with the Health Ministry to implement the program. And that turned out to be one of the most successful things we've ever done. Now that I think back, I remember being sent in the summer of 1966 to CDC in Atlanta to brief a group of field officers who were to be stationed in Africa. These people turned out, in most cases, to be the staff of the Smallpox-Measles Program. Yet the Smallpox-Measles Program, per se, was a surprise ... And, as with the embryonic Smallpox-Measles Program, one often had a frightening degree of latitude because no one else could focus on such matters.[13]

Gilbert's recollection both emphasises the ability of an MFU leader like Grant to put something on the table of international health organisations, and also the 'frightening degree of latitude' local assistant programme officers had in programme initiation. Far from the post-hoc histories that have shown SEP to be inevitable, Gilbert's statement emphasises just how contingent and much of a 'surprise' it actually was. As shown in a USAID memorandum

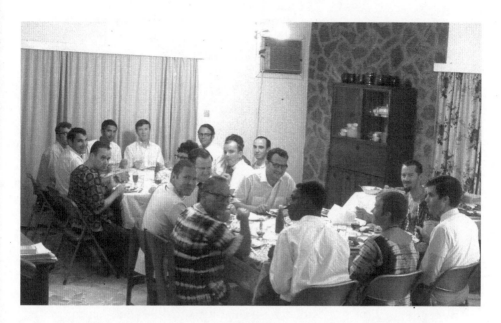

Figure 4.1 | CDC staff dinner, including Frank Grant sitting nearest the camera (1967). Dinner at Anne and Nat Rothstein's house in Lagos, Nigeria. Back table, left to right: Neal Ewen, Tony Masso, Jean Roy, Jay Friedman, John McEnaney, Christopher D'Amanda, Pat Imperato, unknown. Front table, left to right: Mark LaPointe, unknown, CDC short-term physician, unknown, Frank Grant (Ghanaian physician, head of smallpox program in Nigeria), Vicki Jones, David Melchinger, Andy Agle.

in July 1965 and in a memorandum from Donald Henderson to the CDC and the Bureau of State Services in November 1965, USAID and CDC were reluctant to include Ghana in the overall small-pox and measles programme because of concern that the scope of the 'African problem' was too great for 'any one donor'.[14] WHO instigated the programme but it required Grant wanting to talk about smallpox and measles to ensure USAID financial backing. As David Newberry puts it, 'WHO had nearly no contribution the Ghana program' – instead the CDC 'truly depended on vari-ous Christian missionary groups' for both surveillance and treat-ment.[15] There were complex negotiations on the ground and key individuals who by sheer will and force of personality drove the early stages of the programme. The WHO sponsored the initiative, certainly, and they deserve a great deal of credit for empowering people like Frank Grant. Moreover, once the WHO were involved, there were Russians and Japanese medical staff 'who had a long history in Ghana' working alongside the CDC. However, the CDC, with David Newberry supporting the supervision of MFU staff, surveillance, and training, implemented it (as well as, in time, the Expanded Program on Immunization, and campaigns against yaws, yellow fever, and guinea worm).[16] Moreover, it was actually USAID, despite barely getting a look in official histories, who financed it. Coordinating these groups within Ghana and pushing forward with the vague plans of the WHO fell to Frank Grant, who made sure that for Fred Gilbert it would become 'something that wasn't going to go away'. Grant used the landscape of health organisations already available, the contacts he had already made through the malaria eradication programme in the 1950s, and his position within the Ministry of Health to tackle a local measles problem with a set of global solutions. In this way, international health organisations both were agents of change, and were shaped by Grant and Ghana's specific context and motivations.

Grant was so concerned with measles because, before the 1960s, measles control had been neglected in Ghana in favour of yaws and trypanosomiasis. The biggest disease in Ghana in terms of overall incidence in government in the 1930s had been yaws, at 64.84 per cent of total incidence of infectious diseases in 1932–33.[17] In 1947, 10,253 cases of yaws were treated, and between 1951 and 1953 children's hospitals and clinics treated 46,878 cases.[18] Moreover, the anti-yaws campaign begun in 1956 was assisted by the WHO and UNICEF.[19] By 1961, the MFUs' attack phase managed to reduce the incidence of yaws in a given region by 75–90 per cent, though they could not get incidence below 0.5 per cent. Trypanosomiasis had also been given huge funding – £150,000 for an institution in the Northern Territories – in 1951 because of the pioneering work and advocacy of Kenneth Stacey Morris, though by 1961 this was struggling because of the expense of upkeep (tsetse control requires close attention to bush management around rivers and careful coordination of big game and livestock).[20]

Yet measles had been neglected. In 1952, there were 24,949 outpatient cases of measles, with this declining to 8,095 the following year with 476 measles inpatients and twenty-five deaths.[21] Only in 1961 was measles control systematised by the MFUs. That year found incredibly high numbers of children contracting the illness. Surveying a population of 7,515 under fifteen years of age, they found 1,134 cases in children in villages, an attack rate of 15.3 per cent in those communities. From this there were thirty-eight deaths, with a case fatality rate of 3.3 per cent. Most of these, 90.8 per cent, were in the northeast. The MFUs concluded that this was only a 'relative small part of the total which occurred', and if there was an epidemic (as there had been in 1957, in which every community in the extreme North had been attacked), the staff were entirely 'insufficient'.[22] The view of locals that the disease was a 'mild inevitable childhood experience' had 'serious consequences', according to the MFUs. In 1962 they saw 1,366 cases of a total 8,962 children examined and found a 15.2 per cent attack rate, 67.2 per cent complications, and 2.2 per cent fatality, with thirty deaths. This time the survey showed more spread across the North with 40 per cent in the northeast and 45 per cent in the northwest.[23] Internationally, too, measles continued to be ignored, though for the CDC their West Africa programme was always, in fact, a smallpox-measles programme.

Measles was also a far more significant focus for Grant and Ghana because smallpox control had been successful since the early 1920s. The majority of smallpox control was executed by the British colonial state. Except for in the 1940s, when generally the colonial state struggled to implement health programmes because of a lack of resources, they managed to immunise millions of Africans in the Gold Coast between the 1920s and 1950s. This corroborates William Schneider's argument that, while the global eradication effort was necessary to stopping smallpox's continued periodic outbreaks across Africa, those writers such as Fenner and Donald Hopkins who have emphasised this have done so because of their own role in it and have neglected colonial initiatives.[24] By the 1950s in the Gold Coast and Ghana, the colonial state through the MFUs had a lot of the country immunised. In late colonial Gold Coast, smallpox control was a mixture of African health workers and colonial officers, with the MFUs partly operating out of Kintampo. The MFUs began in 1935 in order to tackle sleeping sickness but were soon expanded to other communicable diseases, in 1944 to yaws and 1949 to smallpox.[25] Taking over from G.T. Saunders in the 1940s, the British colonial medical officer Broughton B. Waddy led the MFUs with David Scott.[26] The efforts had begun with Accra in 1919, moved out beyond the capital after this, and in the 1950s began immunising across the North. As Addae has shown, this was a generally successful process, though there were rises in incidence in the 1950s.[27]

It was not only between WHO and USAID that Grant figured as significant; his faith, his experience of diverse forms of Ghanaian culture, and his Methodist identity ensured that he was able to coordinate effectively with missions and local communities. Frank Grant's background in Christian mission and the Ghanaian Methodist church was a key asset to the MFU's smallpox and measles control. One of Frank's colleagues in Ghana, David Newberry from the CDC and USAIDs, recalled that:

> Frank and Mary Grant were deeply religious. Frank's father was the Pastor at the Cathedral ... Working with Frank Grant we held a short prayer session before each day's work. Frank conducted religious training and both he and Mary were parish leaders ... Unlike many African medial officers – Frank and Mary Grant applied their Christian values to everything they did. I traveled to the British System Rest Houses located in every regional area of Ghana. Some of these were local native huts and ill-kept. I never traveled to any such facility that had not recorded Dr. Frank Grant's previous visit![28]

For Grant, professional discipline and technical control were combined with religious mobilisation and social authority. As Paul Greenhough has shown, in East Pakistan there were clashes between international health officials who supported the political and social mobilisation of volunteers in smallpox eradication, against those who believed that this was a dangerous initiative without professional discipline.[29] Grant intermixed both professional and religious identities in order to gain the trust and support of communities during vaccinations. This was critical in the success of campaigns which thrived on local support. Along with medical officers and police telegraphs soliciting smallpox mobility reports, there were also parish priests, local Catholic leadership, and local chiefs who collaborated with the vaccine teams. Churches formed 'groups that supported immunization' and announced the campaigns 'up to the day of the program'. In some contexts, smallpox teams had to navigate and challenge local deities like 'Son Pona – the smallpox God', local 'witchdoctors', and even an old woman following them shouting insults and dancing. Grant negotiated and translated local cultures for the CDC teams as he had already travelled extensively around Ghana with the medical field units – of which he was chief by 1968, in addition to being designated the national (and first Ghanaian) epidemiologist.[30]

It seems that Frank Grant may have imagined his medical mission like that of his father's evangelism. Grant's health work mimicked a Methodist practice of village-to-village evangelism, but with bio-medicine. This connection in health was not unusual and it was one that Grant maintained throughout his work; he combined an understanding of missional Christian theology with 'local beliefs' in order to build relations with a variety of stakeholders in the control of disease. As Newberry explained: 'We had many such conversations (about faith). His beliefs were strictly orthodox but he educated me on the tribal and local beliefs as well. He was the most respectful person that I knew. Frank intimated a persona that commanded respect, trust, likability and a great sense of humor. He was a sort of Ghanaian Abraham Lincoln … There was no hardship he wouldn't suffer for his people, or the poor or the sick'.[31] With Newberry, Grant held a prayer session each day before they began to work.[32]

Grant's professional identity seems to have been formed within a network of Ghanaian graduates who derived models of internationalism from older traditions of medical mission, especially that of Aggrey. Grant regularly created strong connections between the WHO, the CDC, Dutch medical officers, British finance, the government of Ghana, local communities, churches, and mission stations.[33] Grant's style evoked sacrifice, inculturation, accommodation, and faith, and it implicitly contested Nkrumah's reimagining of Aggrey in which missionary Christianity had been downplayed. This form of cross-cultural collaboration and deep involvement in international agencies was a particularly Ghanaian and internationalist vision of what it meant to be a medical missionary. A wave of Ghanaian school and college graduates, trained in foreign universities, who formed a new internationalist elite across the 50s into the 70s, were inspired by Aggrey's missionary internationalism.[34] Notable were the theologian C.G. Baeta and Kofi Busia, leader of the opposition to Nkrumah and prime minister from 1969 until a coup d'etat in January 1972. Both worked actively with international agencies such as the World Council of Churches in the 1960s.[35] Others in the same cohort, who attended a variety of elite colleges, include the Anglican and former secretary-general of the United Nations, Kofi Annan, who started out in WHO as a budget officer in 1962.[36] Mary Grant, Frank's wife, who became Ghana's third woman to qualify as a medical doctor in 1959, led delegations to international conferences, and was the deputy minister of health under Jerry Rawlings.[37] Pioneering Ghanaians like Frank Grant made sense of Africanisation and their place within health work and international diplomacy by building upon earlier imaginaries of development and Christian mission that Nkrumah had not been able to dismantle.[38]

For Grant and the smallpox/measles campaign, connecting with medical missions and an international Christian network was important because of the vital role they played in Ghanaian health care; they could communicate regarding epidemics, distribute health messages, and support MFU activities generally. The contacts with churches and medical missions which David Newberry recollects are backed up in United States government memorandums from the late 1960s. In these there is evidence that Newberry was the smallpox/measles operations officer liaising between Catholic and Protestant medical missions, USAID, the MFUs, and the Ghanaian Ministry of Health to help control a yellow fever epidemic in Northern Ghana.[39] Newberry concluded that 'we truly depended on the various Christian missionary groups and services to support us in both treatment of suspected cases and surveillance'.[40] Grant's role in these emerges too: there is record in the same memorandums of his surveying of yellow fever outbreaks and reporting back from remote areas.[41] Links between USAID, Grant, Foege (who worked in Ghana too), and Ghanaian medical officers were critical to sustain communication about epidemic outbreaks and coordinate effective responses.[42] Mission networks mattered to MFU medicine, and those like Grant and Newberry who could link with them benefitted hugely.

Communication with local communities had been a long-term problem for the MFUs. Sometimes local chiefs were helpful, and other times they actively hindered efforts. Some communities were amenable, but others wanted to dissuade and distract with disinformation. In the 1920s, in the first smallpox control efforts around Accra, Percy Selwyn-Clarke wrote that 'there were cases in which little or no reliance could be placed on the statements made by patients or their friends. Members of the Kroo tribe have a particularly unreliable memory and deliberate misstatements were frequently made in the hope that the health authorities would be led astray, in which case failure to trace the original sources of the disease would result, and the necessary action in the matter with regard to disinfection, isolation, and vaccination of contacts could not be taken'.[43]

By the 1950s, areas in the South had longer-term contact with health authorities and were probably less likely to lead them astray, but expanding immunisation beyond those well-connected areas was complex task. In 1975, Waddy explained in a discussion organised by the Royal Society of Hygiene and Tropical Medicine that, before modern freeze-dried techniques, the MFU practices in the 1940s and 1950s caused terrible ulcers in patients and it was difficult to control reactions: 'A point that has not been mentioned this evening is the acceptability of modern freeze dried vaccines, as compared with the older vaccines. When I was organizing mass vaccination in Ghana, in the 1940's and 1950's, the vaccines (and conceivably the technique) we were using did produce some very severe ulcers. People tended to run away rather than wait to be vaccinated, and one could not entirely blame them'.[44]

As Waddy recalled, word about the negative consequences of vaccination, and thus terror, spread more quickly than the teams could vaccinate. Furthermore, as O.A. Olumwallah and Melissa Graboyes have shown for medical work in East Africa, the legacies of repressive tax policies, military incursions, or broken promises by previous medics and scientists could damage relationships between communities and foreign bodies.[45] While Ghanaians were a part of the teams, the MFUs were not able to find intermediaries in every community and often the damaging side effects of the vaccines caused fear and fleeing.

By contrast, Newberry explains the success the MFUs had in the 1960s in using missions as intermediaries. Missions were often the only contact the communities had with white outsiders before the MFUs arrived: 'The children in these villages would run alongside of our vehicles – shouting ... Father, Father, Father!!! When I asked about this my MFU staff would tell me that the only white person they had seen before me was a Catholic Priest. There were many other protestant and Catholic missionaries operating in the remote interior. The Baptists had a couple of hospitals too'.[46]

Moreover, in a later interview Newberry described how some missionaries were particularly helpful because of their long-term relations with local communities, their knowledge of local customs, and their interest in health care:

> There was a priest in the north West of Ghana who was a White Father out of Canada who totally revolutionized the major tribe in that area ... He came into Ghana way back at the turn of the century by ship and a barge because there was no dock for ships. He trekked upcountry with natives carrying all his belongings. What an amazing person he was! He learned the language and later helped them develop a written language. He loved helping pregnant women who had no assistance other than traditional birth attendants who didn't even practice personal hygiene. So this priest built maternal hospitals and safe delivery facilities. Any time I visited him he would have me help building while we conducted business. I wanted to leave him a fridge so we could store vaccines with him. He pondered that simple request and after several days he turned us down because he said 'He might be tempted to use it for himself'! ... He was such a good man.[47]

Even if this priest was not comfortable even keeping a fridge for vaccines, missions were key points of contact for the MFUs, and connecting with them was indispensable in many areas.

Use of mission networks for international health was not unique to Ghana. In the work of Bill Foege in smallpox control in Eastern Nigeria, it was critical in creating some of the main strategies for effective 'firefighting'. Again, as with Grant, Foege's identifying with both international health organisations and mission made him the ideal intermediary. In his memoirs Foege writes of how he decided that preventative medicine through international organisations was a better option for him than becoming a medical missionary – though he was not fully sure, and instead moved between the two. He began working for the CDC, then became a Lutheran medical missionary before returning to the CDC in 1966 as a consultant for its smallpox operation in Eastern Nigeria. Foege's most famous innovation was the smallpox containment strategy which became the basis for worldwide control and eradication. He describes in his autobiography how, in the latter role, he continued to use missionaries in order to action his eradication plan. As WHO were aware, networks of missionary knowledge were as valuable for smallpox eradicators as networks of hospitals and clinics. There were regular meetings and correspondence in order to combine local, national, and international levels of the programmes. Through missionaries' knowledge of indigenous populations and their expertise in various aspects of health care, they shaped what was imaginable as well as practically possible for smallpox eradication teams. Foege's ability to connect to missionary groups was vital in this. He writes:

> We could use the missionaries' knowledge of market patterns and family patterns to make predictions about high-risk areas for spread, but first we needed to know where the virus was at the moment. Acquiring this type of intelligence would be difficult even in a country like the United States. It seemed absolutely impossible in rural Africa. However, the missionary community's own support system offered an answer. There were no telephones, so every night at 7 P.M., the missionaries turned on their shortwave radios and checked in to make sure that no one was in need of assistance ... missionaries up to some thirty or more miles distant, explained the situation, and, with maps in front of us, divided up the area. We asked each missionary to send runners to every village in his assigned area to ask if anyone had seen cases of smallpox ... [we] were given the precise information we needed ... based on the missionaries' knowledge of where the patients and their families usually travelled, we made some informed guesses regarding other places where the virus was most likely incubating ... In many ways the strategy that stopped the virus was a logical extension of the firefighting principle that I was taught back in the summers of 1956 and 1957.[48]

Missionaries provided the necessary communication capacity for Foege's 'firefighting principle' to actually work and worked closely with him to make it happen. It was missionaries who knew Nigerian travelling patterns and it was missionaries who made the 'informed guesses' about virus distribution. However, it must be noted that in other cases, religious attitudes to biomedicine could directly stop smallpox control, as happened for Foege with the Faith Tabernacle Church in Abakaliki, Nigeria. Some groups were extremely difficult to survey or immunise against smallpox. Medical missionaries' specific models of theology and biomedicine made them key contacts, whereas Pentecostal churches like Faith Tabernacle could sometimes create opposition.

For Foege and Grant, immunisation programmes represented a better version of historic medical mission, not a secular function of international health. International health campaigns have been variously represented in terms of human rights, scientific and technical solutions to problems, and unbiased aid work, as well in many other forms. However, the religious motivation for these campaigns has often been missed. For Foege, working for the CDC was not a rejection of medical missionary work but a proactive improvement on their models which expressed more fully the message of the Christian gospel. Foege originally left missionary work because of its lack of focus on preventative medicine and his concern that churches' 'medical work had become such a useful proselytising tool ... [to] attract people and ... leave them feeling indebted'. He wrote how he found in Dr Wolfgang Bulle, the secretary for the Lutheran Church-Missiouri Synod, an 'unexpected ally'. Bulle encouraged Foege to begin mission in Nigeria, and in 1967 he drew Foege into a conference of theologians and missionary medics at Conoor in India.[49] These conferences organised by the CMC were multiple and included many different missionaries, international health workers, and ministers from all over the world. For example, at the Protestant churches medical conference at Limuru in Kenya in 1970, Foege argued: 'Only when healing is seen as a responsibility of becoming a Christian, part of our redemptive function in the world which needs no other justification, do we possess the freedom to plan our medical work on the basis of the priorities of need rather than the priorities of a church board. When we as a church can see people who need food be assured in advance that not one will be converted and still feed them, we have understood our responsibility as a church'.

Foege was claiming that immunisation, preventative health, and community health care – models lauded in organisations such as the CDC – were actually expressing the 'redemptive function' of the church far better than missions were. He blamed the past lack of smallpox control on the ways in which health care had been directed at individuals and not communities. Measles, too, as for Grant, was tied to this vision for true salvific mission to communities and smallpox control: 'In West Africa 5 to 10 per cent of children die of measles. In some areas 20 per cent of hospital beds are involved in the care of children with measles and measles complications. In the past three years 18 million children have been vaccinated against measles

in West and Central Africa. Although we have not been able to eradicate measles on the budget allotted, we have substantially reduced
death and disease, and we have free hospital beds in the process'.[50]

But this, according to Foege, was only a starting point for a far
wider-reaching agenda in 'community medicine' which missions
needed to begin supporting. He argued that starting simply with
surveillance and 'such things as smallpox, measles, malnutrition and
the price of maize' would lead to missions and health workers being
able to 'obtain the pulse of the community'. Moreover, this would
mean that medical missions would be far more connected to the life
of the church. Foege argued that medical missions should be

> using the local congregation extensively. It has been said that
> community medicine is far too important to be entrusted to the
> medical profession. Our history of medical missions, unfortu-
> nately, bears this out. Even in countries with advanced medical
> care the majority of healing is done by non-professionals. If I am
> sick I may see a professional healer for ten minutes, but it is my
> wife, children, and friends who cover for me, cook my meals and
> provide the support needed while I am a consumer rather than a
> contributor. It may involved the congregation accepting responsi-
> bility in the village, both for their congregation and for others ...
> The congregation can be used in surveillance, as volunteers to
> provide advance publicity, as volunteers in the mechanics of
> assembling people, as a core group to learn and disseminate new
> health information.[51]

This concern built on Foege's success with smallpox and measles
control in which missions had been critical in surveillance. However,
he took it further and showed how this was linked to a greater concern for Christian service beyond the fold. Finally, using phrasing
from the end of Psalm 22 (the psalm which Jesus Christ quoted on
the cross and which Foege linked to future generations remembering
the Lord), Foege concluded that:

> Hospitals in some places may be a luxury which the church
> can afford but the local community cannot afford. It is your
> responsibility to find out. I have taken the risk of offending
> you, but I have taken this risk on behalf of a child who travels
> through life with his potential mental capacity not met because

his mother did not understand the need for protein nor the risk incurred by having another child the next year. I have taken the risk on behalf of the father and mother who lose their child from measles in the shadow of your hospital, I have taken this risk on behalf of children yet unborn.[52]

Foege in certain contexts performed his role within the CDC as that of the technical advisor committed to modernisation. Yet, in this context, he constructs the relationship between mission and development as being vital to expressing the fundamental truths of the gospel. By reassessing historic medical missions through the lens of international health models prevalent in the 1950s and 1960s, Foege challenged the theological foundations of those missions. He argued that their hospital focus neglected malnutrition and the high incidence of communicable diseases such as measles. In doing so, Foege critiqued missions' use of development for direct evangelism because it had come at the expense of communities' need for disease control.[53]

Throughout the smallpox and measles programme, the MFUs and the international health organisations still relied on the infrastructure of medical missions across Ghana. In 1967 the field investigation report that the Ministry of Health in Ghana sent the WHO about the latest smallpox outbreak shows how much missions were still relied on. The report was from the Bawku district, one of the most remote areas of Ghana bordering Burkina Faso and Togo in the northeastern corner. At the time it covered around 1,227 square miles of savanna and had a population of about 180,000. There were four local administrative councils and local authority was in the hands of village headmen and the canton chief. In a poor and isolated rural area, the Basel Mission Hospital in Bawku itself was a towering feature of biomedical, 'modern' life. In order to survey the health of the population the mission hospital was as much an asset as the local authorities. They picked up those who were dying of smallpox in the 1967 epidemic, such as one three-year-old unvaccinated boy whom De Sario records as having died on 8 June in Bawku Hospital. The hospital diagnosed him and his mother who, on the day of the boy's death, also contracted smallpox. In order to obtain information about the spread of the epidemic, the chief of the affected areas had brought it to the attention of the health inspector at Bawku through 'the Sanitary Headman'. However, for the health inspector to do anything he needed to travel, and so had to borrow 'the hospital ambulance, the only means of transport at his disposal' to visit report cases. Information from local headmen was augmented by the regional medical officer of health, who tele-grammed and cabled information to the senior medical officer of health in Accra. It was then De Sario with two US Public Health Service technical advisers who investigated and coordinated the con-trol efforts. Again, this required assistance from the Bawku mission hospital, where 'patients were admitted in the isolation ward ... and treated there'. Overall, there were 2,708 contacts of cases, but of lack of transport made staff surveillance 'impossible'. Local health staff and itinerant Rural Health Services had vaccinated 16,877 people at the point when De Sario arrived; these were surveyed in markets, in schools, and on roads. Vaccination of primary contacts was, De Sario concluded, the primary factor in 'abruptly terminating the spread'. As such, they also disinfected the hospital wards as well as local huts and compounds, but this did not seem to do much.[54] Crucially, the rapid first response was most significant in contain-ing the spread and that relied on help from local authorities, health inspectors, and the mission hospital, before international health offi-cials even arrived.

The very last cases and epidemics of smallpox in Ghana were in 1968. Its success in the mid-1960s had global consequences for smallpox eradication, and for Frank Grant. By 1968 and in contin-ued vaccinations into the 1970s, the layered coordination of MFUs, USAID, the CDC, the WHO, local authorities, the Ghanaian health ministry, and medical missions completed its eradication. When Grant wrote to the WHO Expert Committee in 1964 arguing that an eradication programme be implemented, he claimed that total cover-age could be finished within five years and 'satisfy all WHO require ments'. He was right. He noted that the seventy-five hospitals and forty-six health centres in the country were strategically located in different regions; this, combined with rapid development of roads, meant that a fairly speedy eradication process was possible.[55] In Ghana there were smallpox notifications of ninety-nine in 1959, 139 in 1960, seventy in 1961, and 135 in 1962. Up to this point, since 1951, over half a million vaccinations had been completed annually by the MFUs, but they had not managed to cover most regions. In the yaws campaign, UNICEF had provided vehicles for them to use, as well as having some bicycles and motorbikes. 1967 was the last year of smallpox endemicity in Ghana.[56] By 1968 there were still 144 cases of smallpox reported and in 1968 there were twenty-six (though the number was probably higher as epidemiological information on the 1968 outbreak was not available). However, from 1969 onwards there were zero smallpox cases reported to the senior medical officer of communicable diseases in Ghana. Vaccinations proceeded apace.

Nevertheless, the pattern up to at least 1971 was about a doubling of vaccination efforts from the previous fifteen years. By 1975 there were fifty-seven teams of MFUs working in a system of 110 hospitals, fifty-four urban health centres, and sixty-eight health posts.[57] In 1977, smallpox was declared eradicated in Ghana. The effectiveness of the smallpox campaign in Ghana also had wider consequences. According to Bhattacharya, the successes in Western Africa in the mid-1960s raised the profile of the fight against smallpox in US administrative circles. To make the campaign global it was then extended to India, Pakistan, and Bangladesh.[58] Frank Grant himself, now with personal WHO backing on the smallpox expert committee, travelled to India (as well as Afghanistan, Burma, and Nigeria) to continue the eradication efforts.[59]

Measles was also widely vaccinated and decreasing in incidence in the late 1960s. The campaign began fully in 1967 but then suffered setbacks in the 1970s. Large swaths of children in Ghana were vaccinated in the late 1960s and early 1970s; however, after 1971 the numbers of cases began rising again. During the smallpox/measles programme, between 1967 and 1970 there were 7.3 million smallpox inoculations and 2 million measles immunisations.[60] Between 1971 and 1973, 1,276,643 one-to-four year-olds were vaccinated against measles.

Measles was prevalent and not confined largely to the Upper Regions (as the MFU surveys had suggested) but were spread across Ghana.[61] While this may be because of better recording, another set of data from a different source corroborates some similar rises. The rise itself, rather than the overall numbers, may be more telling of an actual increase in incidence. In the first three months of 1974, 36,000 cases of measles were reported, which was 50 per cent more than the same period in 1972 and 10 per cent more than that in 1973. By 1975 measles cases had risen in contrast to only 275 and 313 acute polio cases in each respective year. Most of these were in children under five: 85 per cent of all cases, as shown by a study of 26,334 cases in the Greater Accra region from 1970 to 1972.[62] By 1977, the

Ghana Health Assessment Project placed malaria first in terms of disease burden and measles second. Between 1973 and 1982, Korle Bu recorded that 8.8 per cent of paediatric admissions were due to measles. Moreover, while measles was part of the Expanded Program of Immunization, in 1985 there was an epidemic with 64,557 cases. Measles was brought under some control, dropping back to 81,788 in 1979 and only 31,470 cases in 1981, returning to 79,184 cases in 1982.[63] In general, vaccination coverage was still low until 1993.[64] As the articles written by Ghanaian health workers at the time often showed, severe malnutrition and kwashiorkor occurred following these measles attacks.

Though smallpox was eradicated, Grant's attempt to tackle measles in Ghana by vaccination was not particularly successful long term. It is hard to know exactly why measles was not controlled given the effective programme tying it to smallpox eradication with the support of the CDC, USAID, and the WHO. Part of the problem was redeployment of MFU units to other emergencies such as the 1970–71 cholera outbreak, which broke up vaccine cycles. Unlike smallpox, which could be eradicated with the surveillance and containment strategy, measles needed high coverage with a fully potent vaccine. National educational campaigns also struggled because of lack of resources and staff. Another issue was probably the increasing realisation of the scale of the problem once surveys had been completed. It was found that measles was present continuously, rather than in separate cycles as in England.[65] Moreover, given that colonial surveys had not recognised how much measles there was, combined with local assumptions about the normality of its prevalence in early childhood, the battle against it was far harder than against yaws or smallpox, which had been widely known. Colonial neglect of the disease ensured that beginning the programme from scratch, even with the boost of placing it in tandem with smallpox eradication, was overly ambitious. This was likely a product of the extractive nature of the colonial state in the Northern Territories where measles was perhaps highest in the Upper Regions, as the MFUs had originally estimated. It was only when the nation-state fully incorporated the North into the development agenda and infrastructure that measles was given the place it desired. Geographies of neglect and extraction in colonial Gold Coast had long-term consequences for inequality and high measles incidence in postcolonial Ghana.[66]

Table 4.1 Smallpox vaccinations in Ghana between 1967 and 1974

Year	Smallpox vaccinations
1967	1,282,550
1968	1,984,308
1969	2,033,128
1970	1,916,342
1971	1,217,357
1972	647,613
1973	354,904
1974	1,037,130

Source: K. Ward-Brew, 'Ghana/Medical Officer at Present Responsible for Smallpox Eradication', World Health Organisation, SE/WP/75.12 (1975), 1–11, accessed in the WHO Institutional Repository for Information Sharing (IRIS).

In the Ghanaian medical culture of the yaws campaign, the neglected disease of measles, and internationally backed smallpox eradication, Ghanaian Christianity and Christian missions figured influentially – but not in ways that were discontinuous with the past. Ultimately, international health planning was one of the disappointments of a postcolonial development era that looked very much like the colonial development era; however, in this case continuity was also success. The 1960s were the high point for WHO and USAID health planning in Africa, when postcolonial African national contexts were seen as ideal for international development programmes through national government strategies. In Ghana there had already been health planning in the first development agenda inaugurated in 1951 under the colonial state and Nkrumah as the leader of government business. This had widened the scope and reach of MFUs that were ultimately responsible for SEP, and also ensured the growth of medical mission.

The second development plan in Ghana that began in 1959 ensured the further expansion of health care, particularly in the

Table 4.2 Data sets of measles cases and deaths in Ghana between 1970 and 1976

Year	1970	1971	1972	1973	1975	1976
Measles deaths (data set 1)	200	361	273			
Measles cases (data set 1)	45,843	94,567	95,529			
Measles deaths (data set 2)		338	273	290		
Measles cases (data set 2)		90,223	95,529	94,918		
Measles deaths (further data)					384	439
Measles cases (further data)					140,821	131,405

Sources: Set 1: J.M. Blankson and Y. Asirifi, 'Measles and Its problems as Seen in Ghana', Health Service Planning, *Ghana Medical Journal* (June 1974): 134–40; Set 2: Measles' *Weekly epidem. Rec./Relevé épidém. hebd.*, no. 45, 49th year (Geneva: World Health Organization, 8 November 1974), 376, accessed in the WHO Institutional Repository for Information Sharing (IRIS), based on *The Ghana Monthly Epidemiological Bulletin* (May 1974); Further Data: Annex II, 'Cases and Deaths of Selected Communicable Diseases in Ghana, 1972–1981' in 'Programme for Production of Vaccines in Africa: UC/RAF/83/088' (Ghana, 5–15 May 1984) 18/370/2GHA/R84, World Health Organization Archives (Geneva, Switzerland); William K. Bosu et al., 'Progress in the Control of Measles in Ghana, 1980–2000', *The Journal of Infectious Diseases* 187, no. 1 (2003): S44–S45.

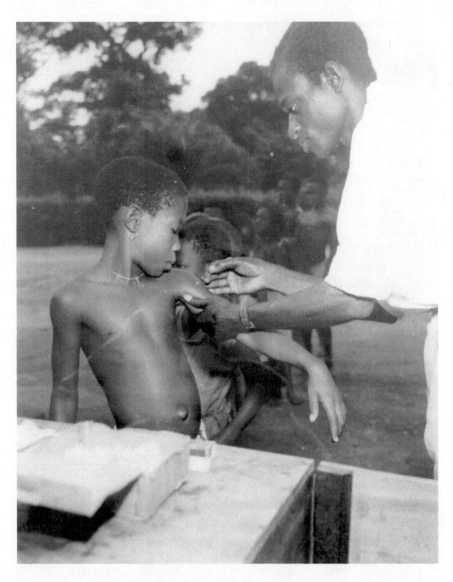

Figure 4.2 | 'Children are vaccinated against smallpox by the Mobile Medical Field Unit working in the Trans-Volta-Togoland Region' (19 October 1954).

South, with the North to be focused on with the MFUs. This was added to with the third development plan in 1963–64. Crucially, where there was increased immunisation and health coverage from WHO-USAID cooperation through national structures in Ghana, it benefitted from older colonial networks, identities and organisations such as the MFUs, and missions and missionary identities. Specifically with immunisation campaigns, medical missions were a key factor in the effectiveness of international health intervention. Ghanaian Christians and international health workers like Grant relied on their links to older medical missions to execute their agendas. At the same time, that colonial neglect of a disease such as measles had lingering ramifications for postcolonial attempts to understand and control it.

Finally, Grant's collaborations with USAID did not stop with measles and smallpox, but extended to elite medical education – a key American concern for influence within Ghana. In the provision of high-level medical education USAID sought to impose its own vision for development, and it used Christian Ghanaian doctors as key contacts. USAID wished to co-opt elite development and ensure its survival amidst the competing priorities of Nkrumah's Ghana. That way, they could influence possible fresh leadership away from Nkrumah. The complexities in these negotiations show further how Christianity and political and human development could mix in various ways. It also shows how, in spite of political turbulence, the US and Christian Ghanaians continued to find in each other helpful allies when the medical school was rebuilt after Nkrumah's downfall. Grant's Christian development vision, mimicking his father's Methodist evangelism and Aggrey's missionary internationalism, was distinct from USAID's narrative of modernization, but their outworking in health programmes and the medical school dovetailed well.[67]

Around 1960–61, the US began to offer funding for a medical school in Nkrumah's Ghana. According to Percy Selwyn-Clarke, a former medical officer, head of smallpox control, and founder of the Gold Branch of the Red Cross, by January 1962 the cost of a hospital attached to the medical school was estimated by the Americans to be around 7.5 million Ghana pounds, with annual recurrent costs of around 1 million Ghana pounds.[68] Long-term, homegrown, medically trained Ghanaians were a key ambition, retaining the talent in which the government had invested and displaying to the world black skins in the white coats of professional medical modernity. This was as much about national identity as practicality. Thus, as the plans proceeded apace and tensions rose, the medical school hit on the raw nerve of independent nationalist self-image and on American Cold War fears.

The medical school was part of the US plans to use development aid to 'influence' Ghanaian politics away from the Soviets. Already by 1960, Nkrumah's socialist leanings were a key concern for American foreign policy makers and diplomats.[69] In 1963, with Nkrumah putting pressure on his relations with the West, the US were still attempting to steer him back to the fold. In a US government report in 1960–61, it was stated at the outset that the 'immediate US objective should be to halt the dangerous drift of Ghana toward the Bloc'. In the $37 million Volta project in Ghana, the US aimed to 'use the increased leverage provided by the Volta project to establish a close working relationship, not only with Nkrumah, but also with his younger officials'.[70] For example, even anti-Western ministers learnt that it could be worth their while to help the US, as it could 'assist its friends in the Ghana Government, so that they are in an improved position to make their weight felt in high government and party circles'. In addition, the hope was to 'influence the next generation of leaders' by emulating the Bloc and seeking out 'potential leaders' in schools, 'cultivating them for the time when they may count'.[71]

The medical school was a key feature of this Cold War strategy, and by 1963 it became the focus of increasingly tense relations with Nkrumah and how to manage him.[72] In the same report in which Volta and strategy in Ghana were discussed, the medical school was explained fully – both its motivations and costs. As the author of the report explained: 'Because of Nkrumah's personal interest in the project it is important that the US carry out its commitment to assist Ghana in the establishment of a medical school'. Until 1963 relations ebbed and flowed between optimism, tension, concern, and outright hostility.[73] USAID even pushed out the Philadelphia group who wanted to contribute five times as much American personnel over twelve years which would cost $18.2 million in staffing alone.[74] According to one government letter to the ambassador from Oliver L. Troxels, charges d'affaires, the economic value was minimal and instead USAID was a useful political strategy to gain an 'American presence' in Ghana.[75] However, in October 1963, the president, John F. Kennedy, backed the medical school funding while also noting that 'this project also seems to me a particularly good example of why we should not make commitments before we know what they really involved'.[76]

However, between 1963 and 1966, the medical school project was terminated and Nkrumah's relationship with the US went from bad to horrendous. Nkrumah feared the CIA and decided that the medical school was a hive of their activity and was being used as a way of spying on him.[77] As a letter from G. Mennen Williams to the assistant secretary of the State Department put it in April 1963: 'We know that Nkrumah believes that the CIA had been actively plotting against him. Given his suspicious nature and tendency to react emotionally, he may conceivably regard Negro American employees of our Government in Ghana as actual or potential CIA agents'.[78]

While the medical school was formally instituted in 1964, its foreign personnel and support was cut off. Even before Nkrumah kicked them out, Oliver Troxels, now counselor of the embassy, wrote in October 1963 to Phillip Narten, officer in charge of Ghanaian affairs in Washington, that 'Ghana has evolved under Nkrumah toward an increasingly unpopular dictatorship of the far left, to the point where we are unlikely to be able to exert any significant constructive influence and where it would be contrary to our long-term interest to be identified with the regime. At minimum we would withdraw from projects marginal to our interest as quickly as possible'.

Within the next couple of years, the US would reduce aid to a bare minimum and rumours still abound as to the extent of their involvement in the coup against Nkrumah in 1966. General Ankrah, who took over the armed forces after Nkrumah, had been in contact with the FBI regularly in the previous year.[79]

After Nkrumah was ousted in 1966, USAID found alternative routes to helping establish the medical school, which built on the work of long-term contacts like Frank Grant and Fred Sai. When in June 1964 the US sponsorship of the medical school was withdrawn, Frank Grant and Fred Sai continued the effort with other notable Ghanaian medics such as Dr Easmon,[80] fulfilling, in a very different way, the dreams of Guggisberg and Aggrey. While Nkrumah's reputation had deteriorated, Grant, Sai, and other key medics were able to continue networking internationally, unhindered by ideological agendas. Quickly after Nkrumah had gone, the medical school was taken up again by USAID.[81] USAID restored its close relationship with the medical school and returned to being the point of contact for international staffing. In June 1969, the *Ghanaian Times* declared triumphantly that thirty-four doctors trained in the Ghana medical school had passed their exams.[82] As with measles and smallpox, the concerns of local Ghanaian doctors, especially Ghanaian Christian doctors, facilitated international health programmes in spite of problems and political blockages in national infrastructure.

RELIGIOUS NETWORKS DISTRIBUTING AID: 1960–83

It was not only Africanising Ghanaian doctors but also new streams of medical mission funding that were linking to and shaping international health. Building on chapter 3, the present section will show how Catholic medical mission became a key actor within this health landscape. In the context of the postwar expansion of Catholic internationalism and the incorporation of Catholicism into the American political mainstream in the early 1960s, USAID made strong links with Catholic medical mission networks in Ghana. It was not only in immunisation but also in food aid that USAID utilised missionary contacts. USAID funded Catholic and Protestant aid networks extensively to maintain and expand their role in Ghana amidst political turbulence.

From 1959 onwards the Catholic Relief Services (CRS) in Ghana had been conducting a food programme with USAID, derived from the 'food for peace' programme Public Law 480 (PL-480). The CRS was a US Catholic aid organisation which was founded in 1943 but reformulated from the 1950s in line with the growth of European Catholic groups such as Memisa and Misereor.[83] PL-480 in many cases was the sale of cheap food, mainly wheat, which resulted in the stockpiling of huge funds that the US government used in a variety of ways. For example, in India some of that money was given to anti-malaria work, green revolution work, and smallpox eradication because of the lack of WHO money.[84] As Nick Cullather has shown, Title I and III of food aid in Asia created a 'crucial source of investment in the industrial sector', up to $400 million a year in India, whereas in Africa it was given for emergency relief.[85] In Ghana, PL-480 provided food commodities distributed through the CRS. After 1980 the US also funded the government of Ghana to produce a PL-480 programme more similar to that in India, with attendant development work using the revenue. This later phase of PL-480 in Ghana added a supply of $12.7 million worth of wheat, corn, and rice, funded by a loan. Under the programme the US gave a loan which was used to buy food from the US, and any proceeds from the sale of those commodities was then put into a counterpart fund in Ghana that funded irrigation projects and the improvement of farm facilities. This amounted to around 85 million cedis, giving the US a 68 per cent share of this counterpart fund and a dominant role.[86]

Andrew Preston's *Sword of the Spirit, Shield of Faith* (2012) shows the significance of religion to American war and diplomacy, especially for the Cold War. Preston has built on Odd Arne Westad's thesis that the Cold War should be approached in a pluralist and internationalist way.[87] This is contrary to the restrictive frame of Anders Stephanson in which after 1963 there was not much of a Cold War to speak of.[88] By contrast, Preston argues in his contribution to these debates in *Uncertain Empire* (2015) that alongside Westad's many Cold Wars which emerged across the world, historians should also emphasise the greater importance of American religion. Preston writes that 'the ebb and flow of American religious conceptions does not explain the Cold War writ large; but it does help, in part, to explain one of its primary components, American behaviour and motivations'. The resurgence of faith between the 1950s and 1970s fused with the ideological and geopolitical pressures of the postwar world: 'In the Cold War ... politics became faith-based and faith became politically based'. Religious liberty, as it had been many times before in American history, returned to the 'heart of American foreign policy' when the Cold War reached its zenith in the late 1950s. However, this did recede in the mid-1960s with the Vietnam War, especially as those on the side of the West were recognised to be at least as brutal as communists in persecuting religious groups.[89]

As Preston also shows, from the early 1960s Catholics were incorporated (though still with some controversy) into the mainstream of American political culture, most apparently with JFK's election victory.[90] Andrew Rotter argues that American Cold War concerns in the late 1940s and 1950s 'mirrored' American Protestants' worries about secularisation, evil communists, and Catholics.[91] However, by the early 1960s this was changing, and with the shift came a greater recognition of the potential for American Catholic networks to benefit development aid and foreign policy priorities. As part of the greater inclusion of Catholicism in US political culture in the early 1960s, the CRS offered USAID a logistical solution based on global Catholic networks and imaginaries which had previously been held at arm's length.

For Ghana, partly as a result of the expansion of West German and Dutch Catholic aid, international Catholic medical mission networks were incorporated into USAID's imaginaries of development and state stabilisation. Through their links to worldwide Catholic mission, the CRS provided USAID with a logistical solution to creating state stability based on a national network of churches and mission clinics. Instead of giving aid directly to the Ghanaian government to prevent it from sliding into communism with all its attendant dangers, USAID could utilise Catholic networks with Title II. This was not restricted to the 1960s or only to Catholic charities, but more widely to NGOs; however, these would not have had the large networks that CRS had. Cullather shows that the Reagan administration actually channelled 'a larger share of food aid through Title II of P.L. 480 ... to Save the Children, CARE and Catholic Relief Services, rather than through Title III to recipient governments ... Title II did not generate a counterpart fund for capital projects as grants under titles I and III did'.[92] The global Catholic network that directly linked the CRS with Misereor and with Catholic medical mission in Ghana changed what was functionally and imaginatively possible for USAID development aid. CRS itself had reformulated in line with European Catholic organisational restructuring, such as through Misereor and the liberalisations of Vatican II in the mid-1960s (which did not include birth control, it is worth noting).[93] CRS was shaped by changes in global Catholicism and, because of shifts in American political culture, USAID could link to these networks.

There was famine and starvation in several areas in the late 1960s, and CRS and USAID combined to tackle this issue with food aid. As John Nott has shown, as a result of starvation in Arabie and Nankon in 1968, the government pleaded with the Christian Council of Ghana to provide relief. The year before, the Catholic Relief Services had struggled to supply Bolgatanga with food during a famine. Again, as Nott's thesis shows, under Kofi Busia between 1969 and 1971 the food deficit increased; between 1963 and 1971 there had been a 38 per cent loss of food imports and the total output of staple crops had decreased massively. The World Bank showed in the Berg Report how between 1969 and 1979 the total production of food and nonfood fell. As Nott argues, malnutrition became an epidemic in the South where access was based on status in relation to the cash economy, and hunger returned viciously to the North, which had been systematically detached from the extractive colonial economy in which the area functioned mostly as a labour reservoir. Political instability, corruption, and environmental issues were exacerbated by long-term 'structural declines in nutrition security' relating to crop transition, the loss of precolonial social securities, and the market dependency of the poor.[94] As the previous section has shown, measles can be added to this cocktail of malnutrition and related diseases. As the state decreased its capacity to provide services across the 1970s, the CRS saw increased attendance at its welfare clinics in tandem with nutrient provision.

The food commodities provided by PL-480 came from the US Agricultural Trade Development and Assistance Act and were way of dealing with US food surplus as well as bolstering America's international agendas. With the CRS, which were monitoring the nutritional status of Ghanaian children (for example, mapping a decline in nutritional status at their child welfare clinics in the early 1980s), USAID had a ready and analytical network for distributing aid in a context of severe deprivation.[95] All this was used to shape Ghanaian society; for example, under Nkrumah they had withdrawn the aid. Title I was seen as an effective means of shaping political change within Ghana. In one USAID report from 1979 on Title I PL-480 they described how 'one of the quickest and most appropriate ways to assist the GCG (Ghanaian Government) in implementing difficult policy changes of the stabilisation plan is through P. L. 480 Title I. USAID's endorsement had been withheld for Title I programs in the recent past because it would have supported the government's country developmental politicals. Now that the new Ghana government is committed to establishing a more development-oriented policy framework, U.S. objections have been withdrawn and a sizeable initial P. L. 480 has been approved'.[96]

Through the CRS and then the government of Ghana, USAID could influence the government when they wanted to. As with the medical school, but here through the CRS, PL-480 was envisioned as a way of manipulating governments and stabilising regimes, while also dealing with excess food stocks within the US. As the report on Title I explained, stabilisation through PL-480 would be successful by attacking inflation from the supply side 'in support of tough demand management', and by increasing the supply of consumer goods in order to reduce social strain.[97]

Aid to the CRS could also be a way of bypassing the government when it did not act in accordance with USAID direction. The overall effect of PL-480 across the 1970s was to help the 'most nutritionally vulnerable groups', who were pregnant and lactating women and children under five years old. As well as CRS and WFP, USAID aimed to complement MIDAS and DRUHS work.[98] By 1971, USAID were proposing giving a $20 million dollar loan to the Ghanaian government for economic development.[99] The next year, in 1972, the US Department of State suspended approval of aid programmes on account of the new regime that seized power in Ghana, abrogating existing debt arrangements.[100] That same year USAID gave $1,039,000 to CRS and $238,000 to the Church World Service for food programmes and maternal and child health. They were spreading their funding carefully and strategically depending on responsiveness to their agendas. In 1973 and 1974 respectively the Church World Service received $203,000, and the CRS funding was raised to $1,554,000 and then $1,543,000.[101] By the beginning of the 1980s, PL-480, the food and material aid programme, was giving between $15 and $20 million annually to Ghana. When relations with government were problematic, USAID took away funding; yet, through Christian medical and aid missions, they continued to impose their agenda on the country by sustaining funding.

Up to 1980, unlike in India, the main PL-480 programme had directly distributed food commodities free of charge through the CRS, using all denominations of missionary networks (Catholic, Protestant, and Pentecostal), and government help. One of the consequences of Vatican II was more ecumenical work under Pope John XXIII's encouragement.[102] In Ghana the CRS was notable in using Catholic mission networks, and evangelical and Pentecostal churches. CRS also worked with the government of Ghana's agencies but only for help with transport and the ports, and this proved to be problematic with great losses of food in the ports. By 1983, the CRS in Ghana directly managed a network of twenty-four hospitals, fifteen stationary clinics, ten mobile clinics, two orthopaedic centres, two Primary Health Care projects, and two family health-care projects. This totalled around 400,000 in patients and 2.5 million outpatients annually.[103] In 1965, the US began supporting this food aid work, giving around a million dollars in support. In 1966 after Nkrumah fell this rocketed to around $7 million dollars, then reaching $14 million by 1968 and peaking at around $19 million dollars in 1968 – it would not be higher than this again until the mid-1980s. In 1977 alone the amount had reached 9,857 metric tonnes of food, worth about $3.9 million, distributed to 202,000 recipients. In 1978 aid rose again to $4.7 million worth of food to around 220,000 people. Through their cross-country network of maternal and child health clinics, preschools, and food-for-work programmes, they were managing to get food from ports to over 400 feeding points. Added to all this was around $3 million of commodity losses, which amounted to around 38.6 per cent of the programme.[104]

By the end of the 1970s, USAID was effectively using the CRS to distribute huge amounts of 'emergency' food relief, but this was not without its problems. According to a USAID report, the Catholic Relief Services PL-480 Title II programme in Ghana was directed toward 'maternal and child health, pre school feeding, food for work and school feeding'. These activities were 'designed and managed by Catholic Relief Services' but 'implemented in the field by many organizations including Missionaries and Government of Ghana agencies'. The CRS monitored the feeding programme, the government of Ghana arranged port handling and transfer from the port, and USAID managed the process and donated the food. The CRS also sold the food packaging, for $43,800 in 1977, in order to produce funds for supporting distribution. During 1977 overall, USAID reported that the US government had delivered 19,386 tonnes of food to the Catholic Relief Services 'for distribution throughout Ghana'. This was duty free and exempt from taxation; moreover, the government of Ghana paid for the transportation. In the same report, USAID were increasingly angry at the CRS because of $3 million in missing food commodities. In 1977, around 20 per cent of the food shipped to Ghana was lost – 3,908 tonnes valued at $1,589,400 in the port and port shortage. In light of these huge losses, USAID heavily criticised the CRS for 'very poorly managed' food distribution. USAID proposed to charge them for any of the commodities not reclaimed and to terminate the programme unless there was significant change.[105] Without insurance CRS had to bear the losses.[106] In another smaller-scale case, USAID found that CRS food was being sold in Achimota markets and so supplies to Achimota chaplaincy were immediately suspended.[107] In another case, food distributed at the Catholic mission at Walewale was deemed not fit for human consumption, and similar issues were found at the Assemblies of God missions at Nasia and Tanga in 1980.[108] Finally, without any explanation, the 1985 Primary Health Care report from St Anthony's Mission Hospital in Dzodze noted that the CRS food distribution stopped due to 'the misbehaviour of the mothers'.[109]

The CRS did benefit from its mission network in improving management and capacity, but the scale of need dogged the organisation. The issue with losses and stealing was not permanent, and the CRS managed to improve commodity accountability after an audit, as well as pursuing loss claims against the government of Ghana for loss at the ports (though USAID pointed out that this did not absolve the CRS).[110] In 1979 USAID gave $4 million worth of food commodities to the CRS, reaching 250,000 people, again through maternal and child health, school feeding, and food-for-work programs.[111] However, general lack of administrative capacity meant that the CRS could not supply 'nutritionally vulnerable groups' with significant short-term aid.[112] This was not restricted to the North; in 1979 the CRS director wrote to USAID to explain that the issues with food distribution in Bolgatanga were actually more widespread: 'The problem at Bolgatanga Assemblies of God Mission is country-wide in our program. Due to source of limitation on our School Feeding category, we programmed this centre for 400 recipients, but unfortunately 1500 recipients are being supported with the Title II food'.

This statement again emphasises that the CRS used Pentecostal (such as mentioned at Nasia) missions as well as Catholic ones to provide food. The mission network was not the issue, the problem was lack of CRS management itself: it was actually from the mission network that the CRS were building itself management. For example, in the same letter, the director explained that the Rev. Father John at Tamale Catholic Mission had just assumed responsibilities over Catholic activities.[113]

After 1979 USAID also began a further PL-480 programme with the national government and exerted pressure through loans instead. Between 1979 and 1980 USAID began a different PL-480 model funded through the government, supplying loans for food amounting to $12.7 million dollars and creating a stockpile which financed irrigation and farming projects.[114] This was separate from the CRS Title I programme because of the 'sensitivity of the whole subject' – perhaps relating to what the CRS saw as government failure in their losses in the late 1970s. In 1979, PL-480 was classed by US officials as at the 'top of the list in per annum dollar of resource transfer'. In that year Title I had transferred $10 million, and Title II had transferred $4.5 million to the CRS and $0.8 million to the World Food Programme.[115] Title I, however, was in food aid, not in 'sales by the United States of food grains to Ghana on a concessional basis'.[116] In addition to this were further shipments of food labelled as Title III which directly aimed to influence Ghanaian government policy in coordination with the IMF. As one USAID report put it, Title III could be used to 'encourage governments to undertake new policy or reform programs not previously agreed to or instituted. Such new reform should flow from the analysis of the CDSS, the country's development plans and our overall A.I.D. strategy of equitable growth'.[117]

In very direct ways Title III was a tool for encouraging Ghanaian policy in the direction of AID priorities. Specifically, Title III (and Title I) aimed to generate the use of 'local currency' and develop 'self-help measures', as well as to improve 'nutritional gaps' and the 'basic food deficit'.[118] Beyond improving self-reliance and the availability of food, Title III aimed to stabilise prices 'while maintain[ing] an incentive to agriculture'. Partly this was based on timing. Title III delivered food at the beginning of the lean season, in order to lower prices for the rural poor and simultaneously incentivise agriculture by providing a grain security scheme.[119] Overall, after the 1980s these targeted development schemes, from PL-480 revenues, were more in line with those conducted in India: they provided for farming and irrigation projects. They were manipulating supply and demand and attempting to construct the ideal liberal Ghanaian citizenry that would help themselves.

Yet, given the heterogeneity of medical mission in Ghana, aid organisations did not only need to use the CRS or Catholic mission, they also could use the Salvation Army, expanding their medical mission work. The World Food Programme and Swiss and Canadian aid work supplied Ghana with milk powder, farming projects, and vitamin tablets through the Salvation Army rather than through the CRS in the late 1970s through into the 1980s.[120] In previous food aid, nurses at the clinics who distributed food around Begoro also 'instructed the women on how best to use it'.[121] The Salvation Army also gained food and medicine from the Christian World Service (USA) and Oxfam in the 1960s, and World Vision International (USA) in 1970.[122] However, in the late 1970s this grew massively with CIDA (Canadian International Development Agency) funding. In 1983, 30 tonnes of milk powder was flown in by the Canadian Air Force, in addition to TEARfund providing a lorry for distribution. Moreover, the US and Dutch Salvation Army provided milk, water, penicillin, and high-protein biscuits. In more sustainable ways, CIDA also provided funding for a young farmers project to improve nutrition and stop slash-and-burn methods. In the next year, the Salvation Army received more than 300 tonnes of food, including 200 tonnes of corn from the World Food Programme, 20 tonnes of tinned fish from CIDA, 3 tonnes of milk powder from Switzerland, 25 tonnes of dried fish powder from Norway, and two container loads of food from the Netherlands. This was not directly to bypass the CRS, as the CRS and the Christian Council also supplied the Salvation Army. Yet, it does show that given the heterogeneity of mission, aid organisations could pick and choose where they supplied food aid and through which denominations they did it. In 1983 alone there were 2,455 deliveries registered at Salvation Army clinics and 389,026 outpatient treatments – large numbers because 'food encourages attendances for antenatal and postnatal care'. The Salvation Army, with SIMAVI of the Netherlands, also helped to build a nutrition centre at Wiamoase clinic. By the end of 1984 the Salvation Army had treated 450,000 outpatients, and their role in distributing food aid had allowed their medical mission work to expand.[123]

It was not only through missions, but also from missions, that food aid was being donated. In 1983 the Danish church gave $146,975 in food relief, and the Seventh-day Adventists fed 1,000 people and gave medicine costing $107,000. World Vision International, the Christian aid organisation, supplied $235,000 worth of relief supplies. The Holy See also gave $10,000. In this, missions and churches were linking into a wider international effort, with Sweden giving $1,035,879 in food and relief, and UNICEF donating 227 tonnes of medicine ($177,247) as well as food items, totalling $1,012,300. As usual, West Germany and the Netherlands gave large amounts: the Germans donated $819,234 in food and relief and the Dutch provided the highest total amount of all organisations and nations with separate donations of $2,036,586 and $2,036,386. There

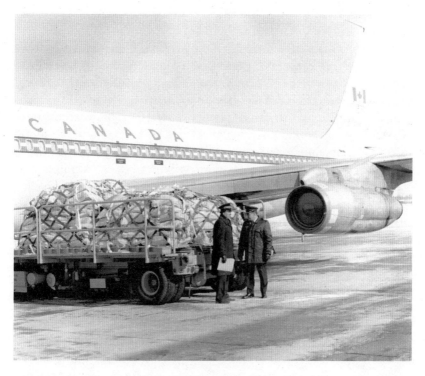

Figure 4.3 | 'Major Mel Bond Asst. Public Relations Officer and Canadian Forces Officer re: Milk Powder Shipment to Ghana'.

was a spread of other nations also donating, with the third-highest being Italy who donated $3,757,500. This was vital because even the £100,000,000 loan the government had obtained from a commercial bank and the $40,000,000 requested from the World Bank for a general import credit was still recorded as not having been enough to deal with the ensuing crisis. The extent of the need was unsurprising given that estimates at the time were of around 900,000 to 1.2 million people, mainly young men, entering the country and increasing the population by around 10 per cent.[124] In this context missions were only one element in a patchwork international response to the chaos.

Outside of the crisis, nutrition generally worsened through the late 1970s and early 1980s, continuing to decline even after structural adjustment and this period of intense foreign aid. As so often is the case, the targeted emergency response to the famine was discontinued once 'normal' circumstances had resumed. Though PL-480 food aid generally did increase across the 1980s. According to records kept by CHAG, between '1975 and 1979 39% of children aged 12–23 months suffered from acute malnutrition, i.e. weight for age roughly less than 77% of the standard (WHO). This percentage is higher now due to the drought, bush fires and worsening economy. In 1980 the average index of food production per capita stood at 74 in comparison 100 in 1969–71. The daily per capita calorie intake was 88% of the requirements (FAO)'.[125]

As Nott shows, nutritional status declined across Ghana in the late 1970s and early 1980s, and in rural Asante kwashiokor was a major concern. After Flight Lieutenant Jerry Rawlings's first revolution in 1979, markets declined and went into almost complete collapse on the eve of structural adjustment in 1983; this was dangerous especially for those who relied upon bought food. Up to 1983 political instability combined with food insecurity to produce 'epidemic malnutrition'.[126] After 1983, malnutrition endured and inequality grew, though the CRS did detect a return to the 1980 level by 1986. Generally, however, there was still malnutrition, with 64 per cent of children underweight in the North and 48 per cent in the South. Food aid could not keep up with the social effects of neoliberal reforms, however much they improved macroeconomic growth. As with measles, malnutrition remained divided along North-South lines, and again limited what foreign intervention could do. There was certainly some impact but again generally the colonial geographies of neglect and extraction continued to determine the shape and depth of malnutrition and famine in 1980s.

A USAID report in 1996 concluded that, between 1965 and 1994, Ghana received $340 million in food aid from the United States, over 50 per cent of the food aid total across this period. It was the sixth-largest recipient of PL-480 and the second-largest of countries receiving PL-480 who were not at war. However, US aid still only accounted for 0.5 per cent of the total food consumption in Ghana. Surveys in 1993–94 showed that wasting, severe food deprivation was found in 10 per cent of Ghanaian children – notably high compared with other sub-Saharan African countries. In addition, 31 per cent of children were classed as 'stunted' – low height for their age. Malnutrition was again notable in the North and 'forest zones'. In spite of improved economic growth between the 1980s and 1990s, agricultural rates did not match population growth, which led to reduction in per capita food production. Nationally, under-fives' mortality was at 131 per 1,000 live births, worse than it had been in the 1930s.[127]

CONCLUSION

As Warwick Anderson has argued, a 'postcolonial approach' to health histories means recognising how 'modern science and bio-medicine are put together, assembled, on the terrain that various sorts of colonialism have worked over'. Anderson contends that 'biomedicine is constitutively colonial: that it derives from colonial practices, becomes a means of managing the colonial aftermath, and functions always in a multiply contested contact zone'.[128] The history of international health in Ghana shows how complex, constructed, and contingent networks negotiated and exchanged within specific contexts. This chapter has shown that long-term colonial geographies of extraction and neglect, and colonial structures of medical mission, were key factors in shaping what international health and development aid could do in postcolonial Ghana.

This chapter nuances the arguments of Stephen Feierman (et al.) and Vihn-Kim Nguyen on the restrictions that are perceived within global health.[129] Feierman argues that power imbalances have led to blockages in global health; however, in the case of medical missions and Christian medicine in Ghana, Africans have been able to circumvent programmes supposedly created in the Global North for their own concerns and priorities. This also nuances Nguyen's arguments about the denial of sovereignty to Africans resulting from the power of 'therapeutic citizenship' in global health regimes. By contrast, as has been shown through the history of medical mission and Christian medicine in Ghana, African actors could be a part of creating global health regimes as well as being subject to them. By managing, empowering, or limiting medical mission and Christian medicine, local actors have effectively manipulated global health programs and refocused them on local priorities since the late 1950s.

It was not only in the Ghana Smallpox Eradication and Measles Control Programme that mission and Christian connections were central to the strategies of US medical aid in Ghana. The effect of missions on USAID was, however, divergent between programmes and particularly between organisations. While Frank Grant used international health priorities to conduct measles vaccinations, which he considered to be the main priority (given Ghana's colonial health legacies), the CRS opened up a global Catholic network and imaginary which shaped the way in which USAID used PL-480. For Grant, this work was related to long-term identities linked to Africanisation, evangelism, and structural inequality. For USAID with its Cold War concerns, influencing and shaping an incredibly turbulent Ghanaian politics required navigating various missionaries and Christian Ghanaian and Christian aid organisations, especially when the national government was hostile. Success in these protracted non-governmental relations with Christian groups enabled USAID to have a complex set of tools and levers for managing the Ghanaian state and Ghanaian health care. The Salvation Army was also a key actor in this landscape, acting as a hub for large-scale foreign aid in the famines of the early 1980s. Catholic mission may have dominated but it was certainly not the only feature of Ghana's landscape of medical mission which international health organisations could utilise.

Within a larger shift in American political culture toward the incorporation of Catholicism in the early 1960s, global Catholic networks became a more significant actor within US development work. As Misereor and Memisa helped to expand Catholic medical mission across Ghana, through the CRS USAID linked into this network and used it for their programmes. While the postwar growth of Catholic medical mission was driven by West German and Dutch development narratives of restoration and claims to humanitarianism and suffering, it also figured in Cold War conflict through connections to the CRS and USAID. It certainly was not determined by these motivations, but it was not entirely detached from them either. Moreover, as the emerging international health community evolved from the late 1960s, the Catholic medical mission network was reconstructed and utilised for even more imaginaries of development in Ghana. Overall, while there were different development narratives and agendas in play within the health landscape in Ghana, shared aims allowed for connections and collaborations.

Shared responses to the emergence of international health organisations was part of a process in which Protestant and Catholic medical missionaries in Ghana (Ghanaians, Europeans, and Americans) began moving into closer coordination in the late 1960s. Adrian Hastings argued that there emerged in the late 1950s a modern leadership of Presbyterian and Methodist African elites, particularly in Ghana. This was a group 'deeply committed to their Protestantism, nationalist through and through yet very moderately so in expression, mildly anxious to reassert the values of traditional religion and culture'.[130] In the context of health care, Presbyterian and Methodist Ghanaian leadership developed in the 1960s with key individuals such as Frank Grant, Mary Grant, Fred Sai, Felix Konotey-Ahulu, Michael Baddoo, and many others. Their Africanisation had a specific tone and conceptual tradition that can be traced back to the creation of development in the 1920s and 1930s. As for Catholic health providers, though the Africanisation of institutional hierarchies remained limited by expatriate control in the 1970s, there were ecumenical shifts, work within international health organisations, membership in the Christian Health Association of Ghana (CHAG), and shared adherence to the Primary Health Care movement, which brought about new relationships amidst decolonisation.

5

Primary Health Care, Global Health, and Medical Mission: Ghana, the WHO, and the World Council of Churches, 1960–2000

A narrative of 'development' and subsequent 'disappointment' has marked the history of postcolonial Africa.[1] This narrative captures the hope and triumphalism of the early years after independence, which gave way to the corruption and poverty of the 1970s and 1980s, and was followed by structural adjustment and neoliberal reform. The history of international health has been structured by this kind of trajectory as well. Ruth Prince describes the 1970s as the period when 'modernization faltered and the vision of public health pursued by the developmentalist state was downscaled'; then the 1980s witnessed 'a decisive shift away from developmentalist African states as aggressive neoliberal policies pushed by Western donors promoted privatization of health services and a dominant model of voluntary provision by humanitarian NGOs'.[2] From the 1970s, Prince argues that interventions focused on emergencies and African states retreated from the 'health for all' goals pursued with the WHO in the 1960s and 1970s, and the Primary Health Care (PHC) goals of the Alma-Ata declaration in 1978 were 'short-lived'. Kelley Lee ties the setbacks for PHC to neoliberalism and the power of the World Bank, which imposed 'greater restrictions on public health spending'. Moreover, she argues that PHC was 'out of step' with the priorities of major donors such as the US who wanted to return to a focus on major diseases such as tuberculosis.[3] Marcos Cueto has further shown how PHC was left behind for the less 'broad and idealistic' selective Primary Health Care (SPHC), with the Rockefeller Foundation identifying more 'cost-effective health strategies' as early as the Bellagio Conference in 1979. This was backed by UNICEF under the leadership of James Grant from 1980.[4]

This chapter will challenge this periodisation and show how medical missions, especially Catholic medical missions, both figured within, continued, and expanded PHC reforms into the 1990s. Vital to understanding medical mission is comprehending how their operation within national contexts was at variance or in conjunction with their international role, and how these matched up in different ways at different times. In the 1970s, medical missionaries were taking up PHC before it was adopted by the WHO, and missions had a role in driving its uptake around the world. By the mid-1970s, PHC was a key part of both Catholic and Protestant missions' work in Ghana. Missions continued their national and international work in PHC detached from international transformations. This was made possible because, on the ground, they were able to weather the storms of neoliberalism and Ghana's decline.

The relationship between mission and development was reconstructed in the 1960s and 1970s by Christians in international health offering new models for performing older missionary ideals. Long-term medical missionary visions of human development were reformulated and critiqued through the CMC and PHC. These offered an alternative to older forms of medical missionary practice, such as hospital construction as described in chapter 1. In doing so they re-expressed the historic relationship between mission and development as being based on flawed conceptions of theology, community, and health care. For both Christian international health workers and missionaries, PHC reconstructed the relationship between mission and development.[5]

The final section of this chapter will show how Catholic medical missions expanded PHC because they were prevalent, they were interested locally in this kind of work, they had continued funding in spite of economic problems in Ghana, and because Misereor supported (and partly financed) the CMC. Furthermore, Catholics in Ghana had an unusually strong relationship with the CMC and with health-care ecumenism. In spite of retrenchment in international health in the 1980s, the transition to PHC within medical mission development work continued beyond Alma-Ata into the mid-1980s at least. WHO continued to link to CMC and medical mission PHC activities through the 1980s. Medical mission provided another forum in which the WHO director-general, Halfdan Mahler, could continue his campaign for a holistic PHC. This was all in the face of the prevailing winds of retreat to SPHC from the original

PHC programme: member states immediately challenged PHC after Alma-Ata, donor agencies backed the technical solution-focused 1979 Bellagio Conference, UNICEF supported SPHC by the mid-1980s, and Mahler lost the support of the WHO bureaucracy.[6] Nevertheless, with the CMC and missionaries, Mahler's vision of the original PHC continued to be promoted in contexts such as Ghana. Showing this complex reality offers the chance to challenge the periodisation of international and global health, further reorienting the history of these concepts away from the presumed centres of their power.

RESILIENT MISSION: MAKING HEALTH AMIDST SCARCITY AND COLLAPSE

Between 1979 and 1983 more than half of Ghana's doctors left the country.[7] As one UNICEF report shows, 8.5 per cent of nurses left in 1982 alone.[8] Between 1960 and 1975 physicians in Ghana had increased from 383 to 1,031, nurses from 1,554 to 6153, midwives from 130 to 4,932, and hospital beds from 5,787 to 12,973. Later in the 1970s many of these trends were quickly reversed. Already by 1975, per capita Ministry of Health spending had fallen from 5.8 cedis per capita in 1974–75 to 4.13 in 1975–76 and 3.27 in 1976–77 (this was against an average of 3.2 per cent population growth annually from 1970).[9] In 1988 the Ministry of Health developed a report on the problems in the health system in Ghana for the National Health Symposium. It opened with an explanation of the disaster of the years between 1979 and 1983, when Ghana began structural adjustment under the military leadership of Flight Lieutenant Jerry Rawlings. The picture was damning. The report described how the extended economic decline in advance of the Economic Recovery Programme 'had a heavy toll on most sectors of national endeavour, but few suffered as much as the health sector ... drug supplies all but dried up; communications between different levels of the health system virtually broke down; and almost no funds were available for essential maintenance of equipment and buildings'.[10]

Moreover, the report argued that the damage was long-lasting, as morale suffered and middle management struggled to implement reforms.[11] As GNP spiralled downwards, declining every year save one between 1972 and 1984, Ghana's health care collapsed and food self-sufficiency plummeted. Between 1975 and 1980, the government only allocated around 3 per cent of its total budget (this compared to 25.5 per cent for agriculture, 21.6 per cent for transport and communication, and 12.6 per cent for education).[12] Real monthly earnings also fell rapidly. In 1983, 2 million Ghanaians returned from Nigeria, adding to the pressure on food stocks from droughts, bush fires, and low production. As the PNDC secretary for finance and economic planning put it in 1985, 'the economic difficulties of the late seventies and early eighties have had serious consequences for the living standards of many Ghanaians, especially on their health and nutrition state ... The sacrifices involved have been in many cases, crushing'.[13]

Using World Bank sources, the UNICEF report showed how for health care the expenditure per capita dropped from 84.9 in 1978–79 to 47.2 in 1979–80, then further to 35.8 in 1980–81 and 22.6 in 1982. Education expenditure followed a similar pattern. Foreign exchange restrictions hindered the import of new equipment in hospitals and clinics. The supply of drugs, bandages, needles, and other health-care basics dried up, in some rural cases being entirely absent for months. Moreover, even before this in 1977–78, only around 30 per cent of the population had access to formal health care. At Korle Bu Hospital in Accra, in 1979 they had an outpatient attendance of 198,000; in 1983 it was 117,000.[14]

The anthropologist James Ferguson has argued that the state's reduction by neoliberal reforms both exacerbated the current political crisis and continued a long history of exploitative colonialism. Following the work of Christopher Clapham, Ferguson argues that aid work actively sucked the life out of governments by offering better salaries and conditions, leaving the state 'hollowed out'.[15] Moreover, the 'privatization plan' was conducted by state officials in their own idiosyncratic ways, leading to the 'criminalization of the state' that Jean-Francois Bayart, Stephen Ellis, and Beatrice Hibou describe.[16] Thus, in this picture, international health organisations were active participants in exploitation and in creating 'separately administered enclaves' connected transnationally and in a point-to-point style. These were formed of oil companies and 'humanitarian hinterlands' – in a sense, both alike in structure. Looking back to the resource extraction methods of King Leopold's Congo, Ferguson argues that this is an advanced form of globalisation and that post-independence Africa's development triumphalism was a short-term blip. Instead, local politics, combined with the international flows of resources, reign supreme. Chiefs, priests, imams, and community leaders acted as gatekeepers to foreigners – which, as Bayart and Ellis have shown, they have been doing for centuries.[17]

In the late 1970s Ghana was forced to abandon a democratic national government infrastructure, and, because of the long-term makeup of the Ghanaian state, the 'humanitarian hinterlands' of medical mission were almost all that was left.[18] Medical missions sustained their care under the emergency rule of a disintegrating Ghanaian state in the late 1970s and early 1980s. There were times when missions offered the only real access to biomedical health care that Ghanaians had. As was the case across the country, missions still lacked resources and had to beg, borrow, and steal to ensure the continued running of their hospitals. However, unlike many other aspects of the health infrastructure, they maintained their staff and external funding streams. As the mid-1980s UNICEF report *Adjustment with a Human Face* showed, in many areas mission hospitals were the only ones still running. Instead of the voluntary sector underpinning or enabling nationalist health services, they had become its only surviving feature: 'The situation in mission hospitals was much better because medical equipment was functioning more efficiently, drugs and medical supplies were more adequate, and the loss in health manpower was less'.[19]

Whereas overall attendances in Ghana almost halved from 7,613,624 in 1979 to 4,468,482 in 1984, the Catholic Hospital at Duayaw-Nkwanta increased attendance in the same period: 40,000 in 1979 up to 49,000 in 1983. Moreover, UNICEF's statistics on malnutrition in under-fives between 1980 and 1984 came from the Catholic Relief Services survey. While Ghana's state and private health care was being wiped out, medical mission was surviving.[20] To nuance Ferguson's model, in Ghana there was not a shift in the relation between humanitarianism and state development back to a pre-1960s, pre-blip form. As the conclusion of this book will emphasise further, the interrelation of religion, health, and development was a continual feature of the Ghanaian state across the twentieth century.

The answer to why and how medical missions could be growing when health infrastructure in Ghana was collapsing all around can be found by looking at the role of continued foreign aid, the stability of mission staff, and the pattern of mission hospitals established in the 1950s and 1960s. As shown in chapters 3 and 4, medical missions were continually funded and supported by US, Dutch, and German aid into the 1980s, so when crises hit, they had support.

While the drug drought hamstrung most hospitals in Ghana, the Christian Health Association of Ghana (CHAG) and other medical mission institutions were able to find foreign sources of drug supplies. CHAG brokered a deal with a Ghanaian state-owned pharmaceutical company to produce drugs for 'church-related hospital and clinics in Ghana from raw materials made available by the Netherlands Government'.[21] In 1983, funded by the Dutch government, GIHOC produced 40 million aspirin tablets, 50 million vitamin B-complex tablets, 5 million anti-TB tablets (paediatric and adult), amongst millions of others drugs. The total cost of materials was 1.2 million cedis; this was at a time when the exchange rate was 2.75 cedis to the dollar, but the exchange rate later fell to 51 cedis to the dollar, making local production very cheap.[22] As Patrick Twumasi wrote in his survey for the Catholic Health Secretariat in 1982, the cost of drugs was extremely high and revenues received by patients' fees and government grants and secondment schemes could not cover expenditure. By this point some of the initial congregations that started medical missions had declined and 'the income of local people, it must be stressed, has not risen proportionately, even though the present patient's fees charged are much higher than before'.[23] The range of external donors, particularly in streams established in the 1950s and 1960s, resulted in mission hospitals being able to sidestep the economic crisis to some extent. Training and personal support, as well as resources, were available in mission hospitals because they had their origins, sources, and networks outside of the context of fragile national governance.

Missions still relied on the local community and national government to support their work, politically, financially, and physically. Twumasi notes that the struggles of impoverished Ghanaians adversely affected missions even with foreign support: 'the important constraints are finance, lack of community support, difficulty in finding local building materials, lack of interest in working in rural areas and thus the difficulty in recruiting health workers, and to find reliable building contractors'.[24]

Local negotiations were critical to missions being able to sustain their health institutions. Access to food and drugs depended on chit systems and bartering at the ports. Foreign donors enabled medical missions to weather the storms of Ghana's economic collapse and structural adjustment in the early 1980s – though they were not islands unto themselves or afloat only on foreign money. Missions had to broker deals with locals and gain access to supply chains that inevitably went through national channels as well as through USAID. When the government went on strike and there was no money, replacing those funding streams could be incredibly hard. Moreover, in a very local sense, the pain and struggle of Ghanaians, both Christian and non-Christian, affected how medical missions were able to operate, from staffing to building contracts. In black markets, missions had to negotiate and bargain to stay above water.[25]

With foreign support and government subventions, mission hospitals were able to survive, but staff and facilities were stretched by increased demand as other areas of the health-care system collapsed. As the annual report for St Michael's Pramso in 1981 explained, the economic problems we are facing in Ghana today are well-known. However there is much help for Mission-hospitals. Our position is not too bad, compared to Government-hospitals and to Institutions without any foreign support'.[26]

The problem was that, with only seventy-five beds, the hospital was founded to serve 50,000 people, but 'moderate fees' and 'the availability of all necessary drugs' were leading to 'alarming' pressure on St Michael's. Notably, because of sufficient transport links, there was an 'increasing number of patients' from Kumasi (28 per cent of 850 patients) and from further afield (24 per cent of 850 patients).[27] St Michael's was surviving because of patchwork of foreign aid and government support. They were receiving 'gifts of expensive drugs and hospital-equipment' from Memisa, services and products from IDA and IMPAS, and equipment and goods transport from Orion – all of which were Dutch organisations. The hospital also received drugs from INTERCARE in the UK and in 1982 from the US Medical Mission Board, and there were donations from Misereor for a desperately needed senior staff bungalow (to house a second doctor). Various local arms of the Catholic Church were also important: the Diocesan pharmacy at Kumasi, the Catholic Service Center in Accra, the CRS in Accra (which gave food and drug supplies in 1982), and the Catholic Secretariat (along with CHAG's representations to the government and initiative deployment). The government of Ghana provided a quarterly grant and the Kumasi Field Unit provided vaccines. This government support, with an additional supplement in 1981, was critical for resolving the 'shaky' financial situation at St Michael's by the middle of the year. As a result, management were able to restart repair and maintenance work which had been put on hold because of struggling to keep up with medical supply expenditure. In 1981 government subventions were 480,000 cedis and patient fees 610,000 cedis. Staff costs were 510,000, medical supplies 110,000.

Increased demands put pressure on mission hospitals, though further resourcing and funding meant that some of the challenges could be met. In 1981 an overall income of 1,090,000 cedis actually left St Michael's with 198,000 in income surplus and enough for 84,000 cedis on repairs. By the end of the year finances at the hospital were 'not all that bad' and there was some hope for a bright hospital building, wards, and surroundings. Overall, with a 40 per cent increase in admissions and 37 per cent increase in visiting patients, in 1981 St Michael's could still survive and even increase child welfare by 60 per cent. However, at times, both its finances and its staff were put under significant pressure by the 'unexpected increase in workload in almost all the departments'.[28] This problem continued in 1982. The danger of 'overworking' the nurses and their staff of sixty-two was a real concern, leading to a reduction in facilities to only children and emergencies on Tuesdays and Thursdays. The major issue was that without improved facilities, the hospital could not house further staff.[29]

Foreign support was vital to mission resilience, as drought, high inflation, and scarcity – in addition to increased patient attendance – both hindered and benefitted different mission work. At the Catholic hospital in Assin Foso in 1982 there was an 'unexpected and substantial increase in OPD-attendance'. The hospital was funded and staffed by the Spanish Congregation of the Sisters Hospitallers of the Sacred Heart of Jesus (as well as several Dutch and German agencies), and had a seventy-four-person staff including two medical officers. In spite of the challenge and difficulty for the staff, there was enough capacity here to cope with the demand, and by the end of the year the hospital had a surplus of 100,800 cedis. It was, the annual report stated, 'now free of debts' and able to finance an urgent 'isolation ward' and two new wells. Moreover, they were able to keep patient fees lower than expected.[30] By contrast, at the St Elisabeth Hospital in the Brong Ahafo region, the annual report of 1983 described how the 'intensive drought and the high inflation, combined with scarcity' and prices (such as fuel) reaching 'incredible' levels, was influencing the functioning of the hospital. The report noted that the local population were mainly farmers living in scattered small villages, many of whom 'lack the basic necessities to live, like good drinking water, good education for their children and good health facilities'. Added to this there was a menigitis epidemic at the end of 1983 (with a 57 per cent mortality rate) and pneumonia cases from Ghanaian returnees from Nigeria who were 'sick and badly nourished'. As a result, there was a big increase in hospital expenditure at the time: within four years the budget doubled twice, which was an increase of 400 per cent. In spite of staff salary increase and necessary renovations, the hospital was able to continue because of financial donors and donated goods, alongside increasing patient fees. The donors included Catholic communities, the Dutch government, the Ghanaian government, the Red Cross, the Catholic Relief Services, and Misereor, as well as drug donations from German, Danish, and US agencies. Amidst all this it is worth noting that there was a drop in OPD attendance because of transport problems and the high cost of living.[31]

Expatriate missionaries also continued to work in Ghana under adverse conditions because of long-term commitments and long-term patterns of continual replacement, whereas Ghanaian doctors, of which there were far fewer new recruits, had more options and more routes out. Many medical missionaries had morally and personally sacrificed as a collective body to 'Africa' and to the mission community or congregation that they lived with permanently. For example, medical mission in the case of MMS nuns was a permanent covenant bond to a religious order and to God. The orders' hierarchical control ensured that local discomfort was seldom the reason for leaving. By contrast, Ghanaian doctors were free to move in and out of different contexts and networks to benefit themselves and others when particular situations became stifling or seemingly impossible. Ghanaians had other networks in the West and around Africa in 1960s, through their training abroad and the openness of the international community to foreign medics (such as Frank Grant who went to work at the WHO Regional Office for Africa in Brazzaville in the late 1970s). Moreover, when European, Australian, and American health systems wanted immigrant doctors, Ghanaian doctors had new options. Medical missions made their decisions about location using a different set of standards and norms of practice. Furthermore, all this was in the context of the relative paucity of trained Ghanaian doctors. Whereas in some mission hospitals (as chapter 3 describes) there was a successive turnover across about

2–3 years of young Dutch doctors and nurses, such a fast-flowing pipeline of Ghanaian medics was simply not available.

Local bonds of companionship as well as hierarchical control could be significant motivators for medical missionaries remaining in Ghana. The longer-term theologies and philosophies that under-pinned the culture of development and health in Ghana – stretching back to the inception of its performance and practice in the 1920s – were ideally suited to a context in which the wider state was collaps-ing. Theologically shaped development ideals did not depend on the strength of state modernity outlined in the 1960s, and they did not go through the same disillusionment and agony of the breakdown of Ghanaian decolonisation's heyday. Instead, religious motivation to make health, which was understood within the cultural framework of Ghanaian developmentalism and voluntarism, endured the dis-appointment of national government failure. In some ways, it actu-ally thrived on the crises and repression that revealed (or perhaps constructed) its distinctiveness. Bartering, negotiating, and making health with limited resources – adopting a stance which combined the shrewdness of snakes and the innocence of doves – was a classic missionary trope rather than an aberration of modernised medical practice. These tropes and local development tradition were being reapplied and reimagined for a new context of repressive military control, protest, and battles over labour rights. In the scarce years of coups and revolutions, European, German, Dutch, American, and Ghanaian medical missionaries were enacting an older imagined community under development's umbrella, within the specific cul-ture of development operating in Ghana, and largely as a part of the formalised voluntary sector.

To nuance this argument, by the late 1980s and into the 1990s there were significant issues for some mission hospitals; some were facing too much demand and others were unable to sustain them-selves amidst continued financial problems. In the late 1980s the Assemblies of God took over the health post at Techimantia in the Sunyani district. By 1988 they had managed to make improvements in infrastructure, such as with a borehole, but serious staffing prob-lems led to a 'strained relationship' with local people, according to a health services report. The nearby Catholic mission hospital, St John of God at Duayaw-Nkwanta, was reducing beds and staff. The report also noted that locally salaries were 'increasingly inadequate to cater for a family's needs', and the minimum wage (170 cedis a day) could not buy more than 'two very simple meals for one person'.[32] At the Catholic hospital in Apam in 1989, the annual report stated at the outset that the hospital had 'inadequate infrastructure' to cover the vast Gomoa district with around 138,000 inhabitants (according to the 1984 census). The report complained that their facility was regarded as a district hospital but had not been converted to that status by the government. There was an increasing influx of patients and an expansion plan was desperately needed. As for financial support, the report explained that the hospital relied on CHAG and the CDC for drug supply, but also relied on credit, which was causing problems because of rapid increases in drug prices and an inability to buy in bulk. Nevertheless, as with so many others, the hospital was sustained by funding from Memisa, Misereor, Horizon Holland, and the Catholic Mission Board, as well as the Catholic Relief Services.[33]

MISSION MAKING GLOBAL HEALTH: CHRISTIAN MEDICAL COMMISION AND PRIMARY HEALTH CARE

One major effect of continued religious motivation to maintain the voluntary health-care sector (amidst wider state failure) was that medical missions who valued PHC could continue working on it on the ground in Ghana, in spite of international retrenchment. Especially significant in this were Catholic medical missions in Ghana. PHC emerged from the WHO and UNICEF's concern in the second half of the 1960s, in the wake of the failure of malaria eradication, to support national health systems rather than focus on disease eradication. In the 1970s there were attempts by the WHO to pin down a definition of Primary Health Care, which had centuries-old connotations of community care and preventative medical work, in order to use it as a rallying cry for equity in health care. Socialist medicine and the Chinese barefoot doctors were used as contextual examples for a declaration which asserted health as a human right, which had social determinants, was the responsibility of government, and was 'not merely the absence of disease or infirmity'.[34] It also incorporated the use of traditional medical practitioners.[35] This section will show how the Christian Medical Commission (CMC), its Ghanaian institution the Christian Health Association of Ghana (CHAG), and medical missions across denominations were a key part of the creation, formation, and sustaining of the PHC movement. Through the CMC and PHC movement, medical missionaries reformulated their conceptions of human development, medicine, and community, with long-term effects.

Many Ghanaian Christian doctors such as Fred Sai, German Catholic medical missionaries in Ghana such as Margaret Marquart, and medical thinkers like Kofi Appiah-Kubi and the Ghanaian Catholic bishop Peter Sarpong were key members of the CMC. The CMC was effectively the health wing of the World Council of Churches (WCC), and it had met all around the world since the mid-1960s to discuss how medical mission was going to change in the light of the end of colonialism and the significance of ecumenism. The WCC itself had roots in the 1930s concern to mobilise Christian democratic nations about nationalism and a key mode of that was through ecumenism, particularly Protestants working with Catholics. The CMC and the German medical mission institution in Tübingen (founded by the Basel Mission) between the 1960s and 1980s were the main settings for debate into Christian medicine, drawing in theologians, doctors, and ministers to discuss how to imagine, survey, and advise the huge amount of mission hospitals that were having to adapt to the end of colonialism. It managed to set up many pilot projects and surveys in coordination with the WHO, particularly within PHC. Other key West African medics attended, too: the Nigerian deputy director of the WHO, T.A. Lambo, was a founding member, and the Sierra Leonean assistant deputy director of the WHO and ordained minister, John Karefa-Smart, was simultaneously the CMC's vice-chairman.[36] As for Ghana, by the late 1970s, the CMC was working with the Church Hospital Association (CHAG, which it had helped to set up), the Christian Council of Ghana, and the National Catholic Secretariat.

Within the context of the CMC, Christian concepts of development were reformulated through cross-denominational perspectives from all around the world – though they struggled to involve Catholics in these early days.[37] The CMC had debates involving voices as various as the Russian Orthodox theologian Metropolitan Anthony Bloom and the Anglican bishop David Jenkins. Catholics were not heavily involved but representatives at the first commission meeting in 1968 were sent through a relationship built with SEDOS. One of the CMC's main innovations was to affirm that the holistic approach to health care had value, that the community could itself have healing properties, and that too much attention on hospital provision by past missions missed these vital elements of the expression of the Christian gospel. A key part of the CMC's aim was to break down the boundary between formal medical mission practice and the life of the church community, but they went even further, attempting to redefine the social units for biomedical mission. Part of the reason for this was because, as the Finnish medical missionary J. Hakan Hellberg put it in a CMC meeting around 1967: 'The modern hospital supported by a functioning society with laws and regulations, transport, education, hygiene and health control is like the apex of a pyramid depending on the underlying structures. If we "export" this highly developed hospital, with its abilities to cure, to a country without these underlying structures, the hospital is a more or less distorted sign of God's healing power'.[38]

Hakan Hellberg argued that Christian medicine had to move beyond the ways in which it had been so far conceived of socially. To confine it to the hospital, even in greater contact with the non-medically trained church community, was to 'distort' the sign of God's healing power. God's healing was attained commonly in an institution such as a hospital which was inaccessible to most. This, Hakan Hellberg asserted, said much about the limited sign of salvation which medical missions were offering; whereas true Christian medicine required understanding the communities already in a 'given area', in order to provide the 'total proclamation of healing and of salvation'. The biomedical dream of 'cure' had to be enriched in Christian medicine to encompass the 'having' and 'not having', now and not yet, tensions of Christian 'healing'. This required going beyond the flock and the hospital.[39] For another CMC contributor, American Lutheran minister Martin H. Scharlemann, this did not exclude technological advance which as in all contributions to human health could be viewed as 'a kind of endowment intended to urge us all to participate with the communion of saints in anticipating and preparing for the prospect (eternity) that lies before us'.[40] But it did mean reimagining how societies and cultures lived in dynamic relation to technological intervention and biomedical structures.

Built into CMC dialogue about development was the importance of community-level health care. This was more than simply ensuring that an individual patient had companionship; the idea was that the unique local communities of belonging themselves had primary importance when it came to the healing of the person. G.C. Harding argued that church groups had 'false collective identification', and that healing could occur by better attention to feelings of belonging: 'a feeling of togetherness, often amounting to collective hysteria, induc[ing] a welcome feeling of "belonging", a feeling which ordinary membership of the congregation may not have been able to supply ... Many of their followers are "healed" of minor disorders simply because they have lost their loneliness'.[41]

Judging what counted as a true community, what was false, and which community mattered for which particular problem of physical or social healing could be very complex in a world perceived to be full of porous borders, bad theology, cults, demagogues, insurgent rebellions, and communism. The only way to deal with such issues in church formation was to keep attempting to explore the problem. In this, sociology was as important as medical science. How God interpreted what was a just community required anthropology as well as biblical insight.[42] As the Anglican bishop Ian Ramsey summarised: 'the saving work of Christ must necessarily be ... contextualised' and the deliverance experience of the hospital must symbolise salvation in every situation, without resorting to 'theological relativity'.[43]

The church congregation itself was proposed as a model community for healing. In order to exemplify the ideal society, Harding and Lambourne argued, the church could function as an experimental group in enacting universal social health and wholeness.[44] There was a communal linkage between doctor and church that made Christian medicine distinct. This could function more prosaically too, with American Presbyterian minister Seward Hiltner suggesting the distribution of materials about health in churches and the encouragement of member physicians.[45] Fred Sai added that the church must help governments provide total population health coverage, even with the danger of being manipulated. The call to help reimagine and extend the limits of the churches' role in health care across diverse contexts – rather than only modelling social or individual health through the medical provisions of hospitals – was vital to both the theologian and the doctor.[46]

For the CMC, PHC embodied a new way of conceiving of medical mission and human development. In *The Quest for Wholeness*, the CMC's most significant publication in 1981, their way of viewing and practising community health was emphasised as their greatest legacy. The report summarised the CMC's most important work: 'While the Church had emphasized personal (individual) salvation, it was now coming to recognize that the uniqueness of the individual most frequently lay in his relationships in community. So, there was a need to recapture the Hebraic concept of corporate salvation and the Pauline version of it as the New Community in Christ ... [thus] solutions must always be developed within a local context'.[47]

How exactly corporate salvation linked with local health-care solutions was hammered out in practice by individual project makers. Crucially, this vision of holistic care expressed the complex theological discussions about salvation, community, and the church in ways that had direct relevance for PHC. They argued that medical mission had focused on individuals confined to hospital beds because historically they had imagined salvation as an individual process of returning to God. The CMC contended that an improved model of salvation should reincorporate the Hebraic tradition of 'corporate salvation' with St Paul's vision of the community as a new creation in Christ. On this basis, an improved model of health care should attend to the local context, to the whole individual (as part of a community), and thus to primary rather than secondary health care. Moreover, by this point Catholics were more closely involved in the CMC, with Margret Marquart included as part of the advisory study group for the work; later she was named as representing the Pontifical Council 'Cor Unum' of the Vatican to the CMC.[48]

The CMC's extensive work with the WHO on the PHC movement led by Director-General Halfdan Mahler testifies to the reach of their theologies of social salvation. As Socrates Litsios has argued, CMC ideas directly influenced the WHO Primary Health Care movement, as the WHO building was literally just down the road. Mahler even required WHO staff to read particular editions of the CMC's magazine *Contact*. Matthew Bersagel Braley also emphasises that the CMC had a major influence on the development of PHC.[49] Part of this was simply because key members of the WHO, such as T.A. Lambo, also worked within the CMC, and because of the closeness of Mahler and the leader of the CMC, James McGilvray. At the Alma-Ata conference in 1978, a group of non-governmental organisations including the CMC presented a statement to the WHO and UNICEF: 'Non-governmental organizations support the view that the promotion of Primary Health Care must be closely tied to a concern for total human development. The totality of human development, and in fact, a holistic view of health encompasses the physical, mental, social and spiritual well-being of the individual ... The integrated approach to human development embodies a concern for "people" rather than merely economic growth'.[50]

Between the 1960s and 1970s, medical missionaries had an active role within and alongside international health organisations. As Litsios showed in his article on the CMC, from the earliest days of the PHC movement in the WHO, the CMC was closely involved.[51] The director-general of the WHO between 1973 and 1988, Halfdan Mahler, is notable for the championing of PHC; crucially, this flagship policy and Mahler's connection with it emerged out of 1960s CMC debates and its later collaboration with the WHO. The CMC was key in the planning and makeup of the 1978 the International Conference on PHC in which the WHO, UNICEF, and others committed to the Alma-Ata declaration concerning the urgent necessity of 'health for all'. In the background document by Kenneth Newell on *Health by the People*, there were comprehensive health projects in Venezuela, Iran, and Niger, and one in in Jakhed, India, financed by the CMC.[52] Still, as Ted Karpf has argued, in spite of its intimacy and significance for policy making, the CMC-WHO relationship in the late 1970s broke down swiftly after Alma-Ata. In the face of pressure from governments on the WHO, the CMC clung to the older, bottom-up principles of PHC which they had formed and piloted in the 1960s and 1970s – those which focused on intersectoral collaboration, community involvement, and a notion of health as wholeness.[53]

In Ghana in the early 1970s, Fred Sai (who had been a key member of the CMC debates) set up a project to express exactly what community medicine, PHC, and social salvation could mean in practice. In many pilot medical projects around the world the CMC's donors and doctors reimagined what community health meant in various settings. One of these was led by Sai at Danfa on the outskirts of Accra in the late 1960s and 1970s. Sai explained his vision behind Danfa to the Presbyterian Church of Ghana in 1971, after having lauded the past work of medical mission: 'every health worker has to be a little bit of a sociologist, a social scientist, in that community, and he should be able to identify the strength and weaknesses of the community, hammer on the strength and minimise the weaknesses … We [the church] have hammered too much at the weaknesses of our colleagues in health care and not brought up enough of their strength … If there is a conflict let us send it to Tubingen and I will be there'.[54]

This speech registers key CMC ideas about the value of community, the role of the church, the importance of ecumenical debate at Tubingen, and the sociological categories that could facilitate better health care. In his actual work at Danfa, Sai expressed this vision of health work in a wide-ranging project that combined family planning with community development and the training of traditional birth attendants. The buildings constructed in the Danfa project were multi-purpose, serving as a venue for weddings as well as vaccinations. The vision was that the community, through owning the health-care work, would contribute to collective belonging. Thus, a new form of medical mission in which salvation was imagined through the healing of social relationships as much as individual physicality was being constructed literally in Ghana. Moreover, Sai continued a similar vision for health care later as president of the International Planned Parenthood Federation, UN programme coordinator, and population advisor to the World Bank.[55]

Given its ecumenical basis as part of the World Council of Churches, the CMC also set up ecumenical health organisations such as the Christian Health Association of Ghana (CHAG); these were considered to be directly tied to PHC. Both Catholics and Protestants were involved in CHAG. CHAG was originally an ecumenical organisation designed to enable medical missions to cooperate across denominational lines and to form a single lobbying power to formalise their relations with government. Its establishment was aided by the CMC who aimed to spread the initiative across Africa.[56] CHAG, with the Catholic Secretariat, was effective at brokering deals with government such as around hospital staff pay. CHAG was funded largely by Memisa, Misereor, CIDA, and Christian Aid.[57] Between 40 and 50 per cent of the costs were funded by the Ministry of Health.[58] CHAG helped to further institutionalise and give direction to the medical mission voluntary sector. According to Wodon, Olivier, and Dimmock, this ensured that missions could 'be represented and negotiate together as a group'. As it was put in the CMC-led Tubingen meeting in 1967 in Legon, CHAG aimed to 'co-ordinate all church-related medical programs both Catholic and Protestant ... [and] represent a united voice in negotiations with the government ... churches should explore new avenues of service in community health as distinct from ... the individualistic approach through curative medicine as practiced in hospitals'.[59]

Crucially, this meant that CHAG encouraged the norms of community and social health that the CMC promoted, such as PHC. By 1985, CHAG had within it fourteen PHC projects related to its institutions. In 1984 it argued that its essential drugs list, one of the key initiatives of CHAG, was directly related to its need to ensure that PHC was effective.[60] Moreover, it had argued in 1983 that 'since PHC ultimately has to serve 70% of the Ghana this should become a very strong ecumenical activity with a separate department in CHAG'. CHAG with its PHC work was aiming to advance 'spiritual and pastoral care for personnel and patients' in CMC terms.[61]

From the 1970s onwards, amidst turmoil in Ghana, missionaries expanded their PHC programmes. By the late 1970s, Ghanaian government had become more haphazard with fewer clear priorities, as military dictatorship ousted Kofi Busia in 1972. The religious and spiritual tastes of the new leaders, such as General Acheampong, were eclectic and inconsistent.[62] Missionaries continued to receive funding from the government but relationships were fractious. Missions focused on their own projects rather than concerned themselves with reforming government. One of those foci was PHC. In Pascal Schmid's work on the Basel Mission Hospital at Agogo, he has shown that they were producing PHC projects by 1978. Before this preventative health care was limited to maternal and child health. However, this did not curtail their highly curative and specialised hospital focus. Crucially, the new Dutch doctor in the mid-1970s and others were keen to promote more PHC: in their view it was a 'happy coincidence' that this was where the government wanted to focus too. It was not financial struggles and dependency on the government (though these existed), but rather changes in background and vision for medical mission, that transitioned Agogo in favour of PHC.[63]

By the early 1980s the Salvation Army was, in all likelihood, also contributing to the growth of PHC. In 1981, 401,694 people attended Salvation Army clinics in Ghana, and they too were doing nutritional work, food preparation, and hygiene demonstrations.[64] Where their work seems to have particularly matched the PHC agenda is in what they described as holistic care: 'The Salvation Army is committed to the Total Person: physical as well as spiritual well-being'. Rather than meaning simply biomedicine combined with preaching, this was related to planting over 35,000 trees, community building, and raising rabbits – all this through funding from

CIDA (Canadian International Development Agency). Moreover, as the previous chapter has shown, the Salvation Army combined food aid and community development with their medical mission.[65] While there is no direct evidence or an explicit 'PHC' label given to Salvation Army activities here, these kinds of definitions and practices are related to those which were being worked out in the CMC. For example, a 1980 paper given at the Salvation Army in Ghana states that 'Salvation is HEALTH – spiritual, physical and mental health'.[66] These were the exact terms of salvation for which the CMC had been contending since the mid-1960s. The Salvation Army were not always in comfortable relationship with these bodies – for example, they suspended their membership regarding the WCC's $85,000 grant of food, clothing, and medicine to the Rhodesian 'liberation families' (the Patriotic Front of Rhodesia) – but in general they were allied.[67] The CMC was vital in shaping the ways in which its member bodies envisioned community health care and they were also critical in creating PHC with the WHO.

CATHOLIC MISSIONS STARTING AND SUSTAINING PRIMARY HEALTH CARE IN GHANA

The most significant actors in PHC, through the CMC and in CHAG in Ghana from the mid-1970s into the 1990s, were Catholic medical missions. Against prevailing international norms, Catholic medical missionaries in Ghana especially supported the WHO director-general Halfdan Mahler and expanded their PHC work in many regions and contexts (though this was not without challenge). Crucially, this section shows the dynamic relation that could exist between visions of development and medical mission practice when medical missionaries themselves moved between the various layers of both international and global health. Again, however, this was limited by changing international politics which were detached from missionaries' concerns about the theological basis of health and development.

From the late 1960s, ecumenical discussions between Catholic and Protestants flourished on the ground in Ghana, beginning with the CMC meeting at Legon in Accra in 1967 that set up CHAG. Partly because of a survey of all mission health institutions in 1966, Catholic, Protestants, and government officials attended the conference in 1967. Following this, not only were Catholics incorporated as key players in CHAG, but Catholics from missions in Ghana became leaders within the CMC. By the 1980s Bishop Peter Sarpong had become one of the CMC's main Catholic consultants and Margret Marquart represented the Vatican for them. For decades previously, Protestant ecumenism could be successful at the grass-roots level; David Maxwell has shown how ecumenical Protestant experience help to construct a broad sense of Luba Katanga identity in the Belgian Congo in the late 1950s.[68] Moreover, in many cases, the context of the mission field had resulted in the playing down of denominational differences. As previous chapters have shown, there was hostility combined with pragmatic cooperation in the Gold Coast between Catholics and Protestants. In the 1970s, ecumenism achieved a different level in Ghana. By the 1980s, 69 per cent of CHAG members were Catholic health institutions.[69] With their links to the CMC and their domination of CHAG, Catholics took a major role in the expansion of PHC in Ghana.

At the same, international ecumenism was critical. Misereor were funding many of the CMC conferences and Catholics were contributing to the journal *Contact*.[70] The wider inclusion of Catholics within international health was partly a result of the end of mandatory habit wearing and the encouragement to ecumenism through Vatican II. Misereor played a key role in the emergence of CMC ecumenism. For example, through CMC to the Christian Health Association of Nigeria (CHAN), Misereor donated 116,707.50 DM between 1974 and 1977.[71] Misereor also donated directly to the CMC throughout the 1970s and 1980s: for example, they gave 50,000 DM for helping continue *Contact* in 1984 and a further 60,000 DM to the CMC for projects in 1985.[72] In Ghana the National Catholic Secretariat was also supportive, reporting in 1979 that they wanted to 'start now, not wait' to begin pilot projects, and (in line with CMC thinking) begin these efforts 'within the concept of the healing ministry with Christian emphasis on the wholeness of man'. Moreover, they wanted to 'work effectively through identifiable Christian groups on the local level' and with CHAG at the national level. For them PHC was about doing Christian ministry in a way that recognised localities' 'particular health priorities' and that worked with a community to 'recognise their health needs'.[73] The Ministry of Health wrote that the cost of PHC would be 'moderate and well within Ghana's means'. They concluded that 'the cost of not instituting the Primary Health Care System will be the continuing high level of unnecessary sickness, disability and death of the people of Ghana'.[74]

It was not only in international health circles but also in national governance and churches that PHC in the late 1970s was appearing to be the solution to a great many problems, particularly regarding communicable disease. Thus, in this case the government provided impetus to the concerns that missionaries had already developed. Furthermore, in 1981 Memisa gave the 'first important drug donations' to CHAG.[75] When ecumenism broke down, as in the Agogo Ecumenical Nurses Training School in the mid-1980s, Peter Sarpong appealed to Memisa to change their approach. When a Catholic Revered Sister was forced out of the Agogo school because her 'life there was like hell' (Presbyterians made her feel that she was on 'alien land'), Sarpong wrote to Memisa asking if they would support a Catholic-only health programme as well. He asked that they make sure that all the eggs were not in the 'one basket' of the ecumenical 'healing community'.[76]

Catholics' work in PHC in Ghana was the result of local and regional factors such as relations with anthropologists and the reading of particular books. Dutch Catholic medical missionaries, as noted previously, were reading works such as *Small Is Beautiful* by E.F. Schumacher, which was internationally significant in arguing for 'community development' models.[77] Local circumstances also ensured that PHC was an interest of particular missions from the mid-1970s. With the Ministry of Health and social welfare, they studied the village, finding that it had adequate food but poor techniques and a lot of malaria. Thus, they began simple clinics and nutrition demonstrations with the assistance of sanitation teams. After that they started training local midwives and community health workers. Part of the reason for this early PHC work was also that a local anthropologist, Mike Warren, had encouraged the missionaries to start a programme to learn from traditional health and traditional midwives.[78]

In seminars, training programmes, and new projects, Catholic medical mission in Ghana took up PHC intensely and promoted, through international health organisations' conferences, what they had already been doing in the mid-1970s through into the 1980s. The missions themselves increasingly were working together, cooperating with CHAG, and setting up Diocesan health committees. At a seminar in Kintampo in 1978, amongst many others, Sisters and Catholic medical missionaries attended and took notes in order to put new PHC initiatives into practice. They studied how to build community leadership and maintain contact with key individuals. In 1978 the Catholics had a conference with USAID on Primary Health Care and community health workers. PHC seminars included medical missionaries and practitioners from across the world discussing how PHC could be possible through mobilising groups and training teams. These projects, which included Ministry of Health workers as well as missionaries, received support from CIDA and USAID. At one PHC conference, sponsored by UNICEF in Madina in October 1978, there were representatives from the Christian Health Association of Ghana, the Catholic Relief Services, USAID, the Peace Corps, the Red Cross of Ghana, and Social Welfare.[79] Catholics took a prominent role in discussions. For example, at Madina there was included a report on PHC promotion at Berekum, where midwifery students were beginning to be trained with an emphasis on the promotion of PHC. There was an under-fives clinic at the hospital and at ten surrounding villages, and immunisation programmes at the department of the hospital itself. There was also supervision of the new Drobo clinic, the Sampa Government Health Center, the Seketia health post (weekly), the Seikwaa dressing station (fortnightly), and the other clinics (when possible). In addition, the Drobo clinic was able to extend further services of the under-five clinic to three outstations. Finally, Berekum was managing the coordination with the activities of the medical field units, the environmental health units, and the leprosy services. Under the banner of international health seminars on PHC, Berekum lauded what it had already been doing with regard to the initiative with government for the previous few years.[80]

Catholic medical missionaries by 1981 were training those who trained PHC workers. Though PHC was falling out of favour in international health circles and being replaced by the more circumscribed SPHC, in Catholic medical mission PHC continued apace. In Nsawam in 1981 a large group of Sisters trained those who were tasked with teaching 'village health workers in the skills of leaders, group dynamics and the use of codes'. The aim was that these Sisters should also be able to 'train the Village Health Worker to use the Psycho-Social method in the Community Health Education Programme'. These programmes were not at all secularised but began with an explanation of the relationship between the church and PHC which registered key concepts from the CMC:

Health care was considered by Christ as part of development process aimed at improving the 'quality of life'. It is essentially a community struggle in which the sick person, with the aid of the human community can be restored physically and psychologically to health to enable him to become an active agent and subject of his own development ... Primary Health Care is increasingly being accepted as the strategy for achieving this objective ... The Church should build awareness among the Community that by making purposeful attempts to link health programmes with Community development programmes and on the efforts of the Community itself, the Church will seek to ensure that the 'quality of life' of the Community is improved ... In conclusion the Church is perhaps the only organization which is based at the very grass roots of the Community and whose selfless, disciplined and well trained leaders have influence with their members and the society of which they are a part. This influence can be the basis for active participation by the people in Primary Health Care.[81]

PHC was imagined as a Christian development project in the form of the CMC, not a way of simply reducing costs or aligning with international or global health trends or coping with a failing state, but of promoting Christ's ministry to the whole human, the whole community, and the whole of humanity. The CMC vision for human development had a direct effect on the way in which USAID-backed Catholic mission conceived of development on the ground in Ghana.

Contrary to what Marcos Cueto has shown for Latin America, in Ghana by 1982 many Catholic medical missions were growing their PHC work rather than retracting it.[82] The Catholic health institutions in 1982 provided many mobile clinics, immunisation, preventative health work, family planning advice, nutritional support, travelling nurses, community health teaching, and village health work. In addition to this there were also a great deal of PHC activities, labelled as such by Catholic records themselves, which begun in 1982 across Catholic medical mission in Ghana. There is some sense that when described as PHC, the initiative was new and was shaping Catholic health by the particular PHC global movement. For example, St Martin's Hospital at Agoryesum described the 'Primary Health Care' it did in the surrounding villagers and separately explained its plans for a 'Primary Health Care programme' in the next five years to train Primary Health Care workers. Furthermore, at Abease Primary Health Care Centre in Sunyani diocese, there was the usual clinic activities of traditional birth attendant (TBA) training and village health worker (VHW) teaching, as well as family planning advice. From this there was a plan to extend 'Primary Health Care to villages within 10 and 20km' but execution was hindered by issues of isolation, personnel, water problems, and transportation.[83] Again the capitalised 'PHC' suggests that the programme was in line with the kind of models laid out in PHC pilot projects in the 1970s, especially work with TBAs, which would have generally been new to Catholic missions given their historic rejection of traditional belief systems. This is not to say the distinctions were cut and dried but that there were some separate visions from older practices.

In 1982, there were many PHC programmes beginning or extending in Catholic health institutions in Ghana. At Apam Catholic Hospital there were also plans to begin health education work combined with PHC within the five years from 1982. At Breman Asikuma, there was a survey begun in order to implement PHC, as well as training of VHWs for three to four years and digging wells across a number of villages as part of a 'long term project'. At St Dominic's Hospital in Akwatia there was already PHC teaching with VHWs and TBAs taught to 'improve upon their traditional services'. At Akim Swedru in Accra there was PHC teaching as well, with family planning advice and TBA teaching. There was PHC work already started at Holy Cross Mobile Clinic in Tamale and it was starting at Wiaga in the Navrongo-Bolgatanga diocese. There was also PHC teaching through extension services from Holy Family Hospital in Techiman. This was being grown because 'the need is concerned with the patients' total care and not just with their diseases. They feel part of the community and are responsive to their needs and desires'. Moreover, this statement, which fit very well with PHC's holistic models, was tied to 'building a sense of Christian Community and care'.[84] PHC functioned well with evangelistic visions for biomedicine – especially those which envisioned stretching out beyond the hospital.

Evangelism was the part of the target of PHC reforms actioned by the National Catholic Secretariat and by Catholic medical missions in Ghana. In a report on a Misereor fund for PHC from the National Catholic Secretariat in 1980, attended by Misereor delegates, one piece noted that a PHC training workshop would be held to make 'the healing activities and influence our priests more effective'. In other cases, while the overall intent of PHC was evangelistic, specific gospel-health links were separated in specific events, apart from bio-medical training. For example, at the conference in a list of health training, village visits, and rural classes, there was a meeting with the 'Berekum District Catechist Society' in which members of the latter would be trained to see the 'relation of health to the Gospel'. In the first two meetings eighteen catechists attended. The goal in the long term was to 'establish a means of linking health education and the Church's role in healing/concern for her people. Link health workers - - catechist - - parishiners [sic] - - sick persons'.[85]

This is not to say that Catholics did not struggle in their efforts to make PHC ideals a reality on the ground. PHC was not perfectly executed in Ghana; there were many issues, such as local community intransigence and lack of cooperation because of scarcity. There were problems mobilising local communities. At the Assin Foso Catholic Hospital there were plans to extend PHC, to train a greater number VHWs, to train TBAs, and to complete a 'district profile and to pre-pare a Village Health Workers Manual'. The issues were not actu-ally in funding or in international support (though they encountered challenges getting a reliable contractor and building materials), but crucially with 'seeking the co-operation of the villages in Primary Health Care work'. PHC had invasive aspects and required commu-nity belief systems and health work to become more intermixed with Christian biomedical practice. This meant that a strict division or a pluralist approach to health in which the community itself could pick and choose its responses to illness or to pregnancy was less possible. PHC involved a further extension of power into Ghanaian lives and this, in Assin Foso at least, was resisted. At St John's Clinic in Akim Ofoase there was also PHC work planned for the following five years, but there was uncertainty about local community partic-ipation: 'the only problem is whether the people will be willing to accept it through their own active participation and involvement'. St Mary's Clinic in New Drobo also noted that PHC had issues with the 'lack of interest of villagers' as well as petrol shortages and bad roads – all of which was linked to the 'difficult times'. In addition, given the significance of close relations with local communities to make PHC effective, some of the problems harked back to when mis-sions depended far more on local communities.[86] For example, at a PHC project from Berekum, one incident was recorded in which the Sister in charge, Sister Camillus, infuriated an Ashanti community to the extent that they tried to harm her by traditional means: the MMS found that 'some of the patients had put the juju' on her, and when she left to go on an annual holiday, they attributed it to their power.[87]

There were also resource issues, conflicts, and a lack of missionary staff who were keen to work outside of established clinics and hospitals. There were difficulties with mobilising missionaries themselves. In other cases, such as at St John of God Hospital in Duayaw Nkwanta, the issue with setting up PHC was that there were not enough staff who wanted to work in places where 'modern facilities are lacking or non-existent': their report explained that 'there are no good schools and there is a lack of recreational facilities. There is also a lack of appropriate housing'. In contrast to the kinds of rural mission in the extreme Northern Territories explored in chapter 1, PHC for Catholic missions in 1982 was difficult because of its reliance on local communities who did not have the resources to support staff who were used to working in hospitals. However, for Holy Family Hospital at Berekum, the problem was not unwilling staff but 'the exodus of skilled personnel to other countries', as well as issues with water, roads, electricity, and communication – but these were not problems specific to PHC. The mobile clinic at Kandiga in Navrongo-Bolgatanga diocese also noted lack of petrol hindering its PHC efforts.[88] Similarly, the two PHC projects that the CRS was running in 1983 had to be curtailed and training suspended as a result of the refugee problem.[89]

The government of Ghana did support the Catholic PHC projects in critical ways, though lack of financial capacity meant restricted support. One of the key Misereor-supported PHC projects was St Anthony's Hospital in Dzodze between 1977 and 1983, which was planned to be taken over by the government in 1980 but German funding had to be extended. By 1985, the government was financing the staffing costs for eleven workers, including six community health nurses, but could not cover the needed improvements in equipment. There was one Ghanaian government-seconded nurse and successive Sisters-in-charge from the Netherlands. In one year the team carried out monthly maternal-child health clinic sessions in eleven villages, health education talks at schools, home visits in Dzodze town, mass immunization, leprosy control, and malnutrition clinics. Notably, the scheme also facilitated the government's Expanded Programme of Immunization (EPI) in the Ketu district of 25,000 people, as they were the only mobile clinic. Furthermore, the PHC team trained eighteen village health workers (VHW) between 1981 and 1982, although they found it was very difficult to keep them working: by 1985 only two VHWs were continuing to work and 'in fact selling of medicine seemed their only occupation'. The 1986 report noted that the VHWs had not seemed to understand the PHC concept and were just young people 'looking for a profitable business'. Nevertheless, PHC schemes created committees and groups that combined forces with traditional birth attendants, chiefs, 'herbalists', and teachers.[90]

In other cases Ghanaian government support of PHC was restricted by local communities' preference for curative health. In Sunyani district, the Ghanaian government was able to fund PHC activities in thirty-one villages and by 1988 had trained twenty-four TBAs, and in 1989 started training ten community health workers. All this was alongside 'intensification' of CHW supervision, World Vision-assisted nutrition workshops, and seven preventative health workshops. However, the report noted with some frustration: 'the aspirations of the communities are often more geared towards having a clinic with curative care rather than the comprehensive package which we try to offer'.[91] Furthermore, the Assin Foso PHC scheme which had a combined Catholic mission-government management team also had to close two of their community clinics temporarily in 1984 because of 'the peoples' lack of interest to construct toilets, despite numerous discussions with them'.[92]

PHC could be crowded out by long-term established patterns increasingly draining funding from new initiatives, or it could force missions to adapt their historic theologies. As the Ministry of Health wrote, 70 per cent of Ghanaians could not access the service and needed PHC.[93] In the same report as PHC was lauded, the National Catholic Secretariat accepted 1 million DM from Misereor to ensure that urgent staff housing would be built.[94] Some PHC projects were produced, such as at Berekum, but those were situations in which mission hospitals were already stable. In other cases, the priority was simply to sustain the services already being provided. On the other hand, some missions adapted in spite of difficulties. Older theologies around the dangers of traditional medicine could be eclipsed in favour of continuing PHC within limited resources. For example, the Catholic bishop Lodunu of Keta-Ho diocese in 1982 argued that PHC should be intensified even though resources were strained. He explained that this meant that Catholic health institutions needed to cooperate with traditional healers to meet the needs of the people. Working with traditional healers was one of the early challenges to historic missionary medicine made in the debates of the CMC. Fred Sai at the Presbyterian conference in 1971 had challenged them by arguing that traditional healers did the work of God in looking after the dying in places where medical missions could not venture.[95] In 1982, in debates over funding for PHC, these CMC theologies were being supported in order to make PHC work and continue to improve efficient local community health care.[96] Concerns about medical missionary survival and choices around adaptation shaped the extent to which PHC was possible.

Often the Ghanaian state paid lip service to PHC but were unable to actually execute it. Missions cannot be categorised in the same manner as NGOs that contributed to the struggles of African states in the 1980s; they were bound up with its long-term structural weaknesses and strengths. PHC was, in many ways, a luxury that some missions were able to afford, whereas in many cases the Ghanaian state was unable to even entertain it. Whereas the streams of USAID (which was pro-PHC from the beginning) going to Berekum allowed them to produce PHC in the early 1980s, funding was not similarly available to the Ghanaian government in rural areas. The formal voluntary sector strengthened its ties with each other in the 1980s around PHC and ecumenism, and continued to draw from foreign funding, whereas the military government of Ghana had less capacity or perhaps less interest in innovating.

PHC struggled within Ghana's overall economic decline and the long history of structural inequalities in Ghanaian health care. Unfortunately, there are not the statistics to show whether Ghanaians' health actually benefitted from the continuation of PHC or how much health improved generally. Throughout the 1970s, malaria, tuberculosis, and many other diseases were increasing by tens of thousands each year. Measles rose from 94,870 in 1971 to 131,405 in 1976, infectious yaws from 12,747 in 1971 to 71,765 in 1976, TB from 5,605 in 1971 to 6,174 in 1976, pertussis (whooping cough) from 14,664 in 1971 to 22,348 in 1976, and malaria from 75,062 in 1971 to 443,410.[97] It must be noted this could be the result of far better detection of diseases instead of an actual rise in incidence. However, given the size of the rises, particularly malaria, at a time when the state was struggling to monitor even its own employees and capital hospitals, it seems likely that these were real increases and not hugely skewed by better recording. Other health indicators are also not available. Whether the trends suggested by communicable diseases were turned around or not in the 1980s is a question that sadly cannot currently be answered. Given the decline in state and private health institutions and the exodus of doctors and nurses, missions may have had much success with PHC locally, but the overall picture was probably one of continued problems into the 1990s. Pascal Schmid corroborates this conclusion on PHC, showing that by 1990 rural infant mortality was still double that of urban infant mortality, and that more than 70 per cent of Ghanaians lived over 8 kilometres from any health care facility.[98] In Bawku in the 1970s, child welfare figures were increasingly annually, with 98,692 attendances in 1975 and 117,717 by 1980. Antenatal cases went up from 24,247 in 1975 to 31,937 in 1980, and deliveries also improved from 196 in 1975 to 416 in 1980. At the same time, their access to vaccines was irregular.[99] Locally, where there was medical mission, PHC provision could show signs of biomedical coverage and some suggestions of successful improvement in health.

All this Catholic missionary PHC work (alongside various other actors and agencies) challenged prevailing norms in international and global health in the 1980s and the 1990s. After Alma-Ata in 1978, the attitude to medical missions within international health soured. While their national role in Ghana and PHC ministry was being strengthened, medical missions' influence on international health policy, such as in the WHO, was curtailed. The CMC and missionary organisations truncated their role in global health to single-issue campaigns. Most importantly, in the 1980s they shifted from promoting PHC to AIDS policy and using medical mission contacts across Africa to tackle the emerging AIDS crisis. In the 1980s there was a rupture between international health organisations and the medical missions. However, in Ghana, in which the role of medical mission did not diminish, those receiving German and Dutch aid were heavily involved in PHC work.

The ability of medical missionaries and the CMC to continue their PHC work in the 1980s suggests limits to the significance of this transition away from it. In his article on the shift from PHC to SPHC, Marcos Cueto argues that PHC had much of its basis in the work of the CMC, particularly from its members Carl Taylor and John Bryant. However, the challenge was partly to its idealism, especially from the new head of UNICEF, James Grant. Under Grant's leadership, 'UNICEF began to back away from a holistic approach to Primary Health Care ... Grant believed that international agencies had to do their best with finite resources and short-lived local political opportunities'. Grant's father was a doctor at the Rockefeller mission hospital in China, and in some senses, this alternative vision came out of another, adaptationist model of medical mission. With Halfdan Mahler not having the support of the WHO bureaucracy, his crusade for PHC floundered.[100] However, while this was the picture in the highest echelons of international health power, it misses what was happening on the ground. Given that Catholic missions in Ghana had their own streams of funding, and in their nutritional efforts (part of PHC) were supported by USAID, they were able to continue their own version of PHC without UNICEF or WHO backing. As the preceding chapters have demonstrated, both global and international health could be limited both in their interventions and their retractions by the processes already in motion within national and denominational contexts. The original impetus given to the Catholic missions in the late 1970s could not simply disappear. The lack of resources was certainly an extreme issue, but vision and ideas had less to do with international health politics in Geneva than historians often suggest. Moreover, in the CMC itself, until they were forced into focusing on the AIDS crisis, there were a number of PHC projects jointly worked on with UNICEF and the WHO well into the 1980s.[101]

Outside the visible centres of power, in smaller global health organisations and in Ghana, PHC and ecumenism was alive and well. In 1981, the joint WHO/CMC Standing Committee agreed to study PHC in Zimbabwe.[102] In 1982 there was another standing committee meeting in which PHC in southern Africa, Andean countries, and anglophone West Africa was discussed with the former CMC member, with Hakan Hellberg attending as a representative for the WHO.[103] In 1984 the WHO/CMC Standing Committee on Primary Health Care agreed that there would be immunisation efforts, pharmaceutical programmes, and in India guinea worm reduction.[104] While these initiatives may not seem like hallmarks of PHC, the ones discussed in the WHO/CMC Standing Committee in 1986 were far more closely aligned. They agreed to jointly finance seed money (possibly with the World Bank and UNDP) for country projects in Sierra Leone, the Marshall Islands, Togo, and Guinea Bissau, amongst others, with district level committees consisting of church, government, and WHO representatives.[105] In a joint statement with Halfdan Mahler in 1986 they emphasised the ongoing commitment to 'health for all as a basic human right … embodied [in the] promotion and support of health systems based on Primary Health Care'. This was followed by a commitment to a framework for a review including joint government/WHO/CMC teams.[106] The CMC also continued with the WHO: in Ghana they funded and developed a hospital called Nazareth with fourteen surrounding clinics which combined spiritual, social, and physical healing, and elaborated PHC aims within this specific context.[107] The final recorded meeting of this Standing Committee, which, as the records suggest, continued to support PHC, was in 1990, when the 'spiritual aspect of healing and wholeness' was emphasised. However, in this meeting the WHO representatives 'admitted that they were well able to make technical statements, but that often they were trying to tackle the problem with the wrong tool. It was felt that CMC might have the right tool, and that care (rather than intervention), coping with suffering and dying, and spiritual healing were more essential'.[108]

After this the records suggest some curtailing of the WHO/CMC closeness with regard to meeting on care and PHC. It seems that the CMC directed its attention to the AIDS crisis, to essential drugs, and even to polio eradication.[109] Activities reports and annual meeting reports of the CMC show a similar trajectory, from year-on-year attempts with the WHO, the NGO group, and UNICEF to start and survey PHC, to a slow-down in the late 1980s (with the exit of Mahler from the WHO). Yet, the long continuation in the records up until this point should challenge, even in a circumscribed way, the bigger picture of the 'failure' of PHC. Instead, it seems that on the ground and within its original architects' groups, PHC was continuing to have effect on global and national health.

CONCLUSION

Overall, medical missions sustained their role in the Ghanaian state, and in both international and global health across the 1980s and into the 1990s. They were able to continue their formal state voluntary sector role in spite of economic difficulties and the exodus of Ghanaian doctors. Thus, medical missions continued to promote and practise PHC in spite of dominant international health actors turning away from the model. Crucially, in contrast to previous chapters' analysis of medical mission and development, medical missionaries in Ghana directly deployed the new conceptualisations of community, humanity, and health care that were built into PHC because of their active involvement in the CMC.

Particularly significant in PHC work were CHAG and Catholic missions, given their growth and sustained funding shown in the previous two chapters. By the 1980s, over two-thirds of the members of CHAG were Catholic. Through the Misereor-backed CMC and the success of ecumenism in Ghana, Catholic medical mission was creating PHC across Ghana. They were not heavily involved in the earliest stages of CMC discussions, but Catholics were part of CHAG from 1967, which led to a much greater role in the CMC. Thus, Catholics in Ghana took an active though nuanced role in the formation of PHC, though this was complicated by divisions around key issues and because of difficulties with resources in the lean times. For global health, the consequence of their work was that Mahler had another forum in which to encourage PHC and realise some of its potential in the face of prevailing trends. While the emergence of global health did not determine the expansion of Catholic medical mission in Ghana, which was related to postwar West German and Dutch visions of development, through CHAG and the CMC it did shape the way in which it was imagined and practised. In the lean times of Ghana in the 1980s, medical missions were a vital feature of the health landscape. They had survived, they had renewed, and they had adapted, but they were also heterogenous still: missions were spread in particular areas and in particular ways, as a result of long-term processes of colonial and postcolonial development. This would continue into the 1990s and sustained in new health contexts – such as the national social health insurance schemes – in the 2000s.

Overall, by 2015, faith-based organisations were providing 40 per cent of Ghanaian national health services with fifty-eight hospitals, 104 health centres, and ten training facilities.[110] By 2012, CHAG, now semi-nationalised, was still largely Catholic. The new National Health Insurance Scheme (NHIS) contributed to the expansion of mission services and attendance numbers across mission facilities, though it did also have many reimbursement issues.[111] Possibly due to its fast-track NIHS accreditation scheme, CHAG benefitted from this change, growing by 120 facilities from a basis of 180 in 2015; half of these facilities were already established prior to 2013.[112] As Annabel Grieve and Jill Olivier argue, whether it was CHAG's effectiveness in this regard or 'sectoral solidarity' in the face of NHIS problems and changes, faith-based providers demonstrated again their 'decades-long presence, endurance (resilience) and adaptability' across all kinds of upheaval, including in the latest challenges of the twenty-first century.[113] As a result, the story of how medical mission infrastructure continues to relate to global health is being still worked out.

Conclusion: Religion, the Ghanaian State, and the Future of Global Health

The typical post-1980s picture of hollowed-out African administrations with 'humanitarian hinterlands' was not an aberration of an original nationalist modernity; for Ghana, it was the operating system of a swiftly made state.[1] British rule in the Gold Coast was condensed into a few decades. Development and health were produced in fits and starts until the 1920s when the colonial government, in conjunction with missions, J.E.K. Aggrey, and international agencies, sought to generate a model colony in only eight years. In the 1940s and 1950s, using a diverse array of Christian missions, the pattern of development set in the 1920s was imbricated formally into the late colonial state as a voluntary sector. From independence in 1957, Kwame Nkrumah's radical decolonisation agenda could not dismantle this architecture; instead he and many other senior Ghanaian politicians in this period bolstered medical mission. The voluntary sector infrastructure was enhanced and extended further between the 1950s and the 1990s by a range of international, national, and transnational religious actors. A variety of countries unevenly and inconsistently created religious health in Ghana in ways that were disconnected from the 'global community'. Strikingly, new streams of funding and staff emerged, especially from West Germany and the Netherlands, holding visions for European postwar renewal and German reunification. This network, its financing, and its personnel (particularly successive Dutch doctors and nurses), lasted across crises, regime changes, and economic crashes. The making of the Ghanaian state in the twentieth century was a compressed, rapid, and contradictory process in which religion was, and still is, critical to health and development.

The implications of this case for understanding global health and development are numerous; this conclusion will be divided into four key aspects. First, colonial decisions had lasting effects for independent rule, such as with regard to state authority and its continued tension with democratic ideals. African states need to be understood on their own terms, rather than limited by European typologies. Second, Ghanaians and expatriate missionaries had agency to shape global health – this partly through navigating the nuances of the state and international actors. Third, European states and actors have used postcolonial states to make national imaginaries and identities, and even to create 'reverberating' sites of humanitarianism that could restore the unity of European nations. Finally, as seemingly opposing groups have collaborated over development and negotiated its grand narratives, frequently the experiences of those who created health on the ground were contrary to the aims of governments and funders. Overall, the historic complexities of postcolonial state and transnational authority are critical for global actors to comprehend in order to make health in the present.

First, the makeup of postcolonial African state authority, shaped by the sequalae of colonial decisions, is in complex tension with democratic ideals. By embracing faith-based care in its health infrastructure, Ghana followed a model unlike that of European twentieth-century statecraft, with some similarities to US voluntarism. As Elisabeth Clemens puts it in *Civic Gifts*, contrary to the normative picture of a European state as a 'centralized, bureaucratic, autonomous public authority', governance in the United States has been 'organized through *both* public institutions and private organizations'.[2] American voluntarism created a 'submerged' network in which public and private were linked 'symbiotically'.[3] For Ghana, fragmented national governance is a structural and cultural feature of how development and global health can be practised and imagined. In these power dynamics, religion – organised within the voluntary sector – holds a key role. A structure of delegated governance, largely democratically unaccountable and 'extraverted', and in which gatekeepers were empowered by links to external resources, was made vital to the functioning of the Ghanaian state.[4] Using this basis in voluntary services and wider religious networks, international health campaigns were structured and executed, especially when severe resource limits disempowered other aspects of the state.

The consequences of voluntarist state formation would be worth further historical investigation, as would the question of whether this governance architecture can be seen a series of lasting 'exceptions' to national sovereignty or to democratic rule.[5] At the outset in analysing these networks, it is important to recognise that supposed challenges to national sovereignty are not a condition of a twenty-first century 'post-Westphalian' order. In David Fidler's recent piece on the WHO and COVID-19, he argues that it was in the aftermath of the post-Westphalian new world order following SARS in 2003 that 'WHO member states empowered WHO to challenge sovereignty'. By 2020, he argued, the WHO had encountered limits to that sovereign challenge as governments demanded that it follow policies respecting their national interests.[6] Claire Hooker also uses this concept to analyse how, after SARS and the post-Westphalian changes to global health governance, WHO figured in the creation of borders and even the extension of US biosecurity concerns.[7] Part of the problem is that the predominance of a United Nations model of modern states over former imperial or regional subdivisions has hidden some of the transnational structures governance and consigned them to an age before independence. Yet, these complexities still have significant bearing on the present and are not the recent feature that Fidler or Hooker claim.

The delegated state may not actually be a feature of the weakness of Ghana governance but counterintuitively an aspect of its strength. However, this may be changing as some of the sources of voluntarism retreat. As Clemens shows, the delay in creating a centralised bureaucratic state in America should be seen as a strength for a culturally heterogeneous society in which 'circuits of giving' are counterbalanced by patriotism. Voluntarism and democratic principles existed in tension, offering different ways of producing public goods.[8] This created a depth of that which Michael Mann terms 'infrastructural power' well beyond the apparent limits of official institutions.[9] In Ghana, as in America, a rich collaboration formed in which relations between donors and beneficiaries were bolstered, where contribution rather than consent led to solidarity. However, the issue for Ghana is that much of this relied on a range of foreign powers and their postwar national concerns – especially the Netherlands and West Germany. As these concerns change over time and the Catholicism that bore them is in retreat, both their financial sources and the attempt at creating bonds of universal brotherhood are under threat. One question for the future is: will this change be of benefit to the Ghanaian state, will it find alternative means of sustenance, or does it present a serious challenge to the foundations of governance, health, and development? As this question is answered, the level to which Ghanaians are agents in their state's fate will be further revealed.

Second, from within this fragmented state design, Ghanaians and missions were able to manage colonial legacies in tandem with both international and global health interventions – repurposing them, reshaping them, and remaking their meanings. Clemens has argued that the American voluntarist network has been difficult to detect or understand for its citizens.[10] This certainly may be the case; however, for Ghanaians, the sustained role of foreign missionary development and voluntary sector aid was not received passively. Across a century of making development, a specific culture of its practice and performance was formed, reformed, and contested locally. In the postcolonial state, the role of missions was battled over by rival political actors; missions could be seen simultaneously as an impediment to Africanisation or the vital structures from which a decolonised state was going to develop. Depending on their physical location and symbolic place in the culture wars over development, missions could be hounded out of their houses or directly funded by the government. Within the boundaries of earlier colonial formulations, Ghanaians remade the meaning and practices of the voluntary sector, development, aid, and religious mission, as they directed, initiated, fought over, and led health campaigns.

In this process, Ghanaians and missions changed how both international and global health were understood and managed not just in their own country, but around the world. The voluntary sector enabled missions, Ghanaians, and the Ghanaian state to adopt global health initiatives that inspired international initiatives or cut against prevailing international trends. In the 1960s, Frank Grant was able to drive forward smallpox and measles control and eradication in Ghana, before leading similar efforts with the WHO in many other countries. In other cases, the voluntary sector enabled aid programmes, such as with regard to USAID and PL-480, to have the logistical support necessary to make food distribution possible. Through the 1980s and 1990s, missions experimented with and expanded Primary Health Care provision in Ghana, with some government support. While work is still yet to be done on how this infrastructure navigated the early twentieth century, what is abundantly clear is its continued relevance.

Third, through the voluntary sector and the fragmentation of the Ghanaian state, European states and actors have used postcolonial states to remake national identities and promote national unification. The Netherlands and West Germany dominated religious health in Ghana across the latter half of the twentieth century through Catholic mission and state development aid.[11] As described in chapter 3, in 1964 the German president Heinrich Lübke stated that the aim for aid was that 'the unselfish works' of Misereor would 'reverberate' back upon Germany. Moreover, missionaries and aid workers, 'all who serve sacrificially and cooperatively' and who contribute to aid for the needy, would be working 'simultaneously to restore German unity'.[12] The space opened up by delegated statecraft and the voluntary sector in Ghana offered European countries the chance to use former colonies (to which they had previously little connection) to remake their postwar nationalism through humanitarianism. As ordinary German Catholics fasted in order to fund this aid work, they embodied this process, claiming a place in the narrative of shared human suffering after the Nazis. For the Dutch government and the Dutch Catholic mission organisation Mimesa, the restoration of national identity following the Second World War also contributed to driving health and development funding in Ghana. Again, the fragmentation of the Ghanaian state and the state's inability to consistently produce Ghanaian doctors ensured the continued need and space for Dutch medical staff to sustain hospitals and clinics. Crucially, as Dutch and German development in Ghana shifts, sustains, or begins to die away (especially in the context of the institutional decline of European historic churches), the question looms as to whether the architecture of the Ghanaian state is critically vulnerable or can adapt to changes in the sources of the voluntary sector.

Whether or not the making of health and development did consolidate the restoration of a humanitarian national identity or shared suffering with Europe remains open for debate. Further research on the role of the missionaries of all nationalities in reshaping Europe as permanent returnees, immigrants, or travellers on short-term furloughs may also be instructive in answering questions of future global health. In David Hollinger's work *How Missionaries Tried to Change the World but Changed America*, he argues that returning missionaries promoted multiculturalism and anticolonialism, critiqued Protestant hegemony, and advocated pluralism in American life.[13] Medical missionaries upon leaving Ghana (which many eventually did) became anthropologists, managers, teachers, parents, and doctors, and probably did change the way in which Europe and the United States conceived of postcolonial change. P.W. Kok noted in 1998 that Memisa accounted for half of the annual number of Dutch health-care workers in developing countries, and with many physicians returning, there was great benefit for the Netherlands. 6 to 10 per cent of physicians practising in the Netherlands had worked in developing countries, gaining 'rich experience in providing care in areas of scarce resources', knowledge of tropical diseases, and 'social skills'.[14] As for Christian Ghanaian doctors, they also challenged conceptions of African identities, empire, faith, race, and medicine in the places they travelled. Moreover, along with institutional decline, the immigration of new religious communities to Europe in the 'blessed reflex' and cultural changes across global churches perhaps have shifted the ways in which aid is spent and how it relates to states.[15]

Finally, in navigating the cultures of religion, health and development have contained surprising conjunctions between seemingly opposing groups, unusual hierarchies, and identities, as well as contrasts between experiences and the grander narratives of their meaning, and unresolved contests over memory, race, and time. In the historic connections between religion, global health, and development, power emanated from many different sources and cut in a variety of directions. As Christopher Clark puts it: 'Not all power is governmental'.[16] Power has many sources and directions; it is, in Ulinka Rublack's account, 'in flux, it disperses, becomes localised and in doing so changes its character'.[17] Attempts to create identities through funding and managing development and health in Ghana did not match up with experiences of making health on the ground. Rival agencies and groups were able to use the concept of development as an umbrella for diverse aims and agendas. Furthermore, amidst these connections, missionaries, communities, and politicians challenged and reinterpreted the meanings of global health projects, food aid, and medical programmes.

Understanding the relationship between religion, global health, and development requires attention to power and the historical cultures it has formed. John Blevins has argued that scholars in the rapidly expanding field of study between religion, global health, and development have 'oversold their case' when detailing the 'trusted, sustainable, and effective efforts' of religiously motivated initiatives. The neglect of and hostility toward religion, especially problematic in the Ebola crisis in Sierra Leone, Liberia, and Guinea in 2014–16, certainly needs to sit alongside the negative effects of religious stigmatization in HIV and AIDs campaigns.[18] For Ghana, there is also still much research to be done on how the dominance of Catholic mission has affected labour rights, reproductive rights, and other critical areas of health provision. Blevins critiques the field specifically for having been hindered by 'positivistic' and 'instrumentalist' approaches, which focus on concrete measurables and metrics, rather than recognising the varied effects of religion. Instead, he calls for a social historical analysis in which the truth about the 'collusion with power and violence' reveals the 'complexities and contradictions' and 'tragedy and tenacity' in religion's position in health and development.[19] This certainly resonates for the case of twentieth-century Ghana in which power dynamics were not only in individual relations between missionary doctors and their patients, but also in tenacious structural and cultural ways that formed the postcolonial state. Whether this process was a 'tragedy' or the creation of an infrastructural strength – or both – is yet to be decided.

In analysing the long-term processes of religion, the state, and decolonisation, the aim is not that there will simply be a better comprehension of where we have come from in global health and development, but a far clearer picture of where we are going and how we are to approach that future. Awareness of complex historical processes offers the opportunity to engage stakeholders in ways that do not fit with simplistic conceptions of African states or religions, that go beyond the most powerful donors of special projects, and that seek to collaborate beyond the borders of the most visible groups and networks. It can enable us to establish multi-sector, multi-lateral, and multi-layered global health initiatives, which challenge the divides of sacred and secular, religious and scientific, and donor and recipient. It can also provide us the opportunity to face up to the long-term patterns which ensure that the majority of the world's population still have poor access to health. It could allow us to reconsider our global relations and ultimately address the historic processes of exploitation, extraction, wealth, power, and status that continue to sustain injustice.

Catholic Health Services in Ghana, January–April 1982

This set is not a comprehensive list of all the Catholic medical missions in Ghana in 1982, only those with available data. Misereor itself financed the study and checked over the questionnaires. Statistics and information are sourced from Patrick A. Twumasi, *Survey Report Health Services in Ghana: National Catholic Secretariat January–April 1982* (April 1982, Department of Health, National Catholic Secretariat, Accra), Archives of the National Catholic Secretariat (Accra, Ghana).

Health Institution	Patient fees (%)	Govern-ment grants (%)	Private Subsidies (%)	Private Gifts (%)	Other Sources (%)	Major Donors and Aid
1. Sefwi-Aṣafo Hospital	60	10	15	10	5	– Misereor – Spanish government – 'Campaign against Hunger'
2. Eikwe Catholic Hospital	45	15	8	30	2	– Main Support: Overseas (West Germany) – District chief executive – Private people – Chief and elders of Eikwe
3. Assin-Foso Catholic Hospital	40	20	15		20	– Diocesan executive secretary – MIVA (ambulance) – Misereor (drugs) – Dutch hospital in Holland (drugs and equipment) – IDA (drugs) – Sisters' congregation
4. Apam Catholic Hospital	30	50		20		– Apam Development Committee – Diocesan executive secretary
5. Breman Asikuma Catholic Hospital	47	20	16	16	1	– Diocesan executive secretary – Memisa (medical officers) – Misereor (building staff quarters) – S.R.N. Sisters (recruited from Spain by the Sisters of Charity) – SIMAVI (water pump) – Sisters of Charity (two generators and others)
6. Notre Dame Clinic, Nsawam	95		5			– Catholic Relief Services, Accra – Diocesan executive secretary
7. St Michael's Maternity Clinic, Ntronang	90	10				– Memisa (drugs, transport, generator) – Diocesan executive secretary – Misereor (paid for staff quarters) – Parish priest

Health Institution	Patient fees (%)	Government grants (%)	Private Subsidies (%)	Private Gifts (%)¹	Other Sources (%)	Major Donors and Aid
8. Holy Family Hospital, Nkawkaw	54	32		14		– Chief of Nkawkaw
9. St Joseph's Hospital, Koforidua	40	30	20	5	5	– Diocesan executive secretary – Community individuals – 20% from Spain
10. St Martin's Clinic, Agomanya	68	19	6	7		– Diocesan executive secretary – Donor agency in Germany (drugs) – Local community
11. St Dominic's Hospital, Awkatia	68	22		10		– Ghana Consolidated Diamond Corporation – Mother House of Germany – Government of Ghana
12. Child Welfare Clinic, Akim Swedru	65	33			2	– Diocesan executive secretary – Community health nurses attached to Akim Oda Government Hospital – Terre des Hommes, Switzerland (milk powder)
13. St Joseph Clinic and Maternity Home, Kwahu Tafo	50	10	30	10		– District chief executive – Diocesan executive secretary
14. St John's Clinic, Akim Ofoase	73	10			17	– Diocesan executive secretary – Misereor (staff house, generator, a water tank, and an ambulance) – Memisa (drugs) Inter-care (drugs) – s.v.d. Brother, Austria (drugs)
15. Kpando Catholic Hospital, Kpando	60	30	10			– 'Action Kpando' – Diocesan chief executive – Misereor
16. Dzodze Catholic Hospital	75	20		5		– Germany (drugs) – Holland (drugs) – Diocesan executive secretary

Health Institution	Patient fees (%)	Government grants (%)	Private Subsidies (%)	Private Gifts (%)	Other Sources (%)	Major Donors and Aid
17. Battor Catholic Hospital, Battor	50	25	25			– Local council – District chief executive – Community – Diocesan executive secretary – Germany (financial and material help)
18. Roman Catholic Clinic, Nkwanta	50	40		10		– Misereor – Memisa – Friends in Ireland – Catholic Relief Service, Accra (food) – Diocesan executive secretary
19. Anfoega, Catholic Hospital	66	32	2			– Chief and his elders – Diocesan executive secretary – Memisa – Medical firm (USA) – VALCO fund
20. Mary Theresa Hospital, Dodi-Papase	46	41	15			– Memisa – Misereor – KOOK (Holland) – Wor and Wand (USA) – Areon
21. Abor Roman Catholic Clinic	65	28		6	1	– CHAG – Holland – West Germany
22. St Anne's Maternity Clinic, Donyina	25	33.5	12.5	25	4	– Diocesan executive secretary – Villagers
23. St Joseph's Clinic, Abira, Ashanti	100					– Diocesan executive secretary – Villagers
24. St Patrick's Hospital, Maase-Offinso	40	60				– Local council and district chief executive – Local chief and chairman of the local council

Health Institution	Patient fees (%)	Government grants (%)	Private Subsidies (%)	Private Gifts (%)	Other Sources (%)	Major Donors and Aid
25. St Martin's Hospital, Agroyesum	25	25				– Diocesan executive secretary
26. St Michael's Hospital, Pramso	69	25		1	5	– Diocesan health committee
27. Abease Primary Health Care Centre, Sunyani	64	24				– UNICEF (government grant in the form of drugs supplied through UNICEF and Kintampo) – Local council – District council in Atebubu – District chief executive – Diocesan executive secretary
28. St John of God Hospital, Duayaw Nkwanta	52	39	5	4		– Misereor – Memisa – Several hospitals in the Netherlands – Private person from Europe ('Senior nursing Officers, the part payment of staff salaries and the supplies of drugs and medical equipment and instrument are made possible through their generosity')
29. Holy Family Hospital, Techiman	60.7	24.6	15.7	1.0	8.2	– Techiman local council (2,000,000 cedis for Primary Health Care work) – Hospital advisory board – Diocesan executive secretary – Ministries of Health, Agriculture, Social Welfare, and Community Development – Overseas aid
30. St Mary's Clinic, New Drobo	55	43		2		– Diocesan executive secretary – Holy Family Hospital at Berekum – Diocesan pharmacy – Government of Ghana – Catholic mission, Holland (building a new OPD and a ward with Ghana government)

Health Institution	Patient fees (%)	Govern- ment grants (%)	Private Subsidies (%)	Private Gifts (%)	Other Sources (%)	Major Donors and Aid
31. Nkoran- zaman Catholic Hospital, Nkoranza	38	55		5	2	– Ministry of Health, govern-· ment of Ghana (annual grant) – Memisa (essential drugs) – Misereor (VW LT 35 Kombi bus) – INTERCARE, UK (drugs) – Catholic Medical Mission Board, USA (drugs, bandages, etc.) – St Canisuis Hospital, Holland (medical and surgical supplied) – Simavi (generator)
32. Hwidiem Catholic Hospital, Sunyani	48	50		9	9	– Diocesan executive secretary – External donors from abroad
33. Holy Family Hospital, Berekum, Sunyani	61.6	35.4	2.4		0.6	– Executive secretary of the DGC – Overseas donors (including Misereor, MEMISA, German government)
34. Jirapa Hospital, Wa	3.7	95.15			1.15	– Diocesan executive secretary – British high commissioner to Ghana (equipment and dressing) – Orion, Holland (books) – Diocese of Wa (linens and furnishing) – French ambassador to Ghana (drugs) – Germany (secondhand bed linen) – Dr Cumberbatch, England (dressing and equipment)
35. Dafiema Mobile Clinic, Jirapa	70	25		5		– Diocesan executive secretary – Villagers – Diocesan pharmacy and garage – Medical field units
36. Wa Mobile Clinic	80	20				– Diocesan executive secretary – Villagers – Diocesan pharmacy and garage – Medical field units
37. Eremon Stati Clinic, Jirapa	10	90				– Diocesan executive secretary – Jirapa Hospital
38. Kaleo Static Clinic, Jirapa	75	25				– Diocese – Diocesan pharmacy – Credit Union investment

Health Institution	Patient fees (%)	Government grants (%)	Private Subsidies (%)	Private Gifts (%)	Other Sources (%)	Major Donors and Aid
39. Nandom Hospital, Wa	10	80	5–10	1		– District chief executive – Diocesan executive secretary – Registered herbalist – Memisa (all eye clinic equipment and drugs) – West Germany (vw Kombi bus) – Misereor (mobile eye clinic – Datsun pickup) – SIMARI (financial support for PHC project) – Overseas agency, Canada (45,000 cedis) – Dutch embassy (engine for water pumps, X-ray equipment)
40. West Gonna Hospital, Damongo						– Memisa – Misereor – INTERCARE (USA) – Agencies in Austria, Canada and England – Local council and district chief executive
41. Catholic Clinic, Yendi, Tamale	100					– Rev. Fathers (administrative support, drugs, resources)
42. Chamba Maternity Home	30			70		– Private benefactors
43. Kandiga, Mobile Clinic, Navrongo-Bolgatanga	25	1	65	9		– S.M.I. Sisters – Misereor – (Senior staff quarters, Land Rover) – Medical Mission Institute, Wurzburg, Germany (two senior staff, car, drugs on a continuing basis)
44. Wiaga	20	10	52	10	8	– Local council – District chief executive – Parish priest – Alexian Brothers, Germany – USA and UK (drugs and finance) – INTERCARE, Montreal, Canada – INTERCARE, Leicester, England – Memisa, Holland – SIMARI, Holland – Clinic Care Int., England

Notes

PREFACE

1 Jill Olivier et al., 'Understanding the Roles of Faith-based Health-care Providers in Africa: Review of the Evidence with a Focus on Magnitude, Reach, Cost, and Satisfaction', *The Lancet* 386, no. 10005 (July 2015): 1768.

2 Kabir Sheikh et al., 'Boundary-Spanning: Reflections on the Practices and Principles of Global Health', *BMJ Global Health* 1, no. e000058 (2016): 1–5.

3 This historical work builds upon (with specific critiques) the emerging field of the study of global health which has begun to more broadly define its central term to include various intellectual traditions in medicine and development, private and philanthropic interests, and transnational health movements. There have been explorations of the socio-economic approaches to the health of specific populations, the solutions to technical problems and globalised health security threats, the role of international legal systems in health, goals for both communicable and non-communicable diseases, and the metaphors, visions, and cultural norms of universal and collective action in health improvement. These studies have brought out the tensions in global health between differing national health systems and contexts, between varying experiences and priorities for health, and between rival meanings and performances of 'health' as well as its social determinants. Structural issues, such as the flow of financial resources from the so-called Global North to the Global South, inequalities in knowledge production, and clashes over the power of the pharmaceutical industry have also been brought to the fore. Finally, global health has been distinguished as having a concern for health equity over help or aid, multi-disciplinarity beyond the health sciences, and

the health needs of the whole planet rather than the control of diseases and sanitation across borders alone; Jeffrey P. Koplan et al., 'Towards a Common Definition of Global Health', *The Lancet* 373, no. 9679 (June 2009): 1993–5.

4 As Frederick Cooper and Randall Packard argue, the amorphous quality of the term 'development' is actually what makes it so effective in bringing together diverse interests under one roof; Frederick Cooper and Randall Packard, 'Introduction', in *International Development and the Social Sciences: Essays on the History and Politics of Knowledge*, ed. Frederick Cooper and Randall Packard (Berkeley: University of California Press, 1997), 7, cited in Joseph M. Hodge and Gerald Hödl, 'Introduction', in *Developing Africa: Concepts and Practices in Twentieth-Century Colonialism*, ed. Joseph M. Hodge, Gerald Hödl, and Martina Kopf (Manchester and New York: Manchester University Press, 2014), 2; see also Emma Hunter, 'A History of *Maendeleo*: The Concept of "Development" in Tangayika's Late Colonial Public Sphere', in *Developing Africa*, ed. Joseph M. Hodge, Gerald Hödl, and Martina Kopf, 87–108.

5 Hodge and Hödl, 'Introduction', 1–34.

6 Sanjoy Bhattacharya, 'Global and Local Histories of Medicine: Interpretative Challenges and Future Possibilities', in *A Global History of Medicine*, ed. Mark Jackson (Oxford: Oxford University Press, 2018), 243–62.

7 Katherine Marshall and Sally Smith, 'Religion and Ebola: Learning from Experience', *The Lancet* 386, no. 10005 (2015): e24.

8 On religion's role in improving or harming health, and its relation to power in health and development (discussed especially in the conclusion to this book) see also John Blevins, *Christianity's Role in United States Global Health and Development Policy: To Transfer the Empire to the World* (New York: Routledge, 2019), 5–7, 183–4.

INTRODUCTION

1 They define 'international health' as referring to the control of epidemics through public health policy that extended across national boundaries, such as in the International Sanitary Conferences between 1841 and 1938. By contrast, in their definition, 'global health' is different in approach and scale. Global health 'in general implies the consideration of the health needs of the people of the whole planet as an agenda above the concerns of particular nations'. This definition accommodates the growing significance of non-state actors, though they note that there were times when

'global health' visions existed in WHO and US policy well before the pro-
liferation of NGOs in the 1990s. While their understanding of this distinc-
tion is nuanced, their frequent focus on the WHO and its archives restricts
the possible periodisations of global health; Theodore M. Brown, Marcos
Cueto, and Elizbeth Fee, 'The World Health Organization and the
Transition from 'International' to 'Global' Health', in *Medicine at the
Border: Disease, Globalization and Security, 1850 to the Present*, ed.
Alison Bashford (Basingstoke: Palgrave Macmillan, 2006), 76–7;
Theodore M. Brown, Marcos Cueto, and Elizabeth Fee, 'The World Health
Organization and the Transition from "International Health" to "Global"
Public Health', *American Journal of Public Health* 96, no. 1 (January
2006): 62–72.

2   Theodore M. Brown, Marcos Cueto, and Elizabeth Fee, *The World Health
Organization: A History* (Cambridge: Cambridge University Press, 2019).

3   Sanjoy Bhattacharya, 'Global and Local Histories of Medicine:
Interpretative Challenges and Future Possibilities', in *A Global History of
Medicine*, ed. Mark Jackson (Oxford: Oxford University Press, 2018),
243–62.

4   Ruth J. Prince, 'Navigating "Global Health" in an East African City',
in *Making and Unmaking Public Health in Africa: Ethnographic and
Historical Perspectives*, ed. Ruth J. Prince and Rebecca Marsland (Athens:
Ohio University Press, 2014), 208–30.

5   Tamara Giles-Vernick and James L.A. Webb Jr., eds., *Global Health in
Africa: Historical Perspectives on Disease Control* (Athens: Ohio
University Press, 2013).

6   Paul Wenzel Geissler, *Para-States and Medical Science: Making African
Global Health* (Durham, NC: Duke University Press, 2015).

7   A recent example of a critical, robust challenge to the long-term WHO
official histories of success around smallpox eradication is that of
Bhattacharya and Campani. It also offers historical support for respecting
variations in global health attitudes and 'a willingness to negotiate with
wide-ranging actors on equal terms', showing how enquiry into the past
can effectively inform current global health practice; Sanjoy Bhattacharya
and Carlos Eduardo D'Avila Pereira Campani, 'Re-assessing the
Foundations: Worldwide Smallpox Eradication, 1957–67', *Medical
History* 64, no. 1 (2020): 71–93.

8   A divide across which histories of mission and religious health rarely
extend. For a notable example which links histories of colonial health to
postindependence Malawi, and which shows some of the basis of that
health care in missionary work (though which still emphasises the

government role more strongly in the post-independence period) see Luke
Messac, *No More to Spend: Neglect and the Construction of Scarcity in
Malawi's History of Health Care* (Oxford: Oxford University Press, 2020).

9 For more on the incoherence of twentieth-century European imperialism
and how 'Ghana' itself has to be considered as a category 'whose very
existence in human imagination is a product of history, indeed a history of
connections across large spaces', see Frederick Cooper, *Africa in the
World: Capitalism, Empire and Nation-State* (Cambridge, MA: Harvard
University Press, 2014), 52 and 90; see also Frederick Cooper, *Colonialism
in Question: Theory, Knowledge, History* (Berkeley: University of
California Press, 2005).

10 As it was put in one prominent piece, the 'religious underpinning of
global health work remains undertheorized by scholars and unvoiced by
practitioners': M. Basilico et al., 'A Movement for Global Health Equity?
A Closing Reflection', in *Reimagining Global Health: An Introduction*, ed.
Paul Farmer et al., (Berkeley: University of California Press, 2013), 279.

11 Another notable example is the Nigerian psychiatrist T.A. Lambo, who
was both WHO assistant director-general and a key part of the formation
of the World Council of Churches' Christian Medical Commission; see
James C. McGilvray to Thomas Adeoye Lambo, 'Consultation on the
Subject of Health and Salvation' (12 July 1966), 4215.0.3 World Council
of Churches: Christian Medical Commission, History of the CMC 1-9,
WCC Archives (Geneva, Switzerland); '3. T. Adioya Lambo: Traditional
Healing and Scientific Medicine: Some General Problems of Adjustment',
Master File of Material for Consultation on Health and Salvation'
(Tübingen, 1967), 4215.0.3 World Council of Churches: Christian
Medical Commission, History of the CMC 1-9, WCC Archives (Geneva,
Switzerland). For more on West African leadership in health and inter-
national organisations, see Adell Patton Jr, *Physicians, Colonial Racism
and Diaspora in West Africa* (Gainesville: University of Florida Press,
1996); Matthew M. Heaton, *Black Skin, White Coats: Nigerian
Psychiatrists, Decolonization and the Globalization of Psychiatry*
(Athens: Ohio University Press, 2013); for Ghanaian agency as patients
and assistants, see Jean Allman and Victoria Tashjian, *"I Will Not Eat
Stone": A Women's History of Colonial Asante* (Portsmouth, NH:
Heinemann, 2000).

12 Valentin-Yves Mudimbe, *The Invention of Africa: Gnosis, Philosophy and
the Order of Knowledge* (Bloomington and Indianapolis, 1988), 111–25,
140–52, 185–94, 211–13; Megan Vaughan, *Curing Their Ills: Colonial
Power and African Illness* (Cambridge: Polity Press/Basil Blackwell, 1991),

4, 23, 56–7, 65; see also Nancy Rose Hunt, *A Colonial Lexicon of Birth Ritual, Medicalization, and Mobility in the Congo* (Durham and London: Duke University Press, 1999), 161.

13 Achille Mbembe, *On the Postcolony* (Berkeley and Los Angeles: University of California Press, 2001), 228.

14 Bhattacharya and Campani, 'Re-assessing the Foundations: Worldwide Smallpox Eradication', 71–93.

15 For example, on rumour as historical evidence, see Luise White, *Speaking with Vampires: Rumor and History in Colonial Africa* (Berkeley: University of California Press, 2000); Jan Vansina, *Oral Tradition as History* (Kenya: East African Educational Publishers, 1985).

16 Emma Hunter, *Political Thought and the Public Sphere in Tanzania: Freedom, Democracy and Citizenship in the Era of Decolonization* (Cambridge: Cambridge University Press, 2015), 22–8.

17 Simon J. Potter, 'Webs, Networks and Systems: Globalization and the Mass Media in the Nineteenth- and Twentieth-Century British Empire', *Journal of British Studies* 46, no. 3 (2007): 1621–46; note Potter's reference to Tony Ballantyne, 'Rereading the Archive and Opening the Nation-State: Colonial Knowledge in South Asia (and Beyond)', in *After the Imperial Turn: Thinking with and through the Nation*, ed. Antoinette Burton (Durham, NC: Duke University Press, 2003).

18 Markku Hokkanen, *Medicine, Mobility and the Empire: Nyasaland Networks, 1859–1960* (Manchester: Manchester University Press, 2017), 3–13, 220–7, 235, 240–3, esp. 241.

19 As Hokkanen argues for the recruitment of doctors in the 1930s and 1940s, the fixed racial hierarchies in the state which affected mission emerged over time and were part of a complex process and 'entangled networks' rather than being monolithic; Hokkanen, *Medicine, Mobility and the Empire*, 157–80, esp. 180.

20 Patrick Twumasi and Michael Warren, 'The Professionalisation of Indigenous Medicine: A Comparative Study of Ghana and Zambia' in *The Professionalisation of African Medicine*, ed. Murray Last and Gordon L. Chavunduka (Routledge, 1986); Patrick Twumasi, 'A Social History of the Ghanaian Pluralistic Medical System', *Social Science and Medicine, Part B: Medical Anthropology* 13, no. 4 (December 1979): 349–56; Patrick Twumasi, *Medical Systems in Ghana: A Study in Medical Sociology* (Tema, Ghana: Ghana Pub. Corp, 1975).

21 Barbra Mann Wall, *Into Africa: A Transnational History of Catholic Medical Missions and Social Change* (New Brunswick, NJ: Rutgers University Press, 2015).

22 Pascal Schmid, 'Mission Medicine in a Decolonising Healthcare System, Agogo Hospital, Ghana, 1945–1980', *Ghana Studies* 15/16 (2014): 287–331.

23 Pascal Schmid, *Medicine, Faith and Politics in Agogo: A History of Health Care Delivery in Rural Ghana, ca.1925 to 1980* (Vienna and Zürich: Lit Verlag GmbH and Co. KG, 2018).

24 Especially for those who wish to see detailed maps of the development of CHAG, I can highly recommend looking over this article and its images: Annabel Grieve and Jill Olivier, 'Towards Universal Health Coverage: A Mixed-Method Study Mapping the Development of Faith-Based Non-Profit Sector in the Ghanaian Health System', *International Journal for Equity in Health* 17, no. 97 (2018).

25 K. David Patterson, *Health in Colonial Ghana: Disease, Medicine, and Socio-economic Change, 1900–1955* (Waltham, MA: Crossroads Press, 1981).

26 David Scott, *Epidemic Disease in Ghana, 1901–1960* (Oxford: Oxford University Press, 1965).

27 Stephen Addae, *Medical Histories Volume I: From Primitive to Modern Medicine (1850–2000)* (Accra: Eureka Foundation, 2012); Stephen Addae, *Medical Histories Volume II: Diseases, Medical Institutions, and Biographies* (Accra: Eureka Foundation, 2012); Stephen Addae, *Medical Histories Volume III: Principal Medical Events and Personalities* (Accra: Eureka Foundation, 2012). These editions were accessed by the author in the University of Ghana bookshop and are not widely available.

28 On postcolonial Ghanaian governance and religion, see Rupe Simms, '"I Am a Non-Denominational Christian and a Marxist Socialist": A Gramscian Analysis of the Convention People's Party and Kwame Nkrumah's Use of Religion', *Sociology of Religion* 64, no. 4 (2003): 463–77; John S. Pobee, *Kwame Nkrumah and the Church in Ghana, 1949–1966: A Study in the Relationship between the Socialist Government of Kwame Nkrumah and the Protestant Christian Churches in Ghana* (Asempa, 1988), 49–53, 94–5; Paul Gifford, *Ghana's New Christianity: Pentecostalism in a Globalizing African Economy* (Indianapolis: Indiana University Press, 2004).

29 Jean Allman, 'Phantoms of the Archive: Kwame Nkrumah, a Nazi Pilot Named Hanna and the Contingencies of Postcolonial History Writing', *The American Historical Review* 118, no. 1 (February 2018): 104–29.

30 Frederick Cooper and Randall Packard, 'Introduction', in *International Development and the Social Sciences: Essays on the History and Politics of Knowledge*, ed. Frederick Cooper and Randall Packard (Berkeley:

University of California Press, 1997), 7, cited in Joseph M. Hodge and
Gerald Hödl, 'Introduction', in *Developing Africa: Concepts and Practices
in Twentieth-Century Colonialism*, ed. Joseph M. Hodge, Gerald Hödl,
and Martina Kopf (Manchester and New York: Manchester University
Press, 2014), 2; Hodge also links development as human progress and
industrial productivity in British colonialism in *Triumph of the Expert:
Agrarian Doctrines of Development and the Legacies of British
Colonialism* (Athens: Ohio University Press, 2007), 1–20.

31 Drayton has shown that there was a tradition of agrarian Christian
development knowledge that emerged out of interaction between the
nineteenth-century colonial world and enlightened natural scientific
study; Richard Drayton, *Nature's Government: Science, Imperial Britain
and the 'Improvement of the World'* (Hyderabad, India: Orient
Blackswan, 2005).

32 Robert Shenton and Michael Cowen in their history of development argue
that the concept of development had a specific trajectory formed by the
Saint-Simonians, the Catholic theologian Cardinal Newman, and the
industrial improvement work of Joseph Chamberlain. While their history
suffers from a narrow, unilinear conception of the history of ideas, it still
holds that there were specific traditions of development; Michael Cowen
and Robert W. Shenton, *Doctrines of Development* (Routledge, 1996).

33 Generally, the material focus of the early missions in the Gold Coast was
on conversion, primary education, and basic industries, especially cocoa
production. The first mission doctor, C.F. Heinze of the Basel Mission,
died six weeks after his arrival in 1832. This untimely demise discouraged
any further discussions of a professional medical mission presence until
1865 when a Gold Coast government medical officer pushed the missions
to provide their own doctor, having spent a lot of his time keeping missionaries healthy. After the 1882 health survey of the Gold Coast by the
Basel Mission, Dr Rudolf Fisch was posted to Aburi on the Gold Coast in
1885 and Dr Alfred Eckhardt was posted to Christiansborg in 1887. With
Eckhardt and his nurse dying within four years, Fisch was left responsible
for all missionary health and the fledgling outpatient clinics for locals at
Aburi and Abokobi.

34 In contrast to many African colonies where medical mission was the van-
guard of health, in the Gold Coast the colonial state began medical work
first and missionary medicine was informal. Beginning with the Bowdich
missions to Ashanti in 1817 and again during the war with the Ashanti in
1863 and 1864, the British colonial government had a medical presence
on the Gold Coast. However, until the formal establishment of the colony

in 1874 this was minimal, mostly for the military, and entirely for
Europeans. In 1878 the first civil colonial hospital was founded and more
followed by 1880. Moreover, between the 1890s and the early 1900s, the
British population tripled. In the 1890s there was some concern to
improve sanitation in the towns, with Governor Griffith proposing raising
duties in 1891, but these efforts did not flourish until 1908–12 when the
West African Medical Service (WAMS) began a concerted effort to create
indigenous medical and sanitary services. From 1912, Governor Hugh
Clifford had aimed to extend the medical services to the local populations
beyond administrative stations, and in 1916 he sent his criticism of the
exclusion from basic medicine of tax-paying Africans to the secretary of
state for the Colonies; see Stephen Addae, *Medical Histories Volume I:
From Primitive to Modern Medicine (1850–2000)*, 12–19, 23–4, and
29–33; Noel Smith, *The Presbyterian Church of Ghana, 1835–1960:
A Younger Church in a Changing Society* (Accra: Ghana Universities Press,
1966), 183–9; Clare Pettitt, *Dr. Livingstone, I Presume? Missionaries,
Journalists, Explorers and Empire* (London: Profile Books, 2007). See also
Christoffer H. Grundmann, 'Mission and Healing in Historical Perspective',
International Bulletin of Missionary Research 32, no. 4 (October 2008):
185–8, and the introduction to the key volume, which provides important
regional studies but which does not extend far into the postcolonial world,
David Hardiman, *Healing Bodies, Saving Souls: Medical Missions in Asia
and Africa* (Amsterdam and New York: Rodopi, 2006).

35 Smith, *The Presbyterian Church of Ghana*, 183–9.

36 How these two women fit in the wider landscape of women's medical mis-
    sionary work and the spaces that gender norms could be challenged,
    upheld, or reformed in missionary organisations and in empire would be
    valuable further work, for which there is not adequate space in this study
    to do the subject justice. Gold Coast Mission Council (19 July, 1921–20
    August 1927), 42–97, Gold Coast. Minutes of Mission Council 1918–27,
    D51, Acc. 7548,s Church of Scotland, National Library of Scotland
    (Edinburgh, UK).

37 Margaret Jones, *Health Policy in Britain's Model Colony: Ceylon (1900–
    1948)* (Andhra Pradesh, India: Orient Longman, 2003).

38 There is sadly no detail in Wilkie's diary as to exactly how he assessed
    standards or what came of his reports. Merely the extent of his travelling
    is documented: A.W. Wilkie, Gold Coast. Scottish Mission Record Book
    1918–1938, D55, Acc. 7548, Church of Scotland, National Library of
    Scotland (Edinburgh, UK).

39 'Construction of Hospitals and Dispensaries, 1920–1927', *Gold Coast Colony Legislative Council Debates, no. 1 Session 1927–8*, 135–40, Balme Library, University of Ghana (Accra).

40 'Health', *Gold Coast Colony Legislative Council Debates Session 1916–17* (Accra: Government Press, 1917), 154, Balme Library, University of Ghana (Accra).

41 In Ceylon's colonial government budget, health received a similar priority between 1921 and 1937; Jones, *Health Policy in Britain's Model Colony*, 42, 47, 52–60, 75–8, 152. However, there were exceptions and neglected diseases, people, and places. Jones shows this well in her work on Jamaica. In the Gold Coast, N.J.K. Brukum has shown how medical work and infrastructure generally in the Northern Territories was 'under-developed' throughout the Guggisberg years. See Margaret Jones, *Public Health in Jamaica, 1850–1940: Neglect, Philanthropy and Development* (Kingston, Jamaica: University of the West Indies Press, 2013), and Nana James Kwaku Brukum, 'Sir Gordon Guggisberg and Socio-Economic Development of Northern Ghana, 1919–1927' *Transactions of the Historical Society of Ghana: New Series 9* (2005), 1–15.

42 This was all in the context of an expansion of railways by 233 lines and 250 further lines surveyed, costing £5,948,000. In addition, 3,338 miles of road were built, bringing the amount up to 4,688, and by 1928 the Takoradi harbour opened at a total cost of £3,230,912; Florence M. Bourret, *Ghana: The Road to Independence, 1919–1957* (London: Oxford University Press, 1960), 2; 'Review of Public Health Work, 1920–1927', 3 March 1927, *Gold Coast Colony Legislative Council Debates, no. 1 Session 1927–8*, 185–6, Balme Library, University of Ghana (Accra).

43 Stephen Constantine, *The Making of British Colonial Development Policy 1914–1940* (London: Frank Cass and Company, 1984), 21, 302–4.

44 As Stephen Constantine argues, the pre-First World War West African model of 'limited Imperial government assistance' was the basis for policy making into the 1920s and 1930s. Moreover, he summarises: 'Between the wars, as before 1914, Colonial Office staff expected colonial development schemes to be initiated by colonial governments' and 'Colonial Office permanent staff [still] framed their requests for Treasury financial aid in those traditional terms ... primarily to secure the future financial self-sufficiency of the Territories'. Overall, 'the efficacy of such a strategy inevitably depended on the ability of colonies to raise their own capital'. Stephen Constantine, *The Making of British Colonial Development Policy*, 83, 286–305.

45 This was both a result of the increased cost of commodities and increased
   quantities – for example, in 1920 the value of cotton goods imported
   doubled from the 1919 level to around £4,000,000. This continued with
   the total trade between 1920–26 being double that of 1913–19, and revenue improving by 100 per cent. In spite of a slump in cocoa, revenue
   increased by over £1,000,000 from 1919 to 1920. Moreover, the cocoa
   price recovered and in the 1920s was consistently around £50 a tonne,
   reaching £80 and even £120, compared with an average of £20 to £30 a
   tonne in the 1930s; H.E. Governor Guggisberg, 'A Review of 1920: Speech
   in the Legislative Council', *Gold Coast Pioneer* 1, no. 1 (Accra: February
   1921): 10–11, NEWS8145, NP000449727, British Library (Boston Spa,
   UK). It must be noted that the 1920–23 depression did mean that the
   initial development plan costing £24,000,000 had to be reduced to
   £16,648,848: Florence M. Bourret, *Ghana: The Road to Independence,
   1919–1957* (London: Oxford University Press, 1960), 26–32.

46 One loan was for £4,000,000 at 6 per cent in 1920, another for
   £4,628,000 at 4.5 per cent in 1925. By 1927 colonial debt was at
   £11,000,000; Bourret, *Ghana: The Road to Independence*, 26–32; see also
   Michael A. Havinden and David Meredith, *Colonialism and Development:
   Britain and Its Tropical Colonies, 1850–1960* (New York: Routledge,
   1993), 158.

47 John W. Cell, 'Colonial Rule', in *The Oxford History of the British
   Empire: Volume IV: The Twentieth Century*, eds. Judith Brown and Wm
   Roger Louis (Oxford: Oxford University Press, 1999), 232–55.

48 Wm Roger Louis, 'Introduction', in *The Oxford History of the British
   Empire: Volume IV: The Twentieth Century*, eds. Judith Brown and Wm
   Roger Louis (Oxford: Oxford University Press, 1999), 1–47.

49 The government sent the African Dr Tagoe to take charge of the hospital
   and operating theatre at Dunkwa in 1927. Tagoe was greeted by formal
   protest from Dunkwa's local Europeans. The state demanded that Tagoe
   remain in place in order to 'give the lie direct to any possible assertion by
   ill-advised persons that any British Government shows any racial prejudice
   in dealing with the governed'. At the time, there were only three African
   medical officers out of the sixty-seven total medical staff in the WAMS.
   'The Case of Dr. Edward Tagoe', *Gold Coast Colony Legislative Council
   Debates, no. 1 Session 1927–8*, 188–9, Balme Library, University of Ghana
   (Accra). See also Patton Jr, *Physicians, Colonial Racism, and Diaspora in
   West Africa*, 156–7; Ryan Johnson, '"An All White Institution": Defending
   Private Practice and the Formation of the West African Medical Staff',
   Medical History 54, no. 2 (2010), 237–54.

50 Gordon Guggisberg and Alexander G. Fraser, *The Future of the Negro: Some Chapters in the Development of a Race* (London: Student Christian Movement, 1929), 64. The use of the word in this book's title is the subject of intense and important debate. The author has chosen not to use the full title in the text; however, for the sake of clarity and historical accuracy, it is being used in the references.

51 Ibid., 99–100.

52 Hodge, *Triumph of the Expert*, 136–43.

53 Fred Shelford, 'Review: The Future of the Negro by Sir Gordon Guggisberg, K. C. M. G. and A. G. Fraser, M. A.', *African Affairs* 29, no. 113 (London, 1929): 104–5; H.S. Keigwin, 'Review: The Future of the Negro. By G. Guggisberg and A. G. Fraser', *Africa* 4, no. 3 (July 1931): 372–3.

54 Constantine, *The Making of British Colonial Development Policy 1914–1940*, 289; Sam Brewitt-Taylor, 'From Religion to Revolution: Theologies of Secularisation in the British Student Christian Movement, 1963–1973', *The Journal of Ecclesiastical History* 66, no. 4 (October 2015): 797–811.

55 Guggisberg and Fraser, *The Future of the Negro*, 91–2.

56 Ibid., 122.

57 It must be noted the difference between the public outworking of the Phelps Stokes reports and the more hidden challenges made by missionaries to the framing of African gender roles in them. See Andrew E. Barnes, '"Making Good Wives and Mothers": The African Education Group and Missionary Reactions to the Phelps Stokes Reports', *Studies in World Christianity* 21, no. 1 (March 2015): 66–85.

58 Sylvia M. Jacobs, 'James Emman Kwegyir Aggrey: An African Intellectual in the United States', *The Journal of Negro History* 81, no. 1/4 (winter–autumn 1996): 47–61.

59 As James Campbell rightly emphasises, the Phelps Stokes survey was about promoting the Tuskegee philosophy in Africa, not creating new ideas altogether; James T. Campbell, *Songs of Zion: The African Methodist Episcopal Church in the United States and South Africa* (Oxford: Oxford University Press, 1995), 311–12.

60 John Illife, *A Modern History of Tanganyika* (Cambridge: Cambridge University Press, 1979), 338; Y. G-M. Lulat, *A History of African Education from Antiquity to the Present: A Critical Synthesis* (Westport, CT: Praeger Publishers), 36, 214–15.

61 The Rockefeller Foundation itself had strong links to Baptist mission and funded Christian medical education in China; Edward H. Berman, *The Influence of the Carnegie, Ford and Rockefeller Foundations on American*

Foreign Policy: The Ideology of Philanthropy (Albany: State University of New York Press, 1983), 23; John Farley, *To Cast Out Disease: A History of the International Health Division of the Rockefeller Foundation (1913–1951)* (Oxford: Oxford University Press, 2004), 307; Qiusha Ma, 'The Peking Union Medical College and the Rockefeller Foundation's Medical Programs in China', in *Rockefeller Philanthropy and Modern Biomedicine: International Initiatives from World War I to the Cold War*, ed. William H. Schneider (Indiana: Indiana University Press, 2002), 159–84; John R. Stanley, 'Professionalising the Rural Medical Mission in Weixan, 1890–1925', in *Healing Bodies, Saving Souls: Medical Missions in Asia and Africa*, ed. D. Hardiman (Amsterdam an New York: Rodopi, 2006), 115–37; Anne-Emmanuelle Birn and Elizabeth Fee, 'The Art of Medicine: The Rockefeller Foundation and the International Health Agenda', *The Lancet* 381 (2013): 1618–19.

62	Edward H. Berman, 'American Influence on African Education: The Role of the Phelps-Stokes Fund's Education Commissions', *Comparative Education Review* 15, no. 2 (1971): 132–45; Edward H. Berman, 'Tuskegee-in-Africa', *Journal of Negro Education* 48, no. 2 (1972): 99–112; Shoko Yamada, 'Educational Borrowing as Negotiation: Re-examining the Influence of the American Black Industrial Education Model on British Colonial Education in Africa', *Comparative Education* 44, no. 1 (February 2008): 21–37; Kenneth King, *Pan-Africanism and Education: A Study of Race, Philanthropy and Education in the Southern States of America and East Africa* (Oxford: Clarendon Press, 1971).

63	'General Conditions Governing Medical Training of Africans', *Gold Coast Colony Legislative Council Debates Session 1927–8*, 147–8, Balme Library, University of Ghana (Accra).

64	H.E. Governor Guggisberg, 'A Review of 1920: Speech in the Legislative Council', *Gold Coast Pioneer* 1.1 (Accra: February 1921), 10–11, NEWS8145, NP000449727, British Library (Boston Spa, UK).

65	Roger S. Gocking, *The History of Ghana* (Westport, CT: Greenwood Press, 2005), 61; H.E. Governor Guggisberg, 'A Review of 1920', 10–11.

66	Christopher Clark, *Time and Power: Visions of History in German Politics, from the Thirty Years' War to the Third Reich* (Princeton, NJ: Princeton University Press, 2019), 1 and 15.

67	Stephanie Newell, ed., *Marita: or the Folly of Love, a Novel by A. Native* (2002), 1–37, 42–9, 53–75, 93–9, 120–44.

68	Robert Yaw Addo-Fening, 'Christian Missions and Nation-Building in Ghana: An Historical Evaluation', in *Uniquely African: African Christian*

Identity from Cultural and Historical Perspectives, eds. James L. Cox and Gerrie ter Haar (Trenton, NJ: Africa World Press, 2003), 206–7.

69 John D. Nott, *Between Famine and Malnutrition: Spatial Aspects of Nutritional Health during Ghana's Long Twentieth Century, c.1896–2000* (doctoral thesis, University of Leeds, 2016), 121.

70 *Report of the Ministry of Health 1953* (Accra: Government Printing Office, 1953), 29, Korle Bu Teaching Hospital Library (Accra).

71 John Parker, *Making the Town: Ga State and Society in Early Colonial Accra* (Oxford: James Currey, 2000), 170, 184–6, 240–1.

72 Ibid., 170, 184–6, 240–1.

73 On the overlapping discourses of landscape, see also James S. Duncan, *The City as a Text: Politics of Landscape Interpretation in the Kandyan Kingdom* (Cambridge: Cambridge University Press, 1990/2004).

74 Bourret, *The Road to Independence*, 26–35.

75 Oldham was a missionary statesman who was critical in combining government and mission in the interwar years; William E.F. Ward, *Fraser of Trinity and Achimota* (Accra: Ghana Universities Press, 1965), 169; Keith Clements, *Faith on the Frontier: A Life of J. H. Oldham* (Edinburgh: T and T Clark, 1999).

76 Philip J. Foster, *Education and Social Change in Ghana* (London: Routledge and Kegan Paul, 1965), 167; Havinden and Meredith, *Colonialism and Development*, 219.

77 'Tribute from Sir Gordon Guggisberg, 3rd August 1927', *The Gold Coast Leader* (17 September 1927), 8, MFM.MC.1788, British Library (Boston Spa, UK).

78 'Tribute from the Rev. A. G. Fraser. Principal of the Prince of Wales's College, Achimota Gold Coast 3rd August, 1927', *The Gold Coast Leader* (17 September 1927), 8, MFM.MC.1788, British Library (Boston Spa, UK). David Rooney, *Kwame Nkrumah: Vision and Tragedy* (Ghana: Sub-Saharan Publishers, 1988), 23–25.

CHAPTER ONE

1 Stephen Addae, *Medical Histories Volume I: From Primitive to Modern Medicine (1850–2000)* (Accra: Eureka Foundation, 2012), 88–92.

2 'Infant Welfare Centres, 1923–1926', *Gold Coast Colony Legislative Council Debates, no. 1 Session 1927–8*, 191–2, Balme Library, University of Ghana (Accra).

3 Just as Jones has shown with Ceylon, Olumwallah has shown that in

Kenya colonial medical coverage largely extended in reaction to outbreaks
of disease and insanitary problems, drawing the state into intervening
more broadly and intensely. Similar processes occurred in the Gold Coast,
most notably with smallpox control. Missions could be key intermediaries
in these extensions. Osaak A. Olumwallah, *Dis-Ease in the Colonial State:
Medicine, Society, and Social Change among the AbaNyole of Western
Kenya* (Westport, CT: Greenwood Press, 2002), 162–85, 223; John
Lonsdale, 'European Attitudes and African Pressures: Missions and
Government in Kenya between the Wars', *Race* 10, no. 1 (1968): 41–51;
Margaret Jones, *Health Policy in Britain's Model Colony: Ceylon (1900–
1948)* (Andhra Pradesh, India: Orient Longman, 2003), 42, 47, 52–60,
75–8, 152.

4 Togoland was a British protectorate but the Gold Coast government set
up medical work (with missions) and economic development there in the
1920s and 1930s. In 1956 the Volta Region (part of Togoland) merged
with Ghana. 'Public Health', *Report by His Britannic Majesty's
Government on the Administration under Mandate of British Togoland
for the Year 1924* (Submitted to the Council of the League of Nations,
Geneva, 1925), 35; Florence M. Bourret, *Ghana: The Road to
Independence, 1919–1957* (Stanford, CA: Stanford University Press, 1960),
106–111.

5 Markku Hokkanen has shown that between 1891 and 1940 in colonial
Malawi missionaries were considerably involved in government vaccina-
tion campaigns and in treating government officials in rural areas;
Markku Hokkanen, 'The Government Medical Service and British
Missions in Colonial Malawi, 1891–1940: Crucial Collaboration, Hidden
Conflicts', in *Beyond the State: The Colonial Medical Service in British
Africa*, ed. Anna Greenwood (Manchester: Manchester University Press,
2015), 39–63.

6 Gordon Guggisberg and Alexander G. Fraser, *The Future of the Negro:
Some Chapters in the Development of a Race* (London: Student Christian
Movement, 1929), 137–8.

7 A.W. Wilkie, Gold Coast. Scottish Mission Record Book 1918–1938, D55,
Acc. 7548, Church of Scotland, National Library of Scotland (Edinburgh,
UK).

8 Gold Coast Mission Council (19 July, 1921–20 August 1927), 42–97,
Gold Coast. Minutes of Mission Council 1918–27, D51, Acc. 7548.
Church of Scotland, National Library of Scotland (Edinburgh, UK).

9 Rapport 1925, Navrongo (38/12), La Nuova Seria (1893–1938), Archivio
Generale della Sacra Congregazione de Propaganda Fide (Vatican City, Rome).

10 This nuances Benedict Der's historical account of Northern Ghana in
which he argues that it was not until pro-Catholic district commissioners
were installed that the White Fathers could expand; Benedict Der, 'Church-
State Relations in Northern Ghana, 1906–1940', *Transactions of the
Historical Society of Ghana* 15, no. 1 (June 1974): 41–61.

11 Leonide Barsalou, 'Rapport Quinquennial à la sacrée congregation de la
Propagande' (Navrongo, 22 October 1930), La Nuova Seria (1893–1938),
Archivio Generale della Sacra Congregation de Propaganda Fide (Vatican
City, Rome). For more on the White Fathers and how mission related to
colonial government, see C. Lentz, *Ethnicity and the Making of History in
Northern Ghana* (Edinburgh: Edinburgh University Press, 2006), 153–74.

12 K. Atoa Puma, 'The Yearly Anniversary of the Scottish Mission: The
Essence of the Basel Mission Spirit and the Failure of the Scottish Mission
Bluff', *The Gold Coast Independent* (16 February, 1921), 127, MFM.
MC1768, British Library (Boston Spa, UK); similar comments and some
reposts challenging the writers' ability to speak for congregations without
statistics are made in other articles such as: A. Full Communicant, 'Letter
to the Editor', *The Gold Coast Independent* (2 June, 1922), 393–4, MFM.
MC1768, British Library (Boston Spa, UK).

13 A. Communicant, 'Re the Basel Missionaries Return', *The Gold Coast
Independent* (24 February 1923), 129, MFM.MC1768, British Library
(Boston Spa, UK); Samafu, 'Return of the Basel Missionaries', *The Gold
Coast Independent* (21 April 1923), 265, MFM.MC1768, British Library
(Boston Spa, UK); J.H.S. Parry and S. Donkor, Translated: 'Return of the
Basel Missionaries', *The Gold Coast Independent* (22 June 1922), 4,
MFM.MC1768, British Library (Boston Spa, UK).

14 See Jean Allman and Victoria Tashjian, *"I Will Not Eat Stone":
A Women's History of Colonial Asante* (Portsmouth, NH: Heinemann,
2000), 181–210.
Jean Allman, 'Making Mothers: Missionaries, Medical Officers and
Women's Work in Colonial Asante, 1924–1945', *History Workshop
Journal* 38 (1994): 23–47; Allman and Tashjian, *"I Will Not Eat Stone"*;
Shane Doyle, *Before HIV: Sexuality, Fertility and Mortality in East Africa,
1900–1980* (Oxford: Oxford University Press, 2013), 124–7, 260–4.

15 Jeffrey L. Cox, 'Master Narrative of Imperial Missions', in *Mixed
Messages: Materiality, Textuality, Missions*, ed. Jamie S. Scott and Gareth
Griffiths (New York: Palgrave Macmillan, 2005), 3–19.

16 A.W. Wilkie, Gold Coast. Scottish Mission Record Book 1918–1938,
D55, Acc. 7548, Church of Scotland, National Library of Scotland
(Edinburgh, UK).

17 Robert I. Rothberg, 'Plymouth Bretheren and the Occupation of Katanga, 1886–1907', *Journal of African History* 5, no. 2 (July 1964): 285–97. When exchange and reliance were reduced, missionaries often more aggressively stuck to their original norms; Marianne Gullestad, *Picturing Pity: Pitfalls and Pleasures in Cross-Cultural Communication; Image and Word in a North Cameroon Mission* (New York: Berghahn Books, 2007), 275–9.

18 As Michael Jennings has demonstrated with Tanganyika, medical mission began being institutionalised through national ecumenical organisations from the 1930s: Michael Jennings, 'Cooperation and Competition: Missions, the Colonial State and Construction of a Health System in Colonial Tanganyika', in *Beyond the State: The Colonial Medical Service in British Africa*, ed. Anna Greenwood (Manchester: Manchester University Press, 2015), 153–73; A.W. Wilkie, Gold Coast. Scottish Mission Record Book 1918–1938, D55, Acc. 7548, Church of Scotland, National Library of Scotland (Edinburgh, UK).

19 The dispensary at Kpando was set up by the Little Servants of the Sacred Heart (Menton Sisters); Catholic Diocese of Ho, 'About the Diocese', http://hocatholicdiocese.org/.

20 *Gold Coast Colony Report on the Medical Department for the Year 1933–34* (Government Printing Office, Accra, 1934), 39–45, Liverpool School of Tropical Medicine (Liverpool, UK).

21 *Gold Coast Colony Report on the Medical Department for the Year 1935* (Government Printing Department, Accra), 31, Liverpool School of Tropical Medicine (Liverpool, UK).

22 In 1938 the superintendent was dismissed and there were even some issues with National Socialism in the staff. The colonial government, who had effectively competed with Agogo for well-paying patients in the 1930s, closed the hospital anyway in 1940 and detained all the staff except one nurse; Pascal Schmid, 'Mission Medicine in a Decolonising Healthcare System: Agogo Hospital, Ghana, 1945–1980', *Ghana Studies* 15/16 (2012/2013): 287–329.

23 For more extensive work on this area, see Holly Ashford, 'The Red Cross and the Establishment of Maternal and Infant Welfare in the 1930s Gold Coast', *The Journal of Imperial and Commonwealth History* 47, no. 3 (2019): 514–41.

24 The Gold Coast League of Maternity and Child Welfare also contributed to midwife care; 'Maternity and Child Welfare', *Report on the Medical Department for the Year 1933–4* (Accra: Government Printing Office, 1934), 41, Balme Library, University of Ghana (Accra).

25 *Report on the Medical Department for the Year 1936* (Accra: Government Printing Office, 1937), 36, Balme Library, University of Ghana (Accra).

26 *Gold Coast Colony Report on the Medical Department for the Year 1934* (Accra: Government Printing Department, 1935), 28, Balme Library, University of Ghana (Accra).

27 As Kathleen Vongsathorn has argued, medical mission in Uganda resulted in an overemphasis on leprosy relative to other diseases because of its biblical links to the work of Jesus Christ healing lepers; Kathleen Vongsathorn, '"First and Foremost the Evangelist"? Mission and Government Priorities for the Treatment of Leprosy in Uganda, 1927–1948', *Journal of East African Studies* 6, no. 3 (August 2012): 544–60.

28 John Manton has argued that leprosy work was left to missions in northern Nigeria until 1945 when this was institutionalised through a combination of the British Empire Leprosy Relief Association (BELRA) and the colonial government, which previously had focused on more prevalent diseases; John Manton, 'Administering Leprosy Control in Ogoja Province, Nigeria, 1945–1967: A Case-Study in Government-Mission Relations', *Healing Bodies, Saving Souls: Medical Missions in Asia and Africa*, ed. David Hardiman (Amsterdam and New York: Rodopi, 2006), 307–32.

29 In the 1940s the White Fathers did build large facilities for their dispensary, adding casualty, children's, and maternity wards. There was also a leper colony at Nandom, and in 1955 Jirapa was turned into a hospital with government funding; Remigius F. McCoy, M.Afr., *Great Things Happen: A Personal Memoir of the First Christian Missionary among the Dagaavas and Sissalas of Northwest Ghana* (Canada: The Society of Missionaries of Africa, 1988), 243–61; Imoru Egala, 'Orders of the Day', *Gold Coast Legislative Debates, 1955–1956: Ministry of Health* (17 March 1955), 1146.

30 John Manton, 'Global and Local contexts: The Northern Ogoja Leprosy Scheme, Nigeria, 1945–1960', *Historia, Ciencias, Saude* 10, no. 1 (2003): 209–23.

31 John McCracken, 'Church and State in Malawi: The Role of the Scottish Presbyterian Missions, 1875–1965', *Christian Missionaries and the State in the Third World*, eds. Holger Bernt Hansen and Michael Twaddle (James Currey, 2002), 176–93, citing Karen E. Fields, *Revival and Rebellion in Colonial Central Africa* (Princeton, NJ: Princeton University Press, 1985), 41.

32 Correspondence and papers of the Church of Scotland Overseas Council relating to Africa (1965–75), Acc. 9638 Church of Scotland, National Library of Scotland (Edinburgh, UK); Correspondence and reports home, under the auspices of the Church of Scotland's Missionary Partner Scheme of

the Reverend Colin Forrester-Paton, in the Gold Coast, later Ghana, 1954–71, Acc. 11977, Church of Scotland, National Library of Scotland (Edinburgh, UK); Further papers, mainly ca. 1970–1995, but many earlier, relating to Church of Scotland and other Scottish Presbyterian Missions, and Scottish churches abroad, Acc. 12398, Church of Scotland, National Library of Scotland (Edinburgh, UK); Colin Forrester-Paton Papers 1939–1994, GB 3189 CSCNWW37, New College Library, University of Edinburgh (Edinburgh, UK); Abraham Adu Berinyuu, ed., *History of the Presbyterian Church in Northern Ghana* (Accra: Asempa Publishers, 1997), esp. 108.

33 Gary Land, *The A-Z of the Seventh-day Adventists* (Plymouth: Scarecrow Press, 2009), 115; The Salvation Army Year Book 1960 (1960), The Salvation Army International Heritage Centre (London, UK), 90–1; John S. Pobee, *Kwame Nkrumah and the Church in Ghana, 1949–1966: A Study in the Relationship between the Socialist Government of Kwame Nkrumah and the Protestant Christian Churches in Ghana* (Accra: Asempa Publishers, 1988), 49–53, 94–5.

34 Barbra Mann Wall, *Into Africa: A Transnational History of Catholic Medical Missions and Social Change* (New Brunswick, NJ: Rutgers University Press, 2015), 33.

35 Stephen Constantine, *The Making of British Colonial Development Policy 1914–1940* (Frank Cass and Company, 1984), 267.

36 Ruth J. Prince and Hannah Brown, 'Introduction: Volunteer Labor – Pasts and Futures of Work, Development, and Citizenship in East Africa', *African Studies Review* 58, no. 2 (September 2015): 29–38.

37 *Volunteer Economies: The Politics and Ethics of Voluntary Labour in Africa*, eds. Ruth Prince and Hannah Brown (Oxford: James Currey, 2016); see also Lauren Graham's review in *The Journal of Modern African Studies* 55, no. 3 (September 2017): 514–16.

38 See also John Stuart, *British Missionaries and the End of Empire: East, Central, and Southern Africa, 1939–64; Studies in the History of Christian Missions* (Grand Rapids, MI: Eerdmans, 2011); Michael Jennings, 'Common Counsel, Common Policy: Healthcare, Missions and the Rise of the "Voluntary Sector" in Colonial Tanzania', *Development and Change* 44, no. 4 (2013): 939–63, esp. 960–1; Michael Jennings, 'The Precariousness of the Franchise State: Voluntary Sector Health Services and International NGOs in Tanzania, 1960s – Mid-1980s', *Social Science and Medicine* 141 (2015): 1–8.

39 Mortimer Epstein, ed., *The Statesman's Year-Book 1943: Statistical and Historical of the States of the World for the Year 1943* (London: Macmillan and Co., 1943), 250.

40 Alan C. Burns, *History of Nigeria* (George Allen and Unwin, 1929/1955), 251–2; first published in 1929, second edition 1936, third edition 1942, fourth edition 1948, fifth impression 1951, fifth edition/sixth impression 1955.
41 Joseph H. Oldham, *Christianity and the Race Problem* (Student Christian Movement, 1924), 263.
42 Burns, *History of Nigeria*, 249–60.
43 Sir Alan Burns Collection of Gold Coast [i.e. Ghana] photographs, 1940s, Ministry of Information, West African Photographic Service, Y30448D, Royal Commonwealth Society Library, University of Cambridge (Cambridge, UK); Joseph M. Hodge, *Triumph of the Expert: Agrarian Doctrines of Development and the Legacies of British Colonialism* (Athens: Ohio University Press, 2007), 136–43; Helen Tilley, *Africa as a Living Laboratory: Empire, Development, and the Problem of Scientific Knowledge, 1870–1950* (Chicago: University of Chicago Press, 2011), 106–7; Sabine Clarke, 'The Research Council System and the Politics of Medical and Agricultural Research for the British Colonial Empire, 1940–52', *Medical History* 57, no. 3 (July 2013): 338–58; David Maxwell, 'From Iconoclasm to Preservation: W. F. P. Burton, Missionary Ethnography and Belgian Colonial Science', in *The Spiritual in the Secular: Missionaries and Knowledge about Africa*, eds. Patrick Harries and David Maxwell (Grand Rapids, MI: Wm B. Eerdmans Publishing Co., 2012), 183, citing Joseph H. Oldham and Hanns Vischer, 'Memorandum on the Place of the Vernacular in Africa Education and on the Establishment of a Bureau of African Languages' (spring 1925), in SOAS, IMC/CBMS, Box 204, cited in W. Young, '"They Had Laid Hold of Some Essential Truths": 'Edwin W. Smith (1876–1957), a Wise Listener to African Voices', in *European Traditions in the Study of Religion in Africa*, eds. Frieder Ludwig and Afe Adogame (Wiesbaden, Germany: Harrassowitz Verlag, 2004), 172.
44 Guggisberg and Fraser, *The Future of the Negro*, 122.
45 Megan Vaughan, *Curing Their Ills: Colonial Power and African Illness* (Stanford, CA: Stanford University Press, 1991), 61–2; Hardiman, 'Introduction', in *Healing Bodies, Saving Souls*, 16–20.
46 Pascal Schmid, 'Mission Medicine in a Decolonising Healthcare System: Agogo Hospital, Ghana, 1945–1980', *Ghana Studies* 15/16 (2014), 287–331, citing James Balfour Kirk, 'Memorandum on the Type of Department Which Will Be Necessary to Implement a Policy of Preventive Medicine of the Gold Coast' (5 July 1943), CSO11.1.646 PRAAD (Accra).

47 Deborah Neill, *Networks in Tropical Medicine: Internationalism, Colonial and the Rise of Medical Speciality, 1890–1930* (Stanford, CA: Stanford University Press, 2012), 5–8.

48 Governor's Despatch, no. 222 of the 26th July 1944, to the Secretary of State for the Colonies (1944) 1–11, access provided by the family of Alan Burns (UK).

49 Pascal Schmid, 'Mission Medicine in a Decolonising Healthcare System'; Stephen Addae, *Medical Histories, Volume 1: From Primitive to Modern Medicine (1850–2000)* (Accra: Eureka Foundation, 2012), 76–90.

50 Governor's Despatch, no. 222 of the 26th July 1944, to the Secretary of State for the Colonies (1944) 1–11.

51 Kenneth Stacey Morris, 'Letter to Ma' (16 September 1939), Box 1, File 2, MSS Afr s 1824; t 34 (1901–65), *Kenneth Stacey Morris: Correspondence and Papers*, NRA 26342 Morris, Bodleian Library, University of Oxford, (Oxford, UK).

52 Ibid.

53 'Appendix II: Revenue and Expenditure: Expenditure by Heads', *Colonial Office: Annual Report on the Gold Coast for the Year 1950* (London: His Majesty's Stationery Office, 1950), 99, British Library (Boston Spa, UK).

54 Kenneth Stacey Morris, 'Letter to Ma' (16 December 1949), Box 1, File 2, MSS Afr s 1824; t 34 (1901–65) *Kenneth Stacey Morris: Correspondence and Papers* NRA 26342 Morris, Bodleian Library, University of Oxford (Oxford, UK).

55 'Provincial Items: Cape Coast: General News', *The African Morning Post* (12 January 1939), 3, MFM.MC1788, British Library (Boston Spa, UK).

56 'Provincial Items: Nkawkaw: State of Affairs is Bad', *The African Morning Post* (17 January 1939), 3, MFM.MC1788, British Library (Boston Spa, UK).

57 'Provincial Items: Kokofu: General News', *The African Morning Post* (17 January 1939), 3, MFM.MC1788, British Library (Boston Spa, UK).

58 'Provincial Items: Mepom: Sanitation is Bad', *The African Morning Post* (18 January 1939), 3, MFM.MC1788, British Library (Boston Spa, UK).

59 'Provincial Items: Mpraeso: Sanitary Inspector to Note', *The African Morning Post* (19 January 1939) MFM.MC1788, British Library (Boston Spa, UK).

60 'Health', *Legislative Council Debates Issue, no. 1* (Session 1939: 14 March 1939), 11–13, Balme Library, University of Ghana (Accra).

61 *Legislative Council Debates Issue, no. 1* (Session 1939: 23 March 1939), 158, Balme Library, University of Ghana (Accra).

62 Nana Hima Dekyi XII, *Legislative Council Debates* (Session 1940: 20 March 1940), 131, Balme Library, University of Ghana (Accra).

63 *Legislative Council Debates* (Session 1941: 18 February 1941), 10–11, C.S.C 450, British Library (Boston Spa, UK).

64 Blay's claim was based on evidence in a newspaper rather than a government enquiry; Robert S. Blay, *Legislative Council Debates* (Session 1941: 26 February 1941), 73, C.S.C. 450, British Library (Boston Spa, UK).

65 Nana Nyarko VII, *Legislative Council Debates* (Session 1943: 3 March 1943), 12–115, C.S.C. 450, British Library (Boston Spa, UK).

66 *Legislative Council Debates* (Session 1944: 13 March 1944), 8, Balme Library, University of Ghana (Accra).

67 *Legislative Council Debates* (Session 1946: 12 March 1946), 6–7, 24–6, Balme Library, University of Ghana (Accra).

68 As Kathleen Vongsathorn has shown for Uganda that such leprosy efforts also constituted 'a system of isolated, in-patient ... care that was limited in scope and reflective not of a goal for the public health ... but rather a vision for the future of Uganda as a "civilised" and Christian country'. Given the obvious links to Christ's ministry of healing outcast lepers, Vongsathorn has noted how 'missionaries wrote often that in healing they were following in the footsteps of Christ, and this was truer of leprosy than other ailments'; Kathleen Vongsathorn, 'Gnawing Pains, Festering Ulcers, and Nightmare Suffering: Selling Leprosy as a Humanitarian Cause in the British Empire, c. 1890–1960', *The Journal of Imperial and Commonwealth History* 40, no. 5 (December 2012): 863–78; Kathleen Vongsathorn, '"First and Foremost the Evangelist?"'

69 'Appendix II: Revenue and Expenditure: Expenditure by Heads', *Colonial Office: Annual Report on the Gold Coast for the Year 1949* (London: His Majesty's Stationery Office, 1950), 91.

70 'Appendix II: Revenue and Expenditure: Expenditure by Heads', *Colonial Office: Annual Report on the Gold Coast for the Year 1950* (London: His Majesty's Stationery Office, 1950), 99, British Library (Boston Spa, UK).

71 'Medical and Health', *Legislative Council Debates* (Session 1949: 15 March 1949), 34–5, C.S.C. 450, British Library (Boston Spa, UK).

72 'Social Services: The Medical Service and the Native Authorities', *Colonial Office: Annual Report on the Gold Coast for the Year 1949* (London: His Majesty's Stationery Office, 1950), 34, British Library (Boston Spa, UK).

73 'Social Services', *Colonial Report on the Gold Coast for the Year 1950* (London: Her Majesty's Stationery Office, 1952), 5 and 36–9, British Library (Boston Spa, UK).

74　Ibid.

75　'Between 1948 and 1952, the price of cocoa rose from £139 per ton to
£300 per ton. The Colony's other exports also enjoyed boom prices, and
government revenue, which was predominantly based on export taxes,
increased over fourfold, from over £11 million to over £42 million'. Roger
S. Gocking, *The History of Ghana* (Westport, CT: Greenwood Press,
2005), 99.

76　Hodge, *Triumph of the Expert*, 208; citing Michael P. Cowen and Robert
W. Shenton, 'The Origin and Course of Fabian Colonialism in Africa',
Journal of Historical Sociology 4, no. 2 (1991), 143–74; Cowen and
Shenton, *Doctrines of Development*, 278–9 and 296–7.

77　'Chapter VII: Social Services: 1. Health', *Colonial Office: Annual Report
on the Gold Coast for the Year 1948* (London: His Majesty's Stationery
Office, 1950), 43–5.

78　William H. Schneider, 'Smallpox in Africa during Colonial Rule', *Medical
History* 53 (2009), 193–227.

79　'Medical and Health', *Legislative Council Debates* (Session 1947: March
1947), 28–9, Balme Library, University of Ghana (Accra).

80　'Medical and Health', *Legislative Council Debates* (Session 1948: 27 April
1948), 26–7, Balme Library, University of Ghana (Accra).

81　'Appendix X: Development and Welfare Schemes Initiated or in Progress in
1949', *Colonial Office: Annual Report on the Gold Coast for the Year 1949*
(London: His Majesty's Stationery Office, 1950) British Library (Boston
Spa, UK). It must be noted that the focus of the colonial government on
yaws, smallpox, and sleeping sickness may have been to do with the relative
ease of tackling these diseases. In the case of yaws it may also have been
related to its similarities to syphilis which was a major concern for many
British colonial officers and missionaries in interwar colonial Africa. On
syphilis and yaws in early colonial Uganda see Shane Doyle, *Before HIV:
Sexuality, Fertility and Mortality in East Africa, 1900–1980* (Oxford:
Oxford University Press, 2013), esp. 123–38.

82　'Medical and Health', *Legislative Council Debates* (Session 1949: 15
March 1949), 34–5, C.S.C. 450, British Library (Boston Spa, UK).

83　*Report of the Commission of Enquiry into the Health Needs of the Gold
Coast: Vol. 5, 1952* (Accra, Gold Coast, 1952), 45–7.

84　Andrew Seaton has noted Maude's significance in the National Health
Service in 'Against the "Sacred Cow": NHS Opposition and the Fellowship
for Freedom in Medicine, 1948–72', *Twentieth Century British History*
26, no. 3 (September 2015): 424–49.

85 *Report of the Commission of Enquiry into the Health Needs of the Gold Coast: Vol. 5, 1952* (Accra, Gold Coast, 1952), 45–7.

86 *Statement by the Gold Coast Government on the Report of the Commission of Enquiry into the Health Needs of the Gold Coast* (Accra, Gold Coast: Government Printing Department, 1952), 5.

87 Stephen Addae, *Medical Histories Volume I: From Primitive to Modern Medicine (1850–2000)* (Accra: Eureka Foundation, 2012), 87–91.

88 Alexis de Toqueville, *Democracy in America*, trans. eds. Harvey C. Mansfield and Delba Winthrop (Chicago: University of Chicago Press, [1835–40] 2000), 491–3.

89 Sir John Maude, *The Place of Voluntary Effort in the National Health Service: Address to the Conference of the British Hospitals Contributory Schemes Association* (Bristol: British Hospitals Contributory Schemes Association, 1948), 5–11.

90 Ibid..

91 de Toqueville, *Democracy in America*, 491–3.

92 Maude, *The Place of Voluntary Effort in the National Health Service*, 5–11.

93 *Statement by the Gold Coast Government on the Report of the Commission of Enquiry into the Health Needs of the Gold Coast* (Accra, Gold Coast: Government Printing Department, 1952), 5.

94 Stuart, *British Missionaries and the End of Empire*, 6–25, 170–91, and 192–9.

95 Susan R. Whyte, 'In the Long Run: Ugandans Living with Disability', *Current Anthropology* 61, no. 21 (2020): S132–S140.

96 Jennings, 'Common Counsel, Common Policy', 939–63, esp. 960–1; Jennings, 'The Precariousness of the Franchise State', 1–8.

97 Emma Hunter, 'Voluntarism, Virtuous Citizenship and Nation-Building in Late Colonial and Early Post-colonial Tanzania', *African Studies Review* 58, no. 2 (2015): 43–61.

98 Guillaume Lachenal and Bertrand Taithe, 'Une généalogie missionnaire et coloniale de l'humanitaire: le cas Aujoulat au Cameroun, 1935–1973', *Le Mouvement Social* 227, no. 2 (2009): 45–63.

99 Elias K. Bongmba, 'From Medical Missions to Church Health Services', in *The Routledge Companion to Christianity in Africa*, ed. Elias K. Bongmba (London and New York: Routledge, 2016), 511.

100 Lynn M. Thomas, *Politics of the Womb: Women, Reproduction and the State in Kenya* (Berkeley and Los Angelese, California: University of California Press, 2003), 201–2.

101 Zambia, British Information Services, Centre Office of Information, Reference Division (1964), 23 and 43.

102 Chengetai J. Zvobgo, 'Medical Missions: A Neglected Theme in Zimbabwe's History, 1893–1957' *Zambezia* 13, no. 2 (1986): 109–18; 'Zimbabwe', in *The Statesman's Year-Book: Statistical and Historical Annual of the States of the World for the Year 1981–82*, ed. John Paxton (The Macmillan Press, 1981), 1637.

103 Joseph Roger de Benoist, *Histoire de l'Église Catholique au Sénégal: Du Milieu du XVe siècle à l'aube du troisième millénaire* (Dakar, Sénégal: Clairafrique and Karthala, 2007), 371.

104 Joseph M. Hodge and Gerald Hödl, 'Introduction', in *Developing Africa: Concepts and Practices in Twentieth-Century Colonialism*, eds. Joseph M. Hodge, Gerald Hödl, and Martina Kopf (Manchester and New York: Manchester University Press, 2014), 1–34.

105 Jennings, 'Common Counsel, Common Policy', 939–63, esp. 960–1; Jennings, 'The Precariousness of the Franchise State', 1–8.

106 Stuart, *British Missionaries and the End of Empire*, 6–-5, 170–91, and 192–9.

107 David Rooney, *Sir Charles Arden-Clarke* (London: Rex Collins, 1982), 15.

108 Ibid., 3, 15–19, 100–1.

109 Adrian Hastings, *A History of African Christianity 1950–1975* (Cambridge: Cambridge University Press, 1979), 35–67, 159–175, and 224–88.

110 The Methodists themselves were given grants from the government totalling £104,245 in 1951 alone; this was the second-largest government contribution from all their overseas income. The largest was Ceylon at £172,632. Of course, these were not just for health care and probably prioritised education; 'New Occasions: The Report of 1951 and the 166th Year of Methodist Missions, Arranged for Use with the Prayer Manual', *Methodist Missionary Society* (May 1952), 52, Archives and Special Collections, SOAS Library and Archives (London, UK).

111 Thomas Hutton-Mills, 'Committee of Supply: Ministry of Health: Expenditure', *Gold Coast Legislative Assembly 1954* (1 March, 1954), 1097–8, Balme Library, University of Ghana (Accra).

112 'Written Answers to Questions Rev. S. G. Nimako to I. Egala: Koforidua Hospital (Expenditure)', *Gold Coast Legislative Assembly Debates 1954* (13 August 1954), 22, Balme Library, University of Ghana (Accra).

113 'General Summary of Administration and Development: Staff and Services II', *Ghana Government Report of the Ministry of Health 1954* (Accra: Government Printing Department, 1957), 1–8.

114 J. Ajarquah to Imoru Egala, 'Written Answers to Questions: Ministry of Health: Mid-Volta Health Services (Grants)', *Gold Coast Legislative Assembly Debates 1956–57 Vol. 1* (22 May 1956), 60.

115 Given that the Colonial Office previously staffed hospitals, whereas the colonies paid recurrent costs as well as grants, it must be noted that the form of the provision medical mission received may have been a result of wider imperial policy. See J. Arjarquah, Emmanuel Adama Mahama, Mumuni Bawumia, and Joseph Dawson Wireko, 'Oral Answers to Questions: Ministry of Health: Missionary Hospitals/Dispensaries at the National Assembly', *National Assembly Debates 1958 Vol. 10* (20 June 1958), 117–18, Balme Library, University of Ghana (Accra).

116 Lionel Acton-Hubbard, 'Graduation at Kwahu Hospital', *British Advent Messenger 67*, no. 12 (8 June 1962): 1–3; Land, *Historical Dictionary of the Seventh-day Adventists*, 115.

117 'Medical Work', *60th Anniversary: The Salvation Army: Ghana Territory, 1922–1982* (1982), 7, Salvation Army International Heritage Centre Archive (London, UK).

118 'Oral Answers to Questions: Ministry of Health: New Dunkwa Hospital', *Gold Coast Legislative Assembly Debates 1953* (5 November 1953), 81–2, Balme Library, University of Ghana (Accra).

119 The struggle to staff hospitals was noted in the 1952 colonial medical department report; *Gold Coast Government Report on the Medical Department for the Year 1952* (Accra: Government Printing Department, 1952), 1–25, Liverpool School of Tropical Medicine (Liverpool, UK).

120 J.G. Awuah to Ferdinand Koblavi Dra Goka, 'Oral Answers to Questions: Berekum Holy Family Hospital (Government Subsidy)', *Gold Coast Legislative Assembly 1956–57 Vol. 1* (27 August 1956), 295, Balme Library, University of Ghana (Accra); Daniel Buadi to Ferdinand Koblavi Dra Goka, 'Oral Answers to Questions: Foso Clinic (Government Grant)', *Gold Coast Legislative Assembly 1956–57 Vol. 1* (27 August 1956), 296, Balme Library, University of Ghana (Accra).

121 Robert Okyere Amuaka-Atta to Ferdinand Koblavi Dra Goka, 'Oral Answers to Questions: Akrokerri Hospital (Government Subsidy)', *Gold Coast Legislative Assembly 1955* (14 November, 1955), 408, Balme Library, University of Ghana (Accra).

122 Christopher Samuel Takyi to Ferdinand Koblavi Dra Goka, 'Oral Answers to Questions: Takyiman Maternity Hospital (Government Subsidy)', *Gold Coast Legislative Assembly 1955* (8 November 1955), 224–5, Balme Library, University of Ghana (Accra).

123 Imoru Egala, 'Orders of the Day: Committee of Supply: Ministry of Health', *Gold Coast Legislative Assembly 1955* (17 March 1955), 1142, Balme Library, University of Ghana (Accra).

124 Emmanuel Adama Mahama, 'Oral Answers to Questions: Damongo Hospital (Ambulance Provision)', *Gold Coast Legislative Assembly Debates 1955* (22 March 1955), 1325, Balme Library, University of Ghana (Accra).

125 Boahene Yeboah-Afari to Thomas Hutton-Mills, 'Committee of Supply: Ministry of Health: Expenditure', *Gold Coast Legislative Assembly 1954* (1 March 1954), 1133–4, Balme Library, University of Ghana (Accra).

126 Editor, 'Evangelism', *Northern Light* 5, no. 7 (July 1955): 7.

127 'News Notes', *West African Advent Messenger: Voice of the West African Union Mission of Seventh-day Adventists* 11, no. 7 (July 1957): 3.

128 'Statistical Report of Seventh-day Adventist Conferences, Missions and Institutions in the World Field for the Year Ending December 31, 1957', *Ninety-Fifth Annual Statistical Report of Seventh-day Adventists 1957* (General Conference of Seventh-day Adventists, Washington, DC, 1957), 2 and 14.

129 'Adventist Doctor for West Africa', *British Advent Messenger: Organ of the British Union Conference of Seventh-day Adventists* (9 December 1955): 7.

130 Albert Floyd Tarr, 'Progress in Our Mission Fields', *Northern Light* 6, no. 6 (June 1956): 2.

131 Ibid., 2.

132 Albert Floyd Tarr, 'Heartening Progress in West Africa', *Northern Light* 9, no. 5 (May 1959): 4–5.

133 Lionel Acton-Hubbard, 'Kwahu Hospital Officially Opened', *Northern Light* 7, no. 12 (December 1957): 6; L. Acton-Hubbard, 'Graduation and Expansion at Kwahu Hospital', *West African Advent Messenger* 16, no. 6–7 (June–July 1962): 3.

134 Ibid., 4.

135 J.M. Bucy, 'Division Committee Highlights, November 6 to 13, 1957: New Gallery Fellowship Day', *Northern Lights: Organ of the Northern European Division* 8, no. 1 (January 1958): 1.

136 Lionel Acton-Hubbard, 'An Interesting Experiment at Kwahu', *Messenger: Voice of the West African Union Mission of Seventh-day Adventists* 11, no. 8 (August 1957): 1–2.

137 Isabel Hofmeyr, 'Inventing the World: Transnationalism, Transmission, and Christian Textualities', in *Mixed Messages: Materiality, Textuality,*

Missions, eds. Jamie S. Scott and Gareth Griffiths (New York: Palgrave Macmillan, 2005), 19–36.

138 Mary Fulbrook and Ulinka Rublack, 'In Relation: The "Social Self" and Ego-Documents', *German History* 28, no. 3 (1 September 2010): 263–72, citing Guido Ruggiero, *Machiavelli in Love: Sex, Self, and Society in the Italian Renaissance* (Baltimore: Johns Hopkins University Press, 2007), 21.

139 Lionel Acton-Hubbard, 'The Light Shines in Kwahu', *The West African Advent Messenger* 10, no. 8 (1 August 1956): 5.

140 Pamela Klassen, *Spirits of Protestantism: Medicine, Healing and Liberal Christianity* (Berkeley: University of California Press, 2011), 18, 102–3.

141 Lionel Acton Hubbard, 'Kwahu Hospital Light Bearers', *The West African Advent Messenger* 12, no. 5 (1 May 1958): 7.

142 Acton-Hubbard, 'An Interesting Experiment at Kwahu', 1–2.

143 In this work, Margaret Shirer became known nationally for producing the first written text of vernacular languages in the North; see 'Life in the Northern Territories: Pressing Problems of Roads, Water', *Daily Graphic* (7 February 1953): 7.

144 Kate Skinner, 'From Pentecostalism to Politics: Mass Literacy and Community Development in Late Colonial Northern Ghana', *Paedagogica Historica* 46, no. 3 (June 2010): 307–23, esp. 311–15.

145 Correspondence and papers of the Church of Scotland Overseas Council relating to Africa (1965–75), Acc. 9638 Church of Scotland, National Library of Scotland (Edinburgh, UK); Correspondence and reports home, under the auspices of the Church of Scotland's Missionary Partner Scheme of the Reverend Colin Forrester-Paton, in the Gold Coast, later Ghana, 1954–71, Acc. 11977, Church of Scotland, National Library of Scotland (Edinburgh, UK); Further papers, mainly ca. 1970–1995, but many earlier, relating to Church of Scotland and other Scottish Presbyterian Missions, and Scottish Churches abroad, Acc. 12398, Church of Scotland, National Library of Scotland (Edinburgh, UK); Colin Forrester-Paton Papers 1939–94, GB 3189 CSCNWW37, New College Library, University of Edinburgh (Edinburgh, UK); Berinyuu, ed., *History of the Presbyterian Church in Northern Ghana*, esp. 108.

146 Correspondence and papers of the Church of Scotland Overseas Council relating to Africa (1965–75), Acc. 9638 Church of Scotland, National Library of Scotland (Edinburgh, UK); Correspondence and reports home, under the auspices of the Church of Scotland's Missionary Partner Scheme of the Reverend Colin Forrester-Paton, in the Gold Coast, later Ghana, 1954–71, Acc. 11977, Church of Scotland, National Library of Scotland

(Edinburgh, UK); Further papers, mainly ca. 1970–1995, but many earlier, relating to Church of Scotland and other Scottish Presbyterian Missions, and Scottish Churches abroad, Acc. 12398, Church of Scotland, National Library of Scotland (Edinburgh, UK); Colin Forrester-Paton Papers 1939–94, GB 3189 CSCNWW37, New College Library, University of Edinburgh (Edinburgh, UK); Berinyuu, ed., *History of the Presbyterian Church in Northern Ghana*, 108.

147 Colin Forrester-Paton, 'Letter to Partners' (2 September 1957), Correspondence and reports home, under the auspices of the Church of Scotland's Missionary Partner Scheme of the Reverend Colin Forrester-Paton, in the Gold Coast, later Ghana, 1954–71, Acc. 11977, Church of Scotland, National Library of Scotland (Edinburgh, UK).

148 Jean Paton, 'Random Personal Memories of Sandema', in *History of the Presbyterian Church in Northern Ghana*, ed. Abraham Adu Berinyuu (Accra: Asempa Publishers, 1997), 126–31; Colin Forrester-Paton, 'Letter to Partners' (8 August 1959), Correspondence and reports home, under the auspices of the Church of Scotland's Missionary Partner Scheme of the Reverend Colin Forrester-Paton, in the Gold Coast, later Ghana, 1954–71, Acc. 11977, Church of Scotland, National Library of Scotland (Edinburgh, UK).

149 Julie Livingston, 'Disgust, Bodily Aesthetics and the Ethic of Being Human in Botswana', *Africa: The Journal of the International Africa Institute* 78, no. 2 (May 2008): 288–307.

150 Though it must be noted that bricolage is almost ever-present in health practice, as Livingston detailed at length; Julie Livingston, *Improvising Medicine: An African Oncology Ward in an Emerging Cancer Epidemic* (Durham, NC and London: Duke University Press, 2012); Leith L. Lombas, *Individualism in Action: An Investigation into the Lived Experiences of Peace Corps Volunteers* (doctoral thesis, University of Colorado, 2011), esp. 61; Michael E. Latham, *Modernization as Ideology: American Social Science and Nation-Building in the Kennedy Era* (Chapel Hill: University of North Carolina Press, 2000).

151 Paton, 'Random Personal Memories of Sandema', 126–31.

152 Robert Duncan, 'Letter to Rev Neil Bernard, Africa Secretary. F. M. C. (6 June 1960), Correspondence and papers of the Church of Scotland Overseas Council relating to Africa (1965–75), Acc. 9638, Church of Scotland, National Library of Scotland (Edinburgh, UK).

153 Justin Willis, 'Chieftaincy', in *The Oxford Handbook of Modern African History*, eds. John Parker and Richard Reid (Oxford: Oxford University Press, 2013), 208–23.

154 Christian Lund, *Local Politics and the Dynamics of Property in Africa* (Cambridge: Cambridge University Press, 2008), 1–67.

155 Rothberg, 'Plymouth Bretheren and the Occupation of Katanga', 285–97; Robert Duncan and Louise Duncan, 'Sandema District (II)', *History of the Presbyterian Church in Northern Ghana*, ed. Abraham Adu Berinyuu (Accra: Asempa Publishers, 1997), 135–41.

156 Colin Forrester-Paton, 'Sandema (1)', *History of the Presbyterian Church in Northern Ghana*, ed. Abraham Adu Berinyuu (Accra: Asempa Publishers, 1997), 108–25.

157 Gullestad, *Picturing Pity*, 275–9.

158 Mary Laven, *Mission to China: Matteo Ricci and the Jesuit Encounter with the East* (London: Faber and Faber, 2011).

159 Benjamin N. Lawrance, Emily L. Osborn, and Richard L. Roberts, eds., *Intermediaries, Interpreters and Clerks: African Employees in the Making of Colonial Africa* (Madison: University of Wisconsin Press, 2008).

160 Jamie S. Scott, 'Penitential and Penitentiary: Native Canadians and Colonial Mission Education', *Mixed Messages: Materiality, Textuality, Missions*, eds. Jamie S. Scott and Gareth Griffiths (New York: Palgrave Macmillan, 2005), 111–34.

161 Duncan and Duncan, 'Sandema District (II)', in Berinyuu, ed., *History of the Presbyterian Church in Northern Ghana*, 135–41.

162 Box 484, 'Report 1958–1959, Navrongo RS1, Rapports and Statistics', A.G.M. Afr., White Fathers Archive (Rome, Italy).

163 This is not to suggest that all conflict was inter-denominational. For example, there were fierce rivalries between Catholic missions such as with the Franciscan Sister of Mary and the White Sisters over episcopate favour in the late 1930s. Amidst these tensions the colonial government was a key player; in this case nuns used government recognition to free themselves from the tutelage of the White Fathers and episcopate control; Jean-Marie Bouron, 'Dominées ou dominantes? Les Soeurs Blanches dans L'Ambivalence des Logiques d'Autorité (Haute-Volta et Gold Coast, 1912–1960)', *Histoire, Monde et Cultures Religieuses* 30, no. 2 (2014): 51–73.

164 'Maternity and Child Welfare', *Report on the Medical Department for the Year 1951* (Accra: Government Printing Department, 1952), 11, Korle Bu Teaching Hospital (Accra).

165 'Birth, Still-Birth, Death, Neonatal, Infantile and Maternal Morality Rates – 1950–1954', *Report of the Medical Department for the Year 1954* (Accra: Government Printer, 1957), 21, 97, Wellcome Trust Library (London, UK).

166 J.K. Donkoh, J.G. Awuah, Dr Ansah-Koi, and Mr Boakye, 'Oral Answers to Questions: Ministry of Health: Maternity Death Rate and Infant Mortality Rate', *Gold Coast Legislative Assembly 1954* (1 March 1954), 1088–90, Balme Library, University of Ghana (Accra).

167 David E. Apter, *Ghana in Transition* (Princeton, NJ: Princeton University Press, 1955/2nd rev. ed. 1963), 40.

168 'Red Cross Clinics', *Report on the Medical Department for the Year 1955* (Accra: Government Printing Department, 1959), 48, Liverpool School of Tropical Medicine (Liverpool, UK).

169 For further information on this issue and how this information was obtained, please contact the author.

170 'Maternal and Child Welfare', *Gold Coast Colony Report on the Medical Department for the Year 1947* (Accra: Government Printing Department, 1948), 4, Korle Bu Teaching Hospital (Accra); 'Kumasi Health Week, 1929–1930: Group of Prize-Winning Babies', *Gold Coast Colony Report on the Medical and Sanitary Department for the Year 1929–1930* (1930), 13–57, Balme Library, University of Ghana (Accra).

CHAPTER TWO

1 David Maxwell, 'Decolonisation', in *Mission and Empire*, ed. Norman Etherington (Oxford: Oxford University Press, 2005), 290–1.

2 See also Adrian Hastings, *A History of African Christianity 1950–1975* (Cambridge: Cambridge University Press, 1979), 224.

3 Mumuni Bawumia was also the father of Ghana's vice-president since 2017, Mahamadu Bawumia.

4 'Distribution of Hospitals, Health Centres and Other Fixed Clinics by the Type of Institution and Region', *Republic of Ghana: Annual Report of the Medical Services of Ghana 1967*, 64, ACS0.1.48, Liverpool School of Tropical Medicine (Liverpool, UK).

5 Maxwell, 'Decolonization', 293.

6 Elizabeth Isichei, *A History of Christianity in Africa: From Antiquity to the Present* (SPCK, 1995), 325–7, 344.

7 Ogbu Uke Kalu, 'Passive Revolution and Its Saboteurs: African Christian Initiative in the Era of Decolonization, 1955–1975', in *Missions, Nationalism and the End of Empire*, eds. Brian Stanley and Alaine M. Low (Grand Rapids, MI: Wm B. Eerdmans Publishing, 2003), 265–77.

8 S.G.D., J. ST. G. Warmann: Regional Services Division, Ministry of Health and Social Welfare, 'Letter to Synod Clerk', (7 July 1961), Further papers, mainly ca. 1970–1995, but many earlier, relating to Church of Scotland and

other Scottish Presbyterian Missions, and Scottish Churches abroad, Acc.
12398, Church of Scotland National Library of Scotland (Edinburgh, UK).

9   Albert Lawrence Kwansa, 'To the Permanent Secretary of the Ministry of
Health', (Accra: 20 February 1959) Correspondence and reports home,
under the auspices of the Church of Scotland's Missionary Partner Scheme
of the Reverend Colin Forrester-Paton, in the Gold Coast, later Ghana,
1954–71, Acc. 11977, Church of Scotland, National Library of Scotland
(Edinburgh, UK).

10 Presbyterian Church of Ghana, 'Medical Work Report 1967/8' (1968),
Correspondence and reports home, under the auspices of the Church of
Scotland's Missionary Partner Scheme of the Reverend Colin Forrester-
Paton, in the Gold Coast, later Ghana, 1954–71, Acc. 11977, Church of
Scotland, National Library of Scotland (Edinburgh, UK).

11 Detailed analysis of the PCG and the Basel Mission can be found in Pascal
Schmid, *Medicine, Faith and Politics in Agogo: A History of Health Care
Delivery in Rural Ghana, ca. 1925 to 1980* (Vienna and Zürich: Lit Verlag
GmbH and Co. KG, 2018).

12 Presbyterian Church of Ghana, 'Medical Work Report 1967/8' (1968),
Further papers, mainly ca. 1970–1995, but many earlier, relating to
Church of Scotland and other Scottish Presbyterian Missions, and Scottish
Churches abroad, Acc. 12398, Church of Scotland, National Library of
Scotland (Edinburgh, UK).

13 Colin Forrester-Paton, 'Letter to Partners' (19 January 1970),
Correspondence and reports home, under the auspices of the Church of
Scotland's Missionary Partner Scheme of the Reverend Colin Forrester-
Paton, in the Gold Coast, later Ghana, 1954–71, Acc. 11977, Church of
Scotland, National Library of Scotland (Edinburgh, UK).

14 Felix Konotey-Ahulu et. al., *Report of the Committee Appointed to
Investigate Hospital Fees* (1971), 27–36, George Padmore Research
Library (Accra).

15 S.G.D., J. ST. G. Warmann: Regional Services Division, Ministry of Health
and Social Welfare, 'Letter to Synod Clerk', (7 July 1961).

16 Robert Duncan and Louise Duncan, 'Sandema District (II)', *History of the
Presbyterian Church in Northern Ghana*, ed. Abraham Adu Berinyuu
(Accra: Asempa Publishers, 1997), 135–41.

17 'Early History of the Presbyterian Mission of Sandema', *Buluk and the
Bulsa*, no. 4 (2005); 'Religion and Missions among the Bulsa', http://www.
buluk.de/.

18 Richard Rathbone, *Nkrumah and the Chiefs: The Politics of Chieftaincy
in Ghana, 1951–1960* (Oxford: James Currey, 2000), 48.

19 Justin Willis, 'Chieftaincy', in *The Oxford Handbook of Modern African History*, eds. John Parker and Richard Reid (Oxford: Oxford University Press, 2013), 208–23.

20 J. G. Awuah to Ferdinand Koblavi Dra Goka, 'Oral Answers to Questions: Berekum Holy Family Hospital (Government Subsidy)', *Gold Coast Legislative Assembly 1956–57 Vol. 1* (27 August 1956), 295–6, Balme Library, University of Ghana (Accra).

21 Christopher Samuel Takyi to Ferdinand Koblavi Dra Goka, 'Oral Answers to Questions: Ministry of Health: Techiman Holy Family Dispensary', *Parliamentary Assembly* (27 June 1957), 1415, C.S.C. 450 British Library (Boston Spa, UK).

22 Christopher Samuel Takyi to Kodzo, 'Oral Answers to Questions, Mission Hospitals (State Aid)', *Parliamentary Assembly Debates* (28 July 1961), 836–7, C.S.C. 450 British Library (Boston Spa, UK).

23 Patrick A. Twumasi, *Survey Report Health Services in Ghana: National Catholic Secretariat January–April 1982* (April 1982, Department of Health, National Catholic Secretariat, Accra), 42–6, 66, National Catholic Secretariat (Accra).

24 'Holy Family Hospital, Berekum, Gold Coast (Ghana) 1948–1967', 195–6, MMS Archive, Fox Chase, (Philadelphia, USA).

25 Maxwell, 'Decolonization', in Etherington ed., *Mission and Empire*, 285–306; David Maxwell, 'Post-colonial Christianity in Africa', in *The Cambridge History of Christianity*, vol. 9, *World Christianities c.1914–c.2000*, ed. Hugh McLeod (Cambridge: Cambridge University Press, 2006), 401–21; Twumasi, *Survey Report Health Services in Ghana*, 192–8.

26 'Issues, Problems, and Priorities of the Health System in Ghana: Background Paper Prepared by the Ministry of Health, for the National Health Symposium, State House, Accra, June 7–8, 1988' (Ministry of Health, Accra, 31 May 1988), 1, National Catholic Secretariat (Accra).

27 David Rooney, *Kwame Nkrumah: Vision and Tragedy* (Ghana: Sub-Saharan Publishers, 1988), 23–5.

28 For similar processes in a different time period and culture see Alexandra Walsham, 'Historiographical Reviews: The Reformation and the "Disenchantment of the World" Reassessed', *The Historical Journal* 51, no. 2 (2008): 497–528, citing Robert W. Scribner, 'The Impact of the Reformation on Everyday Life', in *Mensch und objekt im mittelalter und in der frü hen neuzeit* (Osterrichische Akademie der Wissenshaften, Philosphisch-Historische Klasse Sitzungsberichte, vol. 568, Vienna, 1990), 315–43.

29 Robert Yaw Owusu, *Kwame Nkrumah's Liberation Thought: A Paradigm for Religious Advcoacy in Contemporary Ghana* (Eritrea: African World Press, 2006), 137; Colin Forrester-Paton, 'Letter to E. C. Bernard (African and America Secretary) copy to WFM and T. S. Colvin' (1 December 1961), Ghana Treasury and Secretary 1955–1961, Correspondence and reports home, under the auspices of the Church of Scotland's Missionary Partner, Acc. 11977, Church of Scotland, National Library of Scotland (Edinburgh, UK).

30 Ahmad A. Rahman, *The Regime Change of Kwame Nkrumah: Epic Heroism in Africa and the Diaspora* (New York: Palgrave Macmillan, 2007), 102.

31 Ebenezer Obiri Addo, *Kwame Nkrumah: A Case Study of Religion and Politics in Ghana* (Maryland: University Press of America, 1997/1999), 65–8.

32 Rupe Simms, '"I am a Non-Denominational Christian and a Marxist Socialist": A Gramscian Analysis of the Convention People's Party and Kwame Nkrumah's Use of Religion', *Sociology of Religion* 64, no. 4 (2003): 463–77.

33 Ibid.

34 Florence M. Bourret, *The Road to Independence, 1919–1957* (Stanford, CA: Stanford University Press, 1960), 150.

35 This election was based on around 30 per cent of the adult population and is covered extensively in other histories; see Roger Gocking, *The History of Ghana* (Westport, CT: Greenwood Press, 2005), 99–104.

36 Harris W. Mobley, *The Ghanaian's Image of the Missionary: An Analysis of the Published Critiques of Christian Missionaries by Ghanaians 1897–1965* (Leiden: E.J. Brill, 1970).

37 On the 1950s elections, the role of the school-leavers, and the CPP, see Bourret, *The Road to Independence, 1919–1957.*

38 Mobley, *The Ghanaian's Image of the Missionary*, 150, citing K. Nkrumah, *Africa Must Unite* (New York: F.A. Praeger, 1963), xiii, 5, and 22.

39 Mobley, *The Ghanaian's Image of the Missionary*, 150, citing A. Quaison-Sackey, *Africa Unbound* (New York: F.A. Praeger, 1963), 53. The title of Quaison-Sackey's book was in direct reference to Joseph Casely Hayford's attack on imperialism in his work *Ethiopia Unbound* (London: C.M. Philips, 1911), which extensively explored the relationship between mission and colonialism in the Gold Coast.

40 Jon Miller, *Missionary Zeal and Institutional Control: Organizational Contradictions in the Basel Mission on the Gold Coast, 1828–1917* (New York: Wm B. Eerdmans Press, 2003), 29.

41 Jeff D. Grischow, 'Kwame Nkrumah, Disability and Rehabilitation in
    Ghana, 1957–66', *The Journal of African History* 52, no. 2 (July 2011):
    179–99.
42 Jean Allman, 'Phantoms of the Archive: Kwame Nkrumah, a Nazi Pilot
    Named Hanna and the Contingencies of Postcolonial History Writing',
    The American Historical Review 118, no. 1 (February 2018): 104–29.
43 Nkrumah's tensions with the US and how missions figured within these
    will be further elaborated in chapter 4.
44 Lord Mawuko-Yevugah, *Reinventing Development: Aid Reform and
    Technologies of Governance in Ghana* (Farnham, Surrey and Burlington,
    VT: Ashgate, 2014), 62.
45 Obiri Addo, *Kwame Nkrumah*, 67–8, citing K. Nkrumah, *Consciencism*
    (New York: Monthly Press Review, 1964), 13.
46 Rahman, *The Regime Change of Kwame Nkrumah*, 80.
47 Andrew C. Wheeler, 'From Mission to Church in an Islamizing State:
    The Case of Sudan, 1946–64', in *Christian Missionaries and the State in
    the Third World*, eds. Holger Bernt Hansen and Michael Twaddle (Melton,
    UK: James Currey, 2002), 284–99.
48 Stephen Addae, *Medical Histories, Volume 1: From Primitive to Modern
    Medicine (1850-2000)* (Accra: Eureka Foundation, 2012), 76–90.
49 Ferdinand Koblavi Dra Goka to Jatoe Kaleo, 'Oral Answers to Questions:
    Ministry of Health: Health Centres', *National Assembly Debates 1957*
    (3 December 1957), 233, C.S.C. 450, British Library (Boston Spa, UK).
50 B.A. Konu to Ferdinand Koblavi Dra Goka, 'Oral Answers to Questions:
    Ministry of Health', *National Assembly Debates 1957* (30 May 1957),
    333–5, C.S.C. 450, British Library (Boston Spa, UK).
51 Ferdinand Koblavi Dra Goka to B.A. Konu, 'Oral Answers to Questions:
    Ministry of Health', *National Assembly Debates 1957* (30 May 1957),
    333–5, C.S.C. 450, British Library (Boston Spa, UK).
52 'A Time for Ambition' *Ghana Today* 3, no. 2 (London: Published by the
    information section of the Ghana Office, 18 March 1959), accessed at the
    University of Ghana, Accra; 'Health: A Field of Vast Problems', 3.2 *Ghana
    Today* (London: Published by the information section of the Ghana Office,
    18 March 1959), Balme Library, University of Ghana (Accra).
53 This was the historic Presbyterian Church that set up a hospital at Adidome
    and had its roots in the Bremen and Scottish Presbyterian missions.
54 Ferdinand Koblavi Dra Goka, Mr Kodzo and Mr Kusi, 'Oral Answers to
    Questions: Ministry of Health: Worawora Hospital', *National Assembly
    Debates 1957* (28 June 1957), 1472–3, C.S.C. 450, British Library
    (Boston Spa, UK).

55 Ibid.

56 Ibid.

57 Ibid.; John S. Pobee, *Kwame Nkrumah and the Church in Ghana 1949–1966 : A study in the Relationship between the Socialist Government of Kwame Nkrumah, the First Prime Minister and First President of Ghana, and the Protestant Christian Churches in Ghana* (Accra: Asempa Publishers, 1988), 94–5.

58 David Hardiman, 'Introduction', in *Healing Bodies, Saving Souls: Medical Missions in Asia and Africa*, ed. David Hardiman (Amsterdam and New York: Rodopi B.V., 2006), 21.

59 Adrian Hastings, *A History of African Christianity 1950–1975* (Cambridge: Cambridge University Press, 1979), 35–67, 159–75, and 224–88.

60 Maxwell, 'Post-Colonial Christianity in Africa', 410–11.

61 Maxwell, 'Decolonization', 296.

62 Ibid., 285–306.

63 J. Arjarquah, Emmanuel Adama Mahama, Mumuni Bawumia, and Joseph Dawson Wireko, 'Oral Answers to Questions: Ministry of Health: Missionary Hospitals/Dispensaries at the National Assembly', *National Assembly Debates 1958* (20 June 1958), 117–18, C.S.C. 450, British Library (Boston Spa, UK).

64 Alhaji Mumuni Bawumia, *Memoirs of Alhaji Mumuni Bawumia: A Life in the Political History of Ghana* (Accra: Ghana Universities Press, 2004), 142, 164.

65 Ibid., 32–4.

66 Ibid.

67 Ibid.

68 Arjarquah, Mahama, Bawumia, and Wireko, 'Oral Answers to Questions: Ministry of Health: Missionary Hospitals/Dispensaries at the National Assembly', 117–18.

69 Mumuni Bawumia, *Memoirs of Alhaji Mumuni Bawumia*, 32–4.

70 Joseph Emmanuel Appiah, 'Motion: Ministry of Health', *National Assembly Debates 1960* (30 August 1960), 969–74, C.S.C. 450, British Library (Boston Spa, UK).

71 Ibid.

72 Ibid.

73 Richard Rathbone, *Nkrumah and the Chiefs: The Politics of Chieftaincy in Ghana, 1951–60* (Oxford: James Currey, 2000).

74 Gocking, *The History of Ghana*, 123–4, 104–11.

75 Paul Ladouceur, *Chiefs and Politicians: The Politics of Regionalism in Northern Ghana* (Longman Group, 1979), 212–72.

76 Gocking, *The History of Ghana*, 123–4, 104–11; Rathbone, *Nkrumah and the Chiefs*; Allman, 'Phantoms of the Archive', 104–29.
77 Joseph M. Hodge, 'British Colonial Expertise, Post-Colonial Careering and the Early History of International Development', *Journal of Modern European History* 8, no. 1 (April 2010): 24–46.
78 Robert L. Tignor, *W. Arthur Lewis and the Birth of Development Economics* (Princeton, NJ: Princeton University Press, 2006), esp. 250–1.
79 Sabine Clarke, 'A Technocratic Imperial State? The Colonial Office and Scientific Research, 1940–1960', *Twentieth Century British History* 18, no. 4 (1 January 2007): 453–80.
80 James Ferguson, *The Anti-Politics Machine: "Development", Depoliticization and Bureaucratic Power in Lesotho* (Cambridge: Cambridge University Press, 2000), 256.
81 Christopher Samuel Takyi, 'Motion: Ministry of Health', *National Assembly Debates 1960* (30 August 1960), 986, C.S.C. 450, British Library (Boston Spa, UK).
82 Christopher Samuel Takyi, 'Motion: Ministry of Health: Progress Report', *National Assembly Debates 1961* (4 May 1961), 36, C.S.C. 450, British Library (Boston Spa, UK).
83 Daniel Buadi, 'Motion: Ministry of Health' *National Assembly Debates 1960* (30 August 1960), 992, C.S.C. 450, British Library (Boston Spa, UK).
84 Mr Asumda to Jambaidu Awuni, 'Oral Answers to Questions: Health and Social Welfare: Bawku Hospital', *National Assembly Debates 1959* (23 July 1959), 893, C.S.C. 450, British Library (Boston Spa, UK).
85 Ayeebo Asumda to Jambaidu Awuni, 'Oral Answers to Questions: Health and Social Welfare: Bawku Hospital (X-Ray)', *National Assembly Debates 1959* (27 July 1959), 1016, C.S.C. 450, British Library (Boston Spa, UK).
86 Lawrence Rosario Abavana (minister of health), 'Motion: Ministry of Health', *National Assembly Debates 1960* (30 August 1960), 960, C.S.C. 450, British Library (Boston Spa, UK).
87 Joseph Kodzo (ministerial secretary to the minister of health), 'Oral Answers to Questions: Health: Bawku Hospital (Female Ward)', *National Assembly Debates 1961* (27 February 1961), 267, C.S.C. 450, British Library (Boston Spa, UK).
88 Lawrence Rosario Abavana, 'Motion: Ministry of Health: Missions', *National Assembly 1961* (4 May 1961), 350, C.S.C. 450, British Library (Boston Spa, UK).
89 Ibid., 381.

90 J.A. Owusu-Ansah, 'Motion: Hospital Staff Service Conditions', *National Assembly 1958* (29 August 1958), 1944–46, Balme Library, University of Ghana (Boston Spa, UK).

91 K. Yankah, 'Point of Order: A Note on Language in Parliament', *Graphic Online* (8 March 2004), citing *Parliamentary Debates 1965*, 113.

92 Jambaidu Awuni, 'Ministry of Health: Estimates', *National Assembly Debates 1965* (8 February 1965), 851–2, Balme Library, University of Ghana (Accra).

93 Box 686, J.A. Richard to Richard Walsh, Rg A1, 145–213 (1960–62, 1963–65) A.G.M. Afr., White Fathers Archives (Rome, Italy).

94 Ibid.

95 Colin Forrester-Paton to Partners, 'Pressures on the Church in Ghana' (15 March 1962), Correspondence and papers of the Church of Scotland Overseas Council relating to Africa (1965–75), Acc. 9638, Church of Scotland, National Library of Scotland (Edinburgh, UK).

96 Brian Stanley, 'Christianity and the End of Empire', in *Missions, Nationalism and the End of Empire*, ed. Brian Stanley (Wm B. Eerdmans Publishing Co., 2003), 1–11.

97 Maxwell, 'Post-Colonial Christianity in Africa', 417, citing Terence Ranger, 'Introduction', *Evangelical Christianity and Democracy in Africa*, ed. Terence Ranger (Oxford: Oxford University Press, 2006).

98 David Murray, *Bits and Pieces: The Undistinguished Career of David Murray* (unpublished memoir, 2011).

99 Ibid.; B. Baddoo, *To Ghana with Love* (lulu.com, 2012).

100 'Appendices: Table 1A: Registration of Medical and Dental Practitioners in Ghana 1963-67', *Republic of Ghana: Annual Report of the Medical Services of Ghana 1967*, 55, ACS0.1.48, LSTM (Liverpool, UK).

101 'Table 8: Distribution of Hospitals, Health Centres and Other Fixed Clinics by the Type of Institution and Region', *Republic of Ghana: Annual Report of the Medical Services of Ghana 1967*, 64, ACS0.1.48, LSTM (Liverpool, UK).

102 'Maternal and Child Health Services', *Republic of Ghana: Annual Report of the Medical Services of Ghana 1967*, 25 and 64, ACS0.1.48, LSTM (Liverpool, UK).

103 'Control of Communicable Diseases', *Republic of Ghana: Annual Report of the Medical Services of Ghana 1967*, 10, ACS0.1.48, LSTM (Liverpool, UK).

104 Kathleen Vongsathorn, '"First and Foremost the Evangelist"?'.

105 Owusu-Afriyie, 'Ministry of Health: Estimates', National Assembly (8 February 1965), 805, C.S.C. 450, British Library (Boston Spa, UK).

CHAPTER THREE

1 As Corinna Unger puts it: 'Most scholars agree that the initially humanitarian impetus in the aftermath of World War II was marginalized by Cold
War-inspired geostrategic concerns in the late 1940s. Thus, while modernization thinking in many ways constituted a revised and expanded version
of earlier development discourses, its implementation in the form of professional development aid was very much a post-1945 phenomenon'.
Corinna R. Unger, 'Histories of Development and Modernization:
Findings, Reflections, Future Research', *H-Soz-Kult* (12 September 2010).

2 Erez Manela, 'Globalizing the Great Society: Lyndon Johnson and the
Pursuit of Smallpox Eradication', in *Beyond the Cold War: Lyndon
Johnson and the New Global Challenges of the 1960s*, eds. Francis J.
Gavin and Mark Atwood Lawrence (Oxford: Oxford University Press,
2014), 166, citing Akira Iriye, *Global Community: The Role of
International Organisations in the Making of the Contemporary World*
(Berkeley: University of California Press, 2002).

3 Iris Borowy, 'East German Medical Aid to Nicaragua: The Politics of
Solidarity between Biomedicine and Primary Health Care', *História,
Ciêncas, Saúde – Manguinhos* 24, no. 2 (Rio de Janeiro, April–June 2017):
411–28.

4 Douglas Coombs, *The Gold Coast, Britain and the Netherlands, 1850–
1874* (Oxford: Oxford University Press, 1963).

5 Jonathan Roberts, 'Korle and the Mosquito: Histories and Memories of
the Anti-Malaria Campaign in Accra, 1942–5', *The Journal of African
History* 51, no. 3 (2010): 343–65.

6 Niels Brimnes, 'Vikings against Tuberculosis: The International
Tuberculosis Campaign in India, 1948–1951', *Bull Hist Med.* 81, no. 2
(summer 2007): 407–30.

7 Tony Judt, *Postwar: A History of Europe since 1945* (London: William
Heinemann, 2005; London: Pimlico, 2007), 264–7.

8 Thanks to Henning Grunwald for his comments, guidance, and other
advice relating to postwar German politics and the Nazi persecution of
Catholics; any errors are my own.

9 James Hitchcock, *History of the Catholic Church: From the Apostolic Age
to the Third Millennium* (San Francisco: Ignatius Press, 2012), 386.

10 Gregory Witkoski, 'Between Fighters and Beggars: Socialist Philanthropy
and the Imagery of Solidarity in East Germany', in *Comrades of Color:
East Germany in the Cold War World*, ed. Quinn Slobodian (New York:
Bergahn Books, 2015), 80–5.

11 Misereror, 'Geschichte', https://www.misereor.de/; 'Papstdank für die
    Deutsche Fastenspende', *Passauer Neue Press: Niederbayerische Zeitung*,
    Ausgabe Nr. 149 (3 July 1959); Paddy Kearney, *Guardian of the Light:
    Denis Hurley; Renewing the Church, Opposing Apartheid* (New York:
    The Continuum International Publishing Group, 2009); Hermógenes E.
    Bacareza, *A History of German-Phillipine Relations* (National Economic
    and Development Authority-APO Production Unit, 1980), 214.
12 Walter Bruchhausen, 'From Charity to Development: Christian
    International Health Organizations, 1945–1978', *Hygiea Internationalis:
    An Interdisciplinary Journal for the History of Public Health* 13, no. 1
    (December 2016): 121.
13 Witkoski, 'Between Fighters and Beggars', 80–5.
14 Dora Vargha, 'Between East and West: Polio Vaccination across the Iron
    Curtain in Cold War Hungary', *Bulletin of the History of Medicine* 88,
    no. 2 (summer 2014): 319–42.
15 Judith Randel and Tony German, 'Germany', in *Stakeholders: Government-
    NGO Partnerships for International Development*, eds. Ian Smillie and
    Henny Helmich (New York: Earthscan Publications, 1999), 114.
16 Barbra Mann Wall, *Into Africa: A Transnational History of Catholic
    Medical Missions and Social Change* (New Brunswick, NJ: Rutgers
    University Press, 2015), t53.
17 Karel Steenbrink, 'The Power of Money: Development Aid for and through
    Christian Churches in Modern Indonesia, 1965–1980', *Christianity in
    Indonesia: Perspectives of Power*, ed. Susanne Schröter (Berlin: Lit Verlag,
    2010), 109.
18 Hanaan Marwah, 'Institutional Failure or an Unsustainable Foreign Debt
    Burden? Financing and Management of Ghana State-owned Electricity
    Distribution 1960–2002' (ESSHC conference, Belfast, 5 April 2018).
19 Kees Biekart, *The Politics of Civil Society Building: European Private Aid
    Agencies and Democratic Transitions in Central America* (Utrecht:
    International Books; Amsterdam: Transnational Institute, 1999), 67.
20 Steenbrink, 'The Power of Money', 107–9.
21 Ibid., 119–22.
22 Correspondence to author from Béatrice Looijenga (5 October 2017).
23 For further information on how this was obtained, please contact the
    author.
24 Carole Rensch and Walter Bruchhausen, 'Medical Science Meets
    'Development Aid' Transfer and Adaptation of West German
    Microbiology to Togo, 1960–1980' *Medical History* 61, no. 1 (January
    2017): 1–24.

25 John Iliffe, *East African Doctors: A History of the Modern Profession* (Cambridge: Cambridge University Press, 1998), 34, 200–20.

26 Reinhert Kössler, *Namibia and Germany: Negotiating the Past* (Windhoek: University of Namibia Press, 2015), 237.

27 Mattias Egg, *Krankenfürsorge im Spannungsfeld von Medizin, Glauben und Gesundheitspolitik Die Gemeinschaft der Missionshelferinnen, 1952–1994* (Inaugural-Dissertation zur Erlangung des Doktorgrades der Hohen Medizinischen Fakultät der Rheinischen Friedrich-Wilhelms-Universität Bonn, 2015)

28 Christoph Hendrik Müller, *West Germans against the West: Anti-Americanism in Media and Public Opinion in the Federal Republic of Germany, 1949–1968* (Palgrave Macmillan, 2010), 5, 15–16.

29 Barbara Marshall, 'The Democratization of Local Politics in the British Zone in Germany: Hanover 1945–7', *Journal of Contemporary History* 21, no. 3 (July 1986): 414.

30 Ian Turner, 'Denazification in the British Zone', in *Reconstruction in Post-War Germany: British Occupation Policy and the Western Zones, 1945–55*, ed. Ian Turner (Oxford: Berg Publishers, 1989), 11; Marshall, 'The Democratization of Local Politics in the British Zone in Germany', 414, 447.

31 Cas Mudde, *The Ideology of the Extreme Right* (Manchester: University of Manchester Press, 2000), 117.

32 Robert G. Moeller, 'The "Remasculinization" of Germany in the 1950s: Introduction' *Signs* 24, no. 1 (Autumn, 1998): 101–6; Eva Kolinsky, 'Women in the New Germany: The East-West Divide' in *Developments in German Politics* eds. Gordon Smith, William E. Paterson, Peter H. Merkl, and Stephen Padgett (London: Palgrave, Macmillan Publishers Ltd, 1992), 264–80.

33 Melani McAlister, 'The Global Conscience of American Evangelicalism: Internationalism and Social Concern in the 1970s and Beyond', *Journal of American Studies* 51, no. 4, Exploring the History of American Evangelicalism (November 2017): 1197–220.

34 As Cooper puts it: 'To nationalists, a development that would serve African interests required African rule. After independence, new rules could claim a place for themselves as intermediaries between external resources and national aspirations'; Frederick Cooper, *Africa since 1940: The Past of the Present* (Cambridge: Cambridge University Press, 2nd ed., 2019), 127.

35 Beth A. Griech-Polelle, 'Review of S. Brown-Fleming, *Holocaust and Catholic Conscience: Cardinal Aloisius Muench and the Guilt Question in Germany*', *H-German, H-Net Reviews* (September 2006).

36 'Deutschland: Zitate', *Der Spiegel* no. 14, Panorama (31 March 1964): 20.

37 'Lübke würdigt Misereor-Werk der katholischen Kirche: Kundgebung in Köln zum fünfjährigen Bestehen der Aktion gegen Hunger und Krankheit auf der ganzen Welt', *Passauer Neue Press*, Ausgabe Nr. 57 (9 March 1964).

38 'Adveniat: Spenden sehr grosszügig', *Passauer Neue Presse*, Ausgabe Nr. 22 (28 January 1964); 'Bischof Simon Konrad ruft die Katholiken des Bistums Pissau', *Passauer Neue Press*, Ausgabe Nr. 85 (11 April 1962); 'Bischof Simon Konrad ruft die Katholiken des Bistums Pissau', *Passauer Neue Press*, Ausgabe Nr. 80 (4 April 1963); 'Bischof von Essen: An die katholischen Leser dieser Zeitung!', *Passauer Neue Press*, Ausgabe Nr. 298 (27 December 1963)

39 'Deutsche Hilfe für Aufbau des Arbeitsdienstes: 30,000 Arbeitskräfte sollen Strassen und Brücken bauen – Schulungszentrum und Arbeitsgerät erwünscht', *Passauer Neue Press: Niederbayerische Zeitung*, Ausgabe Nr. 190 (19 August 1965).

40 '24. Juni 1963 – Der Deutsche Entwicklungsdienst (DED) wird gegründet', WDR.*de* (24 June 2013).

41 'Fastenopfer brachte 32 Millionen DM', *Passauer Neue Press*, Ausgabe Nr. 93 (23 March 1959); 'Papstdank für die Deutsche Fastenspende', *Passauer Neue Press: Niederbayerische Zeitung*, Ausgabe Nr. 149 (3 July 1959); 'Vierte Misereor-Kollekte: Köln', *Passauer Neue Press*, Ausgabe Nr. 47 (26 February 1962); '"Misereor" Aktion angelaufen: Bonn', *Passauer Neue Press*, Ausgabe Nr. 75 (30 March 1962); 'Pallaeur Nachrichten: Haute beginnt die Fastenaktion', *Passauer Neue Press*, Ausgabe Nr. 49 (27 February 1963); 'Wieder Fastenaktion: Aachen', *Passauer Neue Press*, Ausgabe Nr. 51 (01 March 1963); 'Misereor will die Not in aller Welt lindern: Die Fastenaktion soll eine Botschaft von Gottes Ordnung sein', *Passauer Neue Press*, Ausgabe Nr. 62 (14 March 1963); 'Fastenopfer wird eingesammelt: Aachen', *Passauer Neue Press*, Ausgabe Nr. 76 (30 March 1963); 'Ein Tropfen auf einen heissen Stein? Wider Sammlung für die Fastenaktion "Misereor"', *Passauer Neue Press*, Ausgabe Nr. 76 (30 March 1963); 'Neue Fastenspende: Köln', *Passauer Neue Press*, Ausgabe Nr. 33 (10 February 1964); 'Fastenopfer 1965 erbrachte 46 Millionen', *Passauer Neue Press: Niederbayerische Zeitung*, Ausgabe Nr. 120 (26 May 1965).

42 'Opfer gegen Hunger und Krankheit: Hamburg', *Passauer Neue Press*, Ausgabe Nr. 83 (9 April 1962); 'Hohes Misereor-Ergebnis: Mainz', *Passauer Neue Press*, 85 (10 April 1963); 'Über 3 Millionen DM gespendet: Passau', *Passauer Neue Presse*, Ausgabe Nr. 66 (19 March 1964);

'Deutsche Hilfe für Aufbau des Arbeitdienstes in Ghana', *Passauer Neue Presse: Niederbayerische Zeitung* Nr. 190, Seite 2 (19 August 1965).

43 'Gebefreudigkeit hat night nachgelassen: Misereor-Spenden der Passauer Pfarrelen so gut wie 1963', *Passauer Neue Press*, Ausgabe Nr. 66 (19 March 1964).

44 'Blick in die Welt: Die stille Entwicklungshilfe der Kirchen: Katholische und evangelische Kirchen sommelten 170 Millionen DM für Notleidende in aller Welt', *Passauer Neue Presse*, Ausgabe Nr. 278 (2 December 1961).

45 'Bischöfliches Hilfswerk MISEREOR e.V.: Ghana – Anzahl und Bewilligungssumme de bewilligten Projekte der DAC-Gruppe 1 im Zeitraum 1959–1990', Bischöfliches Hilfswerk MISEREOR e.V. 11.05.2017 ZI: Statistik/En Archiv/MV, Statistik für Herrn Benjamin Walker, Courtesy of Valentin Moser, Misereor Archives (Aachen, Germany).

46 David Maxwell, *Christians and Chiefs in Zimbabwe: A Social History of the Hwesa People, c. 1870s–1990s* (Edinburgh: Edinburgh University Press, 1999), 69–102.

47 R.G. Brooks, 'Ghana Health Expenditures 1966–80: A Commentary', *Strathclyde Discussion Papers in Economics* 80, no. 1 (Glasgow, Strathclyde: University of Strathclyde, 1981): 41, 50.

48 'Ghana Medical Facilities', *Second Ghana International Trade Fair* (1–14 February 1971), 1–27, PRAAD (Accra); 'Appendix 9: Geographical Distribution of Hospitals (1973)', *Ghana* (Department of Health and Social Security, October 1976), The National Archives (Kew, UK).

49 Nathan Samwini, *The Muslim Resurgence in Ghana since 1950: Its Effects upon Muslims, and Muslim-Christian Relations* (Münster: LIT Verlag, 2006), 170–1.

50 'Ghana Medical Facilities', *Second Ghana International Trade Fair* (1–14 February 1971), 9, PRAAD (Accra).

51 Ibid., 18.

52 'Gh.27: Ghana: CHAG's Efforts in Health Care' (August 1984), 1–9, Annexes I-III, SOAS Library and Archives (London, UK).

53 Brooks, 'Ghana Health Expenditures 1966-80', 34–6, 52.

54 For more detail on CHAG and its development, see Annabel Grieve and Jill Olivier, 'Towards Universal Health Coverage: A Mixed-Method Study Mapping the Development of Faith-Based Non-profit Sector in the Ghanaian Health System', *International Journal for Equity in Health* 17, no. 97 (2018).

55 'ICCO' (28 May 1985, DbB/ap), SOAS Library and Archives (London, UK); 'Ghana: CHAG Drug Supply Programme', CMC Pharmaceutical Advisory

Group held at DIFÄM, Tübingen, FRG' (1–2 April 1985), SOAS Library and Archives (London, UK).

56 'Gh.27: Ghana: CHAG's Efforts in Health Care' (August 1984), 1–9, Annexes I-III, SOAS Library and Archives (London, UK).

57 Jambaidu Awuni, 'Ministry of Health: Estimates', *National Assembly Debates 1965* (8 February 1965), 851–2, Balme Library, University of Ghana (Accra).

58 Barbra Mann Wall, *Into Africa: A Transnational History of Catholic Medical Missions and Social Change* (New Brunswick, NJ: Rutgers University Press), 53.

59 'Erste Ausbaustufe des Holy Family Hospitals in Berekum, ZU:130–4/3 Z 1233', *Projekt Nr. 130-009-0001*, DAC 111, *Bewill Jahr 1973, Ghana – Bewilligungen 1959–1980 DAC 1*, Misereor-Archive (Aachen, Germany).

60 'Ausbau Des St. Marten's Hospitals Agroyesum', *Projekt-NR 130-004-0001*, DAC 111, *Bewill Jahr 1961, Ghana – Bewilligungen 1959–1980 DAC 1*, Misereor-Archive (Aachen, Germany).

61 While the document did not specify DM or cedis, it is most likely that this is DM; Ausbau Krankenhaus Errichtung Pflegerinnenschule Kpandu Ghana', *Projekt-NR 130-003-0001 A, DAC 111, Bewill Jahr 1961, Ghana – Bewilligungen 1959–1980 DAC 1*, Misereor-Archive (Aachen, Germany).

62 'Röntgengerät für das Hospital in Assen Foso', *Projekt-NR 130-002-0016A, DAC 111, Bewill Jahr 1975, Ghana – Bewilligungen 1959–1980 DAC 1*, Misereor-Archive (Aachen, Germany).

63 'Construction of Staff Accommodation at Various Health Care Institutions in the Diocese of Accra', *Projekt NR 130-0/4- KH 789* (16 December 1980), *Ghana – Bewilligungen 1959–1980 DAC 1*, Misereor-Archive (Aachen, Germany).

64 'Essential Improvements Fund for the Preparation of Church Health Care Institutions in Ghana for Basic Health Care Work', *Projekt-NR 130-0/31 Z 2891* (1979) *Ghana – Bewilligungen 1959–1980 DAC 1*, Misereor-Archive (Aachen, Germany).

65 'Report of the Auditor to the Department of Health, National Catholic Secretariat on the State of Affairs of the Essential Improvement Fund' (14 July 1986), *Ghana – Bewilligungen 1959–1980 DAC 1*, Misereor-Archive (Aachen, Germany).

66 'Misereor Hospitals' Improvement Fund – Last Payments', *Projekt NR-130 - 0 - 3 NT 2894* (30 December 1981) *Ghana – Bewilligungen 1959–1980 DAC 1*, Misereor-Archive (Aachen, Germany).

67 'Mobile Eye Clinic Nandom Hospital, Annual Report 1981', *Projekt NR-130-7/2* (23 February 1981), *Ghana – Bewilligungen 1959–1980 DAC 1*, Misereor-Archive (Aachen, Germany).

68 'Nandom Hospital: Statement of Accounts: Yearly Report For Year Ending 31st Dec. 81', *Projekt* NR- *190-7-2D* (1980) *Ghana – Bewilligungen 1959–1980* DAC *1*, Misereor-Archive (Aachen, Germany).

69 '3-years Continuation of Preventative-Medical Programme St Anthony's Hospital Dzodze, Volta Region', *Projekt* NR-*130-3/5 C Z 3149* (30 August 1979) *Ghana – Bewilligungen 1959–1980* DAC *1*, Misereor-Archive (Aachen, Germany).

70 Twumasi, *Survey Report Health Services in Ghana*.

71 'Bau eines Krankenhauses in Papase', *Projekt* NR-*130-003-0001I* DAC *111*, *Bewill Jahr 1961*, *Ghana – Bewilligungen 1959–1980* DAC *1*, Misereor-Archive (Aachen, Germany).

72 Gareth Austin, 'Ghana, the Perennial Test-Case in Africa's Dramatic Development History, 1957–2011' (European Social Science History Conference, Belfast, 5 April 2018).

73 Alice Street, *Biomedicine in an Unstable Place: Infrastructure and Personhood in a Papua New Guinean Hospital* (Durham, NC: Duke University Press, 2014), 11–39.

74 Markku Hokkanen, *Medicine, Mobility and the Empire: Nyasaland Networks, 1859–1960* (Manchester: Manchester University Press, 2017).

75 Adrian Hastings, *A History of African Christianity 1950–1975* (Cambridge University Press, 1979), 225–8.

76 James Owusu, 'Opening Address', Report of National Catholic Health Council Meeting (4–7 November 1980), *Ghana – Bewilligungen 1959–1980*, Misereor-Archive (Aachen, Germany).

77 Ibid.

78 Ibid.

79 *Film of the Medical Mission Sisters at Holy Family Hospital, Berekum* (1961), MMS Archive, Fox Chase, (Philadelphia, USA).

80 Note the similarities between this language and that of J.E. Appiah discussed in chapter 2.

81 James Owusu, 'Appeal to the Most Reverend Members of the Hierarchy of Germany for Assistance for Clinics of the Accra Diocese' (6 May 1959), in *Projekt* NR-*130-001-0002 Einrichtung Fuer Das Hospital in Koforidua* DAC *111*, *Bewill Jahr 1959*, *Ghana – Bewilligungen 1959–1980* DAC *1*, Misereor-Archive (Aachen, Germany).

82 S.N. Addo, 'The Village of Death – Agona Abodom', *Daily Graphic* (27 April 1959), 6, in *Projekt* NR-*130-001-0002 Einrichtung Fuer Das Hospital in Koforidua* DAC *111*, *Bewill Jahr 1959*, *Ghana – Bewilligungen 1959–1980* DAC *1*, Misereor-Archive (Aachen, Germany).

83 James Owusu, 'Appeal to the Most Reverend Members of the Hierarchy of Germany for Assistance for Clinics of the Accra Diocese'.

84 Ibid.

85 Ibid.

86 Gottfried Dossing, 'Your Excellency' (12 May 1959), in *Projekt NR-130-001-0002 Einrichtung Fuer Das Hospital in Koforidua* DAC 111, *Bewill Jahr 1959, Ghana – Bewilligungen 1959–1980 DAC 1*, Misereor-Archive (Aachen, Germany).

87 'Zucuhuss Misereor 66,000DM' (4 November 1959), in *Projekt NR-130-001-0002 Einrichtung Fuer Das Hospital in Koforidua* DAC 111, *Bewill Jahr 1959, Ghana – Bewilligungen 1959–1980 DAC 1*, Misereor-Archive (Aachen, Germany).

88 Antoon Konings (7 July 1975), in *Projekt NR-130-001-001 Kpandu* DAC 111, *Bewill Jahr 1959, Ghana – Bewilligungen 1959–1980 DAC 1*, Misereor-Archive (Aachen, Germany).

89 Ibid.

90 A. Van den Ende S.V.D. (16 May 1961), *Projekt NR-130-004-001 Ausbau Des St. Marten's Hospitals Agroyesum 1961* DAC 111, *Bewill Jahr 1959, Ghana – Bewilligungen 1959–1980 DAC 1*, Misereor-Archive (Aachen, Germany).

91 Gottfried Dossing to A. Konings, in *Projekt NR-130-001-0002 Einrichtung Fuer Das Hospital in Koforidua* DAC 111, *Bewill Jahr 1959, Ghana – Bewilligungen 1959–1980 DAC 1*, Misereor-Archive (Aachen, Germany).

92 James Owusu to Gottfried Dossing, 'I acknowledge with a deep sense of gratitude', *Ablage 130-3 1/2* (7 November 1961), in *Projekt NR-130-3/2*, 'Bau lines Krankenhauses in Papase', *Bewill Jahr 1959, Ghana – Bewilligungen 1959–1980 DAC 1*, Misereor-Archive (Aachen, Germany).

93 Gareth Austin, 'Ghana, the Perennial Test-Case in Africa's Dramatic Development History, 1957–2011'; Hanaan Marwah, 'Institutional Failure or an Unsustainable Foreign Debt Burden? Financing and Management of Ghana State-owned Electricity Distribution 1960–2002' (European Social Science History Conference, Belfast, 5 April 2018).

94 James Owusu to Gottfried Dossing, 'Health Centre at Papase' (7 February 1963), in *Projekt NR-130-3/2* 'Bau lines Krankenhauses in Papase', *Bewill Jahr 1959, Ghana – Bewilligungen 1959–1980 DAC 1*, Misereor-Archive (Aachen, Germany).

95 Rotary, 'Mary Theresa Hospital in Dodi Papase (Ghana)', http://www.rotaryleuven.be/diensten/DodiPapaseProject.html.

96 Patrick A. Twumasi, 'Mary Theresa Hospital, Dodi-Papase', *Survey Report Health Services in Ghana: National Catholic Secretariat January-April 1982* (April 1982, Department of Health, National Catholic Secretariat, Accra), 119–23, National Catholic Secretariat (Accra).

97 Mann Wall, *Into Africa*, 56.

98 However, reliance or otherwise on patient fees was only very loosely linked to a mission's location and was connected to a wider set of factors. The significance of patient fees makes it worth considering whether or not some missions had to be positioned in areas where patients had access to cash in order to pay for the service. The appendix shows that the Catholic missions in the Upper East, Upper West, and North were generally more dependent on government grants and in many cases smaller percentages of their funding came from patient fees. At Jirapa, Nandom, and Navrongo-Bolgatanga (all in the North) the patient fees for hospital contributions are paltry compared with those at St Joseph's Clinic in Ashanti and the Holy Family Hospital at Berekum. Northern mobile clinics such as at Jirapa do have a far higher patient fee contribution, and at the clinic at Yendi, 100 per cent of contributions came from patient fees. Perhaps in the North, where the cash economy was less developed because the area had been colonial labour reservoir, patient fees were less reliable, whereas in the South, in Asante and Brong-Ahafo, some missions fared better at relying on clients. Though again, during the 1980s, ready cash was scarce across most of the nation. Overall, however, there is no strong correlation shown in the available data between patient fees as a percentage of overall income and regional location. There was also very little correlation between the size of the population in a 10 km radius from the institution and patient fees percentage. While these may have been factors they certainly cannot be regarded as determining ones. Instead, there was a range of factors such as urban connections, mobility, sizes, foreign funding, and government links in play; location seems to have made only some difference to the makeup of contributions.

99 In some cases in which only the country of origin of aid is listed, unfortunately it is unclear if the funding is from the national government or an aid organisation. The table covers the majority of Catholic medical institutions in Ghana in 1982. Institutions without available statistics were not included.

100 Rensch and Bruchhausen, 'Medical Science Meets 'Development Aid' Transfer and Adaptation of West German Microbiology to Togo, 1960–1980', 1–24.

101 Walter Bruchhausen, 'From Charity to Development: Christian
     International Health Organizations, 1945–1978', *Hygiea Internationalis:
     An Interdisciplinary Journal for the History of Public Health* 13, no. 1
     (December 2016): 117–34.
102 *Ghana – Bewilligungen 1959–1980*, Misereor-Archive (Aachen,
     Germany); Übersicht uber die vom (16 October–31 December 1959),
     Misereor-Archive (Aachen, Germany).
103 Gonzalo Navarro Sanz, 'Catholic International Cooperation: Social
     Research in the Society of Jesus', in *The Politics of Academic Autonomy in
     Latin America*, ed. Fernanda Beigel (Farnham, Surrey, and Burlington, VT:
     Ashgate Publishing, 2013; New York: Routledge, 2016), 119–34.
104 J.M. Spanjer, 'Medical Activities under Adverse Conditions: Memisa
     Medicus Mundi', *Ned Tijdschr Geneeskd* 136, no. 18 (May 1992):
     888–90.
105 P.W. Kok, 'Memisa: From Medical Missionary Action into a Medical
     Relief Organization', *Ned Tijdschr Geneeskd* 142, no. 51 (December
     1998): 2800–3.
106 'Allemagne', *International Cooperation for Habitat and Urban
     Development: Directory of Non-Government Organisations in* OECD
     Countries (Development Centre of the Organisation for Economic
     Cooperation and Development, 1996), 175–6.
107 Mattias Egg, *Krankenfürsorge im Spannungsfeld von Medizin, Glauben
     und Gesundheitspolitik Die Gemeinschaft der
     Missionshelferinnen, 1952–1994* (Inaugural-Dissertation zur Erlangung
     des Doktorgrades der Hohen Medizinischen Fakultät der Rheinischen
     Friedrich-Wilhelms-Universität Bonn, 2015), esp. 188.
108 Thank you to Paul Jenkins for direction here; any errors are my own.
109 St Michael's Hospital, Pramso (Ashanti) Ghana: Annual Report 1969
     (1969), 2, MMMP 17508, Memisa archives, Katholiek Documentatie
     Centrum (Nijmegen, Netherlands).
110 St Elisabeth Hospital, Ghana: Annual Report 1983 (1983), 1, MMMP
     17513, Memisa archives, Katholiek Documentatie Centrum (Nijmegen,
     Netherlands).
111 James C. McGilvray, 'Appendix II', *Health Is Wholeness* (German Institute
     for Medical Mission, Tübingen, Gesamtherstellung: Breklumer Druckerei
     Manfred Siegel, 1981), 146.
112 Ruth Kutalek, 'Interview with Sjaak Van Der Geest', *Viennese
     Ethnomedicine Newsletter* 5, no. 3 (2003): 18–22.
113 St Michael's Hospital, Pramso (Ashanti) Ghana: Annual Report 1981

(1981), 1, MMMP 17508, Memisa archives, Katholiek Documentatie Centrum (Nijmegen, Netherlands); St Michael's Hospital, Pramso (Ashanti) Ghana: Annual Report 1982 (1982), 1, MMMP 17508, Memisa archives, Katholiek Documentatie Centrum (Nijmegen, Netherlands).

114 St Anthony's Hospital, Dzodze, Ghana: Preventative Health Scheme/ Primary Health Care Annual Report 1985 (1985), MMMP 17503, Memisa archives, Katholiek Documentatie Centrum (Nijmegen, Netherlands); St Anthony's Hospital, Dzodze, Ghana: Programme Report on Maternal and Child Care and Preventative/Primary Health Care Activities (1986), MMMP 17503, Memisa archives, Katholiek Documentatie Centrum (Nijmegen, Netherlands).

115 St Anthony's Hospital, Dzodze, Ghana: Annual Report 1980–81 (1981), MMMP 17507, Memisa archives, Katholiek Documentatie Centrum (Nijmegen, Netherlands); St Anthony's Hospital, Dzodze, Ghana: Annual Report 1982–83 (1983), MMMP 17507, Memisa archives, Katholiek Documentatie Centrum (Nijmegen, Netherlands).

116 St Anthony's Hospital, Dzodze, Ghana: Annual Report 1986 (1986), MMMP 17503, Memisa archives, Katholiek Documentatie Centrum (Nijmegen, Netherlands).

117 Assin Foso Catholic Hospital, Ghana: Annual Report 1982 (1982), 1, MMMP 17506, Memisa archives, Katholiek Documentatie Centrum (Nijmegen, Netherlands).

118 Nkoranzaman, Ghana: Annual Report 1982–83 (1983), MMMP 17507, Memisa archives, Katholiek Documentatie Centrum (Nijmegen, Netherlands).

119 Nkoranzaman, Ghana: Annual Report 1982–83 (1983), MMMP 17507, Memisa archives, Katholiek Documentatie Centrum (Nijmegen, Netherlands).

120 St Elisabeth Hospital, Ghana: Annual Report 1983 (1983), MMMP 17513, Memisa archives, Katholiek Documentatie Centrum (Nijmegen, Netherlands).

121 This included: 'Foundation "Vrienden van Dzodze", Almelo, Holland … Messrs Veldt Heerhugowaard, Beekman Bledel, van Alem Gennep … Foundation 40 MM, Venhuizen, Holland … Pupils R.C. School Primary School, Purmurend, Holland … Pupils School for the Blind, Grave, Holland'. Plus, the US Catholic Medical Mission board gave drugs (ibid).

122 Mohammed Abudulai, ed., St Theresa's Hospital and Health Services Newsletter (July 1987), MMMP 17507, Memisa archives, Katholiek Documentatie Centrum (Nijmegen, Netherlands).

123 Catholic Hospital Apam, Ghana: Annual Report 1989–90 (1990), MMMP 17513, Memisa archives, Katholiek Documentatie Centrum (Nijmegen, Netherlands).

124 St Elisabeth Hospital, Hwidiem, Brong Ahafo, Ghana: Annual Report 1989 (1989), MMMP 17513, Memisa archives, Katholiek Documentatie Centrum (Nijmegen, Netherlands).

125 St Anthony's Hospital, Dzodze, Ghana: Programme Report on Maternal and Child Care and Preventative/Primary Health Care Activities (1986), 3–5, MMMP 17503, Memisa archives, Katholiek Documentatie Centrum (Nijmegen, Netherlands).

126 Emma Hunter, *Political Thought and the Public Sphere: Freedom, Democracy and Citizenship in the Era of Decolonization* (Cambridge: Cambridge University Press, 2015), 10.

CHAPTER FOUR

1 Sanjoy Bhattacharya, 'Global and Local Histories of Medicine: Interpretative Challenges and Future Possibilities', in *A Global History of Medicine*, ed. Mark Jackson (Oxford: Oxford University Press, 2018), 243–63.

2 Sanjoy Bhattacharya, 'International Health and the Limits of Its Global Influence: Bhutan and the Worldwide Smallpox Eradication Programme', *Medical History* 57, no. 4 (October 2013): 461–86; Frank Fenner et al., *Smallpox and Its Eradication* (Geneva: World Health Organization, 1988).

3 Benjamin N. Lawrance, Emily L. Osborn, and Richard L. Roberts, *Intermediaries, Interpreters and Clerks: African Employees in the Making of Colonial Africa* (Madison: University of Wisconsin Press, 2008).

4 The term 'international health', which was more prominent in this period by actors, will, for the sake of historical accuracy, supplant 'global health'.

5 Joseph M. Y. Edusa-Eyison, 'The History of the Methodist Church Ghana' (The General Commission on Archives and History: The United Methodist Church, archives.gcah.org, 2011): 12–13.

6 USAID had a changing relationship to modernization theory between the 1950s and 1980s. For research on state stabilisation, stages of growth, modernization theory, and development aid, see David C. Engerman et al., *Staging Growth: Modernization, Development and the Global Cold War* (Amherst and Boston: University of Massachusetts Press, 2003); Nils Gilman, *Mandarins of the Future: Modernization Theory in Cold War America* (Baltimore: Johns Hopkins University Press, 2003); Michael E.

Latham, *Modernization as Ideology: American Social Science and "Nation Building" in the Kennedy Era* (Chapel Hill and London: University of North Carolina Press, 2000).

7 Sanjoy Bhattacharya, *Expunging Variola: The Control and Eradication of Smallpox in India 1947–1977* (New Delhi: Orient Longman Private Limited, 2006).

8 Bhattacharya, 'International Health and the Limits of Its Global Influence'.

9 Sarah Cook Runcie, 'Mobile Health Teams, Decolonization, and the Eradication Era in Cameroon, 1945–1970' (doctoral thesis, Columbia University, 2017).

10 Monica Saavedra, 'Politics and Health at the WHO Regional Office for South East Asia: The Case of Portuguese India, 1949–61', *Medical History* 61, no. 3 (July 2017): 380–400.

11 Correspondence with author, David Newberry (19 September 2015).

12 Ibid; Correspondence with author, David Newberry (4 October 2015).

13 Fred E. Gilbert interviewed by William Haven North (The Association for Diplomatic Studies and Training, Foreign Affairs Oral History Project: Foreign Affairs Series, adst.org/wp-content/uploads/2018/02/Ghana.pdf, 4 September 1997), 10–11.

14 Fenner et al., *Smallpox and Its Eradication*, 856, 858.

15 Correspondence with author, David Newberry (19 September 2015).

16 Ibid.

17 'Infective Diseases Total Incidence, 96480', *Gold Coast Colony Report on the Medical Department for the Year 1931–32* (Government Printing Office, Accra, 1932), Balme Library, University of Ghana (Accra).

18 *Report on the Medical Department for the Year 1947* (1948), 6, Korle Bu Teaching Hospital Library (Accra); *Report of the Ministry of Health 1953* (1954), 81, Korle Bu Teaching Hospital Library (Accra).

19 *Annual Report of the Medical Field Units 1962* (1962), 15, Korle Bu Teaching Hospital Library (Accra).

20 *Medical Field Units Annual Report, 1961* (1961), 17–18, Korle Bu Teaching Hospital Library (Accra).

21 *Report of the Ministry of Health 1953* (1954), 79, Korle Bu Teaching Hospital Library (Accra).

22 *Medical Field Units Annual Report, 1961* (1961), 20, 92, Korle Bu Teaching Hospital Library (Accra).

23 *Annual Report of the Medical Field Units 1962* (1962), 33, Korle Bu Teaching Hospital Library (Accra).

24 It is mentioned in Fenner's volume that Ghana was the only country in which the MFUs spread across the whole country, the authors did

recognise the postcolonial MFU contribution; Fenner et al., *Smallpox and Its Eradication*, 868; William H. Schneider, 'Smallpox in Africa during Colonial Rule', *Medical History* 53 (2009): 193.

25 'Wider World: Health Services in Ghana', *The Lancet* (21 July 1962): 142–4.

26 David Scott, *Epidemic Diseases in Ghana, 1901–1960* (Oxford: Oxford University Press, 1965).

27 'Graph 1: Annual Notification of Smallpox in Ghana, 1901–1962', *Annual Report of the Medical Field Units 1962* (1962), Korle Bu Teaching Hospital Library (Accra); Stephen Addae, *Medical Histories Volume II: Diseases, Medical Institutions, and Biographies* (Accra: Eureka Foundation, 2012), 323–33.

28 Correspondence with author, David Newberry (19 September 2015).

29 Paul Greenough, '"A Wild and Wondrous Ride": CDC Field Epidemiologists in the East Pakistan Smallpox and Cholera Epidemics of 1958', *Ciência & Saúde Coletiva* 16, no. 2 (2011): 491–500.

30 Gilford A. Ashitey, *An Epidemiology of Disease Control in Ghana 1901-1990* (Accra: Ghana Universities Press, 1994), 4-6; Correspondence with author, David Newberry (19 September 2015); Correspondence with author, David Newberry (4 October 2015).

31 Ibid.

32 Ibid.

33 Ibid.

34 In the conclusion to his large work on the church in Africa, Adrian Hastings described this group as heralding a 'new age of the African Church' in spite of the realities which surrounded them in the late 1950s; Adrian Hastings, *The Church in Africa, 1450–1950* (Oxford: Oxford University Press, 1994), 604–5.

35 John S. Pobee, 'Baëta, Christian G(oncalves) K(wami) (1908–1994): Presbyterian Church Ledaers from the Gold Coast', in *Biographical Dictionary of Christian Missions*, ed. Gerald H. Anderson (New York: Macmillan Reference, 1998), 38–9. In exile Busia completed research on mission as a part of series of World Council of Churches publications; Kofi Abrefa Busia, *Urban Churches in Britain: A Question of Relevance* (London: Lutterworth Press, 1966). Graduate networks, especially from Achimota, published biographies, conducted commemorations, and even created street names, all in Aggrey's honour, and in doing so battled over his legacy.

36 Annan's Anglicanism and spiritual beliefs were an important feature of the 'ethical framework'and 'moral authority' he brought to his global role;

Courtney B. Smith, 'Politics and Values at the United Nations: Kofi Annan's Balancing Act' in *The UN Secretary-General and Moral Authority: Ethics and Religion in International Leadership*, ed. Kent J. Kille (Washington, DC: Georgetown University Press, 2007), 299–337.

37 'Achievement of Past Students', *Wesley Girls High School* (wesleygirl.edu. gh/achievementpast-students, September 2016); General News of Monday 'Former PNDC secretary Mary Grant is dead', *Ghana Web* (GhanaWeb.com, 19 September 2016).

38 Thank you to the Grant family, particularly Anna Mary, Francis, and Mary Grant, for their support. There is not scope within this book to fully cover how the diverse array of Achimota alumni relate to Aggrey's legacy, or how other eminent schools and colleges in Ghana have formed post-graduate networks and international diasporic connections in dialogue with past eminent teachers and students. Further work on this would be illuminating, especially in relation to the University of Ghana and other kinds of tertiary education development. Suffice it to say here that the Achimota oft-repeated statement that graduates go out to be 'living waters to a thirsty land' (echoing Jesus Christs words in the Gospel of John) is one of the many foundational principles that appears to still shape the lives and work of this globally influential community.

39 From David Newberry (operations officer, Ghana Smallpox/Measles Program, USAID/Accra) to R. Cashin (director USAID/Ghana, Accra), 'United States Government Memorandum: GSMP Upper Region Yellow Fever Activities' (1 December 1969) RG 0286 United States Department for International Development, USAID Mission to Ghana/Education Division, Entry# P 347: Subject Files 1969–1974, United States National Archives II (Maryland, USA).

40 Correspondence with author, David Newberry (4 October 2015).

41 David Newberry, D. Dix, and C.A. Herron, 'Report of a Meeting Held on Saturday, December 13 in the Office of the S.M.C. (C.D.) Accra, to Discuss the Current Yellow Fever Problem' (22 December 1969), 3, RG 0286 United States Department for International Development, USAID Mission to Ghana/Education Division, Entry# P 347: Subject Files 1969–1974, United States National Archives II (Maryland, USA).

42 From C. A. Herron (medical officer, SMP/Ghana) to R. Cashin (director, USAID/Ghana), 'United States Government Memorandum: Yellow Fever Problem, 1969–1970' (3 January 1970) RG 0286 United States Department for International Development, USAID Mission to Ghana/Education Division, Entry# P 347: Subject Files 1969–1974, United States National Archives II (Maryland, USA).

43 Percy Selwyn-Clarke, *A Monograph on Smallpox in the Negro and Negroid Tribes of British West Africa, with Special Reference to the Gold Coast Colony* (London: John Bale Sons and Danielsson Ltd, 1921).

44 Keith R. Dumbell and Farida Huq (with Broughton B. Waddy), 'Epidemiological Implications of the Typing of Variola Isolates', *Transactions of the Royal Society of Tropical Medicine and Hygiene* 63, no. 3 (1975): 307.

45 Osaak A. Olumwallah, *Dis-Ease in the Colonial State: Medicine, Society, and Social Change among the AbaNyole of Western Kenya* (Westport, CT: Greenwood Press, 2002); M. Graboyes, *The Experiment Must Continue: Medical Research and Ethics in East Africa, 1940–2014* (Athens: Ohio University Press, 2015).

46 Correspondence with author, David Newberry (4 October 2015).

47 Ibid.

48 William H. Foege, *House on Fire: The Fight to Eradicate Smallpox* (University of California Press; reprint edition, 2012), 56–7.

49 Ibid., 29.

50 William H. Foege, 'The Practice of Community Medicine', in *Health Is Wholeness The Limuru Conference, Protestant Churches Medical Association and Lutheran Institute of Human Ecology* (Printed by Kenya Litho Ltd, Nairobi, February 1970), John Hopkins University Archives (Baltimore, USA).

51 Ibid.

52 Ibid.

53 For more on William H. Foege, see John Blevins, *Christianity's Role in United States Global Health and Development Policy: To Transfer the Empire to the World* (New York: Routledge, 2019).

54 V. de Sario (Epidemiological Division, Ministry of Health, Ghana), 'Field Investigation of an Outbreak of Smallpox at Bawku, Ghana: May–October 1967', World Health Organisation WHO/SE/69.8 (archived at WHO Library 19 September 1969), 1–10, accessed in the WHO Institutional Repository for Information Sharing (IRIS).

55 Francis Chapman Grant, 'Smallpox Eradication in Ghana', World Health Organization, paper presented at the meeting of the Expert Committee on Smallpox, Geneva (14–20 January, 1964), 1–7, accessed in the WHO Institutional Repository for Information Sharing (IRIS).

56 Fenner et al., *Smallpox and Its Eradication*, 1083.

57 K. Ward-Brew, 'Ghana/Medical Officer at Present Responsible for Smallpox Eradication', World Health Organisation, SE/WP/75.12 (1975),

1–11, accessed in the WHO Institutional Repository for Information Sharing (IRIS).

58 Bhattacharya, 'International Health and the Limits of Its Global Influence', 461–2.

59 Grant became the deputy director of Medical Services, continued to work with USAID and WHO on many other disease control and eradication projects, and latterly was a consultant to Global 2000's fight against guinea worm; see Ashitey, *Disease Control in Ghana*, 6. According to Fenner's volume on SEP, Grant was the WHO smallpox eradication consultant for Burma in 1970 and from 1965 had assisted I. Arita in Burma, Afghanistan, Mali, and Nigeria, as well as working on the national programme in Ghana; Fenner et al., *Smallpox and Its Eradication*, 408, 432.

60 David Newberry to E.G. Beausoleil, 'Memorandum: A Review of the Plan "A Primary Health Care Strategy for Ghan" and Recommendations for the Medical Field Unit Participation' (2 August 1978) I8/370/2GHA/R58, World Health Organization Archives (Geneva, Switzerland).

61 J.M. Blankson and Yaw Asirifi, 'Measles and Its Problems as Seen in Ghana', Health Service Planning, *Ghana Medical Journal* (June 1974): 134–40.

62 'Measles', *Weekly Epidem. Rec./Relevé épidém. hebd.*, no. 45, 49th year (Geneva: World Health Organization, 8 November 1974), 376, accessed in the WHO Institutional Repository for Information Sharing (IRIS), based on *The Ghana Monthly Epidemiological Bulletin* (May 1974),

63 Annex I, 'Morbidity and Mortality in Ghana, 1978–1982', in 'Programme for Production of Vaccines in Africa: UC/RAF/83/088' (Ghana, 5–15 May 1984) I8/370/2GHA/R84, World Health Organization Archives (Geneva, Switzerland); Annex II, 'Cases and Deaths of Selected Communicable Diseases in Ghana, 1972–1981' in 'Programme for Production of Vaccines in Africa: UC/RAF/83/088' (Ghana, 5–15 May 1984) I8/370/2GHA/R84, World Health Organization Archives (Geneva, Switzerland).

64 William K. Bosu et al., 'Progress in the Control of Measles in Ghana, 1980–2000', *The Journal of Infectious Diseases* 187, no. 1 (2003): S44–S45.

65 Blankson and Asirifi, 'Measles and Its Problems as Seen in Ghana', 134–40.

66 On structural inequalities see John D. Nott, 'Between Famine and Malnutrition: Spatial Aspects of Nutritional Health during Ghana's Long Twentieth Century, c.1898–2000' (doctoral thesis, University of Leeds, 2016).

67 Again, for the debate on the relation between development, Cold War strategy, and US modernization theory, see Engerman, *Staging Growth*; Gilman, *Mandarins of the Future*; Latham, *Modernization as Ideology*.

68 Percy Selwyn-Clarke, 'A Ghana Journey: The Selwyn-Clarke Report', *Medical Care* 1, no. 1 (January–March, 1963), 60.

69 'Annex 1: UK-Ghana Economic and Military Ties', Sanitized Copy, Central Intelligence Agency (CIA) Office of Central Intelligence (18 December 1965) FOIA Policy – 17276 Plot to Overthrow President Kwame Nkrumah, Washington University Archives (Washington, DC, USA), 5; William Haven North interviewed by Charles Stuart Kennedy (The Association for Diplomatic Studies and Training Foreign Affairs Oral History Project Foreign Assistance Series, 18 February 1993).

70 Ambassador Trimble and R.C. Huffman, cc. Mr Gebelt, 'Proposed Department Position re.PL-480 Program for Ghana' (9 October 1962), 1–2, Admin – Communications, Correspondence with Chief of Mission, RG0059, Department of State, Bureau of African Affairs, Office of the West African Affairs, ca.1960–1985, Entry# A1 3112A, Records relating to Ghana, United States National Archives II (Maryland, USA).

71 U.S. Programs in Ghana, 1–10, esp. 7. (1960–61), 14.A.1 Internal Security Assessment, RG0059, Department of State, Bureau of African Affairs, Office of the West African Affairs, ca.1960–1985, Entry# A1 3112A, records relating to Ghana, United States National Archives II (Maryland, USA).

72 Again, for the debate on the relation between development, Cold War strategy, and US modernization theory, see Engerman et al., *Staging Growth*; Gilman, *Mandarins of the Future*; Latham, *Modernization as Ideology*.

73 Acting Secretary, 'Memorandum for the President, Subject: Relations with Ghana', 1–2 14.A.1 Internal Security Assessment, RG0059, Department of State, Bureau of African Affairs, Office of the West African Affairs, ca.1960–1985, Entry# A1 3112A, records relating to Ghana, United States National Archives II (Maryland, USA); From S. G. Gebelt to Ambassador Trimble, 'Possible Pressure on Government of Ghana', United States Government Memorandum (29 January 1963) RG0059, Department of State, Bureau of African Affairs, Office of the West African Affairs, ca.1960–1985, Entry# A1 3112A, records relating to Ghana, United States National Archives II (Maryland, USA); O.L. Troxel Jr (counselor of the embassy) to P.C. Narten (officer in charge, Ghanaian Affairs, Department of State, Washington, DC), The Foreign Service of the United States of America (Accra, 26 September 1963) POL – Political Affairs and Rel., 1-0 Positive and Negative Factors/

Developments in Ghana, RG0059, Department of State, Bureau of African
Affairs, Office of the West African Affairs, ca. 1960–1985, Entry# A1
3112A, records relating to Ghana, United States National Archives II
(Maryland, USA); SODEFRA were a French firm who were also building a
textile mill in Tanzania: Said Adejumobi and Adebayo O. Olukoshi, *The
African Union and New Strategies for Development in Africa* (New York:
Cambria Press, 2008), 190.

74 P.C. Narten to Ambassador Trimble, 'Medical School for Ghana: United
States Government Memorandum' (1 August 1963) POL – Political Affairs
and Rel., 1-0 Positive and Negative Factors/Developments in Ghana,
RG0059, Department of State, Bureau of African Affairs, Office of the
West African Affairs, ca.1960–1985, Entry# A1 3112A, records relating to
Ghana, United States National Archives II (Maryland, USA); William
Cattell Trimble and Mr Tasca, Medical School in Ghana (19 July 1963),
1–2 POL – Political Affairs and Rel., 1-0 Positive and Negative Factors/
Developments in Ghana, RG0059, Department of State, Bureau of African
Affairs, Office of the West African Affairs, ca.1960–1985, Entry# A1
3112A, records relating to Ghana, United States National Archives II
(Maryland, USA).

75 O.L. Troxel (charges d'affaires) to William Cattell Trimble (Department of
State, Washington, DC)','Country Assistance Program Book' (18 November
1963), Admin – Communications, Correspondence with Chief of Mission,
RG0059, Department of State, Bureau of African Affairs, Office of the West
African Affairs, ca.1960–1985, Entry# A1 3112A, records relating to
Ghana, United States National Archives II (Maryland, USA).

76 John Fitzgerald Kennedy (White House, Washington, DC), 'Memorandum
for D. E. Bell, Administrator for the Agency for International
Development' (8 October 1963), Health and Medical Care HLTH 9
Medical Education and Training RG0059, Department of State, Bureau of
African Affairs, Office of the West African Affairs, ca.1960–1985, Entry#
A1 3112A, records relating to Ghana, United States National Archives II
(Maryland, USA); W.C. Trimble to Mr Tasca, 'Trial of the Accused
Ghanaian Cabinet Ministers', United States Government Memorandum
(12 March 1963), 1–5 RG0059, Department of State, Bureau of African
Affairs, Office of the West African Affairs, ca. 1960–1985, Entry# A1
3112A, records relating to Ghana, United States National Archives II,
Maryland, USA).

77 What is certain is that the State Department was doing psychological assess-
ments of Nkrumah; L.C. Beck to W.C. Trimble, 'Transmittal of

Psychological Study of Kwame Nkrumah', United States Government
Memorandum (27 November 1963): 'Kwame Nkrumah Assessment
Supplement: Juju', in *Kwame Nkrumah: A Psychological Study* (June 1962)
POL 17, Diplomatic and Consular Representation, Ghana Ambassador:
RG0059, Department of State, Bureau of African Affairs, Office of the West
African Affairs, ca. 1960–1985, Entry# A1 3112A, records relating to
Ghana, United States National Archives II (Maryland, USA).

78 Gerhard Mennen Williams to the Secretary, 'Steps to be Taken in Regard
to the Recent Attacks against American Negros in the Ghanaian Press –
Approval Requested', Department of State Assistant Secretary (18 April
1963) RG0059, Department of State, Bureau of African Affairs, Office of
the West African Affairs, ca.1960–1985, Entry# A1 3112A, records relating to Ghana, United States National Archives II, Maryland, USA).

79 Federal Bureau of Investigation, US Department of State, Communications
Section, Urgent to Director 12 from New York 2P, 'Proposed Assassination
of Kwame Nkrumah' (11 June 1965) FOIA Policy – 17276 Plot to
Overthrow President Kwame Nkrumah, George Washington University
Archives, Washington, DC); Memorandum for Deputy Director of Central
Intelligence (25 February 1966) FOIA Policy – 17276 Plot to Overthrow
President Kwame Nkrumah, George Washington University Archives
(Washington, DC, USA).

80 'Memorial and Thanksgiving Service for the Late Dr. Francis Grant', 6–37.

81 E. Gilliatt to File, 'Aid to the Ghana Medical School (University of Ghana)
(Meeting of Mr. Ghebo, Registrar of the Medical School, Mr F. E. Gilbert
and Miss Elinor Gilliatt on Monday, 12 August 1968 at Mr Ghebo's
Office at Korle Bu', Memorandum (14 August 1968) FY69 Ghana
Medical School, RG0059, Department of State, Bureau of African Affairs,
Office of the West African Affairs, ca.1960–1985, Entry# A1 5179, records
relating to Ghana 1964–1975, United States National Archives II
(Maryland, USA).

82 '34 Ghana Trained Doctors Pass Out', *The Ghanaian Times* (27 June
1969), 1, FY69 Ghana Medical School, RG0059, Department of State,
Bureau of African Affairs, Office of the West African Affairs, ca.1960–
1985, Entry# A1 5179, records relating to Ghana 1964–1975, United
States National Archives II (Maryland, USA).

83 Walter Bruchhausen, 'From Charity to Development: Christian
International Health Organizations, 1945–1978', *Hygiea Internationalis:
An Interdisciplinary Journal for the History of Public Health* 13, no. 1
(December 2016): 117–18.

84 Sanjoy Bhattacharya, 'Global and Local Histories of Medicine: Interpretative Challenges and Future Possibilities', in *A Global History of Medicine*, ed. Mark Jackson (Oxford: Oxford University Press, 2018), 258–9.
85 Nick Cullather, *The Hungry World: America's Cold War Battle against Poverty in Asia* (Cambridge, MA: Harvard University Press, 2010), 257–8.
86 Abeeku Essuman-Johnson, 'Influencing a Country's Political and Economic Decision Making with Food: The Case of Ghana', *Research Review* NS 7.1 and 7.2 (1991): 45–60.
87 Andrew Preston, *Sword of the Spirit, Shield of Faith: Religion in American War and Diplomacy* (New York: Knopf, 2012); Odd Arne Westad, 'Exploring the Histories of the Cold War: A Pluralist Approach', in *Uncertain Empire: American History and the Idea of the Cold War*, eds. Joel Issac and Duncan Bell (Oxford: Oxford University Press, 2012), 51–61.
88 Anders Stephanson, 'Cold War, Degree Zero', in *Uncertain Empire: American History and the Idea of the Cold War*, eds. Joel Isaac and Duncan Bell (Oxford University Press, 2012), 19–51.
89 Andrew Preston, 'The Spirit of Democracy: Religious Liberty and American Anti-Communism during the Cold War', in *Uncertain Empire: American History and the Idea of the Cold War*, eds. Joel Isaac and Duncan Bell (Oxford University Press, 2012), 141–64.
90 As Preston puts it: 'It is no small irony that one of the least religious presidents should have been the agent of such profound religious change'; Preston, *Sword of the Spirit, Shield of Faith*, 502–3.
91 Andrew Rotter, *Comrades at Odds: Culture and Indo-US Relations, 1947–1964* (Ithaca, NY: Cornell University Press, 2000), 234.
92 Cullather, *The Hungry World*, 257.
93 Bruchhausen, 'From Charity to Development', 117–34.
94 John D. Nott, 'Between Famine and Malnutrition: Spatial Aspects of Nutritional Health during Ghana's Long Twentieth Century, c.1898–2000' (doctoral thesis, University of Leeds, 2016), 186–7, 265–70.
95 Ibid., 283.
96 FFPO W.M. Carter, P.L. 480 Title I (19 January 1979), 1–5, RG 0286 Agency for International Development, USAID Mission to Ghana/ Education, P 348, Subject Files: 1978–1985, United States National Archives II (Maryland, USA).
97 Ibid.
98 Ibid.

99 Points Regarding Ghana's Economic Development: Ghana's Performance, J.D.S. Tempel (3 December 1971), RG 0286 Agency for International Development, USAID Mission to Ghana/Education, P 347, Subject Files: 1969–1974, United States National Archives II (Maryland, USA).

100 Talking Points Concerning Ghanaian Repudiation of Selected Suppliers Credits, 2, FN 14 Ghana Debt (debt rescheduling) (January-March), Ghana 1972 (RG 0286 Agency for International Development, USAID Mission to Ghana/Education, P 347, Subject Files: 1969–1974, United States National Archives II (Maryland, USA).

101 Ghana: New Resource Commitments by Area of Concentration Annex B RG 0286 Agency for International Development, USAID Mission to Ghana/Education, P 347, Subject Files: 1969–1974, United States National Archives II (Maryland, USA).

102 Preston, *Sword of the Spirit, Shield of Faith*, 509.

103 K. Ward-Brew to regional director, 'AFRO - Memorandum: G-7 Primary Health Care: Catholic Relief Services' (25 August 1983), 57, 'Economic Assistance to Ghana – Report of the Multi-Agency United Nations Mission to Ghana' G2/27/5/GHA, World Health Organization Archives (Geneva, Switzerland).

104 US Agency for International Development, 'Report of the Re-Examination of the Catholic Relief Service P. L. 480 Title II, Food Program in Ghana' (7 July 1978), RG 0286 Agency for International Development, USAID Mission to Ghana/Education, P 348, Subject Files: 1978–1985, United States National Archives (Maryland, USA).

105 US Agency for International Development, 'Report of the Re-Examination of the Catholic Relief Service P. L. 480 Title II, Food Program in Ghana' (7 July 1978), RG 0286 Agency for International Development, USAID Mission to Ghana/Education, P 348, Subject Files: 1978–1985, United States National Archives II (Maryland, USA).

106 FFPO: W.M. Carter (Food for Peace officer) to Rev. W.M. Campbell (program director, Catholic Relief Services), 'Determination of the Value of Claims on P. L. 480 Title II Commodities' (24 January 1979), RG 0286 Agency for International Development, USAID Mission to Ghana/Education, P 348, Subject Files: 1978–1985, United States National Archives II (Maryland, USA).

107 W. Rastetter to Rev. J.T. Addy, 'Suspension of Food Program' (14 August 1978), RG 0286 Agency for International Development, USAID Mission to Ghana/Education, P 348, Subject Files: 1978–1985, United States National Archives II (Maryland, USA).

294 Notes to pages 178–9

108 S. Sugri to Father-in-Charge, Catholic Mission, Walewale, 'Comments on Foodstuff Inspected at the Catholic Mission at Walewale' (27 July 1979), RG 0286 Agency for International Development, USAID Mission to Ghana/Education, P 347, Subject Files: 1969–1974, United States National Archives II (Maryland, USA); The Rev. Pastor, Assembly of God Church, Tanga to Ministry of Health, Environmental Health Division, 'Soy-Fortified Sorghum Grits Certificate of Assembly of God Church – Tanga' (29 June 1980), RG 0286 Agency for International Development, USAID Mission to Ghana/Education, P 348, Subject Files: 1978–1985, United States National Archives II (Maryland, USA).

109 St Anthony's Hospital, Dzodze, Ghana: Programme Report on Maternal and Child Care and Preventative/Primary Health Care Activities (1986), MMMP 17503, Memisa archives, Katholiek Documentatie Centrum (Nijmegen, Netherlands).

110 US Agency for International Development, 'Report of the Re-Examination of the Catholic Relief Service P. L. 480 Title II, Food Program in Ghana' (7 July 1978), RG 0286 Agency for International Development, USAID Mission to Ghana/Education, P 348, Subject Files: 1978–1985, United States National Archives II (Maryland, USA).

111 I.D. Coker (mission director) to J.L.S. Abbey (commissioner for economic planning) (18 January 1979), RG 0286 Agency for International Development, USAID Mission to Ghana/Education, P 348, Subject Files: 1978–1985, United States National Archives II (Maryland, USA).

112 FFPO W.M. Carter, P.L. 480 Title I (19 January 1979), 2, RG 0286 Agency for International Development, USAID Mission to Ghana/Education, P 348, Subject Files: 1978–1985, United States National Archives II (Maryland, USA).

113 Rev. W.M. Campbell (director) to W.M. Carter (Food for Peace officer, USAID Mission/Ghana), 'Inspection Reports' (7 March 1979), RG 0286 Agency for International Development, USAID Mission to Ghana/Education, P 348, Subject Files: 1978–1985, United States National Archives II (Maryland, USA).

114 Essuman-Johnson, 'Influencing a Country's Political and Economic Decision Making with Food', 45–60.

115 FFPO W.M. Carter, 'Memo: Projects Worthy of Visit by U. S. Officials' (18 September 1979), RG 0286 Agency for International Development, USAID Mission to Ghana/Education, P 348, Subject Files: 1978–1985, United States National Archives II (Maryland, USA).

116 FFP W.M. Carter, I.D. Coker (director) to G. Harley (commissioner for transport), 'Priority Berthing for U. S. Food Commodities' (31 August

1979), RG 0286 Agency for International Development, USAID Mission to Ghana/Education, P 348, Subject Files: 1978–1985, United States National Archives II (Maryland, USA).

117 'Memorandum: USAID Title III' (22 August 1979), 4, RG 0286 Agency for International Development, USAID Mission to Ghana/Education, P 348, Subject Files: 1978–1985, United States National Archives II (Maryland, USA).

118 Auditor General, USAID Audit Report 3-641-78-6, 'Report on the Examination of the Catholic Relief Services PL 480 Title II Food Program in Ghana' (7 July 1978), RG 0286 Agency for International Development, USAID Mission to Ghana/Education, P 348, Subject Files: 1978–1985, United States National Archives II (Maryland, USA).

119 FFPO W.M. Carter, P.L. 480 Title I (19 January 1979), 1–5, RG 0286 Agency for International Development, USAID Mission to Ghana/ Education, P 348, Subject Files: 1978–1985, United States National Archives II (Maryland, USA).

120 'Major Mel Bond Asst. Public Relations Officer and Canadian Forces Officer re: Milk Powder Shipment to Ghana', The Salvation Army International Heritage Centre (London, UK); 'Ghana', The Salvation Army Year Book 1981 (St Albans: Campfield Press, 1981), 130–1, The Salvation Army International Heritage Centre (London, UK); 'Ghana', The Salvation Army Year Book 1982 (St Albans: Campfield Press, 1982), 126–7, The Salvation Army International Heritage Centre (London, UK).

121 'Ghana', The Salvation Army Year Book 1963 (London: Salvationist Publishing and Supplies Ltd, 1963), 90–1, The Salvation Army International Heritage Centre (London, UK).

122 'Ghana', The Salvation Army Year Book 1970 (London: Salvationist Publishing and Supplies Ltd, 1970), 121–3, The Salvation Army International Heritage Centre (London, UK).

123 'Ghana', The Salvation Army Year Book 1984 (St Albans: Campfield Press, 1984), 118–21, The Salvation Army International Heritage Centre (London, UK); 'Ghana', The Salvation Army Year Book 1985 (St Albans: Campfield Press, 1985), 124–5, The Salvation Army International Heritage Centre (London, UK); 'Ghana', The Salvation Army Year Book 1986 (St Albans: Campfield Press, 1986), 124–5, The Salvation Army International Heritage Centre (London, UK).

124 Annex 1, 'Emergency Assistance', K. Ward-Brew to regional director, 'AFRO – Memorandum: G-7 Primary Health Care: Catholic Relief Services' (25 August 1983), 25, 66–7, 'Economic Assistance to Ghana

– Report of the Multi-Agency United Nations Mission to Ghana' G2/27/5/
GHA, World Health Organization Archives (Geneva, Switzerland).

125 'Gh.27: Ghana: CHAG's Efforts in Health Care' (August 1984), 6–7,
Annexes I–III, SOAS Library and Archives (London, UK).

126 Nott, 'Between Famine and Malnutrition' (doctoral thesis, University of
Leeds, 2016), 190–200.

127 J. Lieberson et al., CDIE Impact Evaluation: United States Agency for
International Development: Food Aid in Ghana: An Elusive Road to Self-
Reliance (PN-ABY-237, no. 3, 1997).

128 Warwick Anderson, 'Introduction: Postcolonial Technoscience', Social
Studies of Science 32 nos. 5–6 (Sage Publications, October–December
2002): 643–58; Mary Louise Pratt, Imperial Eyes: Travel Writing and
Transculturation (London and New York: Routledge, 2008), 7; Gilbert M.
Joseph, 'Close Encounters: Toward a New Cultural History of U.S.–Latin
American Relations', in Close Encounters of Empire: Writing the Cultural
History of U.S.–Latin American Relations, eds. Gilbert M. Joseph,
Catherine C. Legrand, and Ricardo D. Salvatore (Durham, NC: Duke
University Press, 1998), 3–46, cited in Saavedra, 'Politics and Health at the
WHO Regional Office for South East Asia', 380–400; Warwick Anderson,
'Where Is the Postcolonial History of Medicine?' Bulletin of the History of
Medicine 72, no. 3 (fall 1998): 522–30.

129 Stephen Feierman et al., 'Anthropology, Knowledge-Flows and Global
Health', Global Public Health 5, no. 2 (March 2010): 122–8; Vihn-Kim
Nguyen, The Republic of Therapy: Triage and Sovereignty in West Africa's
Time of AIDS (Durham, NC: Duke University Press, 2010).

130 Hastings, The Church in Africa, 604–5.

CHAPTER FIVE

1 On development and 'disappointment', including emphasis on the struggle
of 'cultural and spiritual institutions' to survive and handle 'disillusionment', see Frederick Cooper, Africa since 1940: The Past of the Present
(Cambridge: Cambridge University Press, 2002), 91–132, esp. 130.

2 Ruth J. Prince, 'Introduction: Situating Health and the Public in Africa;
Historical and Anthropological Perspectives', in Making and Unmaking
Public Health in Africa: Ethnographic and Historical Perspectives, eds.
Ruth J. Prince and Rebecca Marsland (Athens: Ohio University Press,
2014), 1–27.

3 Kelley Lee, The World Health Organization (WHO) (New York: Routledge,
2009), 78–85.

4 Marcos Cueto, 'The ORIGINS of Primary Health Care and SELECTIVE Primary Health Care', *American Journal of Public Health* 94, no. 11 (2004): 1864–74.

5 This new approach has been possible through the analysis of previously unexamined papers in the Misereor archives in Aachen, the National Catholic Secretariat in Accra, the archives of the Medical Mission Sisters in Philadelphia, and the archives of the World Council of Churches in Geneva. Comparing the caches in these various depositories enables the evidencing of historical arguments which go beyond the simplistic narratives of international organisations or national governments alone. It also offers the possibility of challenging common historical categories of 'development' which have not taken into account the complexity of the term's production across many contexts and by many actors, especially in the postcolonial period.

6 Nitsan Chorev, *World Health Organization between North and South* (Ithaca, NY: Cornell University Press, 2012), 82–5.

7 'Issues, Problems, and Priorities of the Health System in Ghana: Background paper prepared by the Ministry of Health, for the National Health Symposium, State House, Accra, June 7–8, 1988' (Ministry of Health, Accra, 31 May 1988), 1, National Catholic Secretariat (Accra).

8 UNICEF, Accra, 'Adjustment Policies and Programmes to Protect Children and Other Vulnerable Groups in Ghana', in *Adjustment with a Human Face Vol. II: Country Case Studies*, eds. Giovanni A. Cornia, Richard Jolly, and Frances Stewart (Oxford: Oxford University Press, 1988), 93–125.

9 Appendix 11 – Primary Health Care Strategy For Ghana – Ministry of Health, report on the Primary Health Care Conference: The Role and Function of NGOs/Ghana (18–20 October 1978, Madina) sponsored by UNICEF, 4215.5.11 Other Organisations 11–12 NGO Primary Health Care, Christian Medical Commission, Archives of the World Council of Churches (Geneva, Switzerland).

10 'Issues, Problems, and Priorities of the Health System in Ghana'.

11 Ibid.

12 'Gh.27: Ghana: CHAG's Efforts in Health Care' (August 1984), 1–9, SOAS Library and Archives (London, UK).

13 UNICEF, Accra, 'Adjustment Policies and Programmes to Protect Children and Other Vulnerable Groups in Ghana', 93.

14 Ibid., 93–125.

15 James Ferguson, 'Seeing Like an Oil Company: Space, Security, and Global Capital in Neoliberal Africa', *American Anthropologist* 107, no. 3 (2005): 377–82.

16 Ibid.

17 Jean-François Bayart and Stephn Ellis, 'Africa in the World: A History of Extraversion', Centenary Issue: A Hundred Years of Africa, *African Affairs* 99, no. 395 (April 2000): 217–67.

18 James C. Scott, *Seeing Like a State: How Certain Schemes to Improve the Human Condition Have Failed* (New Haven and London: Yale University Press, 1998), 223–61.

19 UNICEF, Accra, 'Adjustment Policies and Programmes to Protect Children and Other Vulnerable Groups in Ghana', 101–2.

20 Ibid., 93–125.

21 'Visit to Ghana by R. Amonoo-Lartson' (25 May–6 June 1985), 5–6, Country Files, Ghana 1–6, Christian Medical Commission, 4215.3.10, Archives of the World Council of Churches, Geneva, Switzerland.

22 Ibid.

23 Patrick A. Twumasi, 'Catholic Health Policy and Organization of the Department of Health, National Catholic Secretariat', *Survey Report Health Services in Ghana: National Catholic Secretariat January–April 1982* (April 1982, Department of Health, National Catholic Secretariat, Accra), 16–17, National Catholic Secretariat (Accra)

24 Ibid., 16.

25 For further information on this issue and how this information was obtained, please contact the author.

26 St Michael's Hospital, Pramso (Ashanti) Ghana: Annual Report 1981 (1981), 1, MMMP 17508, Memisa archives, Katholiek Documentatie Centrum (Nijmegen, Netherlands).

27 Ibid., 1–3.

28 Ibid.

29 St Michael's Hospital, Pramso (Ashanti) Ghana: Annual Report 1982 (1982), 1, MMMP 17508, Memisa archives, Katholiek Documentatie Centrum (Nijmegen, Netherlands).

30 Assin Foso Catholic Hospital, Ghana: Annual Report 1982 (1982), 1, MMMP 17506, Memisa archives, Katholiek Documentatie Centrum (Nijmegen, Netherlands).

31 St Elisabeth Hospital, Ghana: Annual Report 1983 (1983), 1–4, MMMP 17513, Memisa archives, Katholiek Documentatie Centrum (Nijmegen, Netherlands).

32 Sunyani District Health Services: Annual Report 1988 (1988), 2–3, MMMP 17506, Memisa archives, Katholiek Documentatie Centrum (Nijmegen, Netherlands).

33 Catholic Hospital Apam, Ghana: Annual Report 1989–90 (1990), MMMP 17513, Memisa archives, Katholiek Documentatie Centrum (Nijmegen, Netherlands).

34 'Declaration of Alma-Ata', *International Conference on Primary Health Care* (Alma-Ata, USSR, 6–12 September 1978), World Health Organization Publications.

35 Margaret Jones and Chandani Liyanage, 'Traditional Medicine and Primary Health Care in Sri Lanka: Policy Perceptions, and Practice', *Asian Review of World Histories* 6 (2018): 157–84.

36 James C. McGilvray to Thomas Adeoye Lambo, 'Consultation on the Subject of Health and Salvation' (12 July 1966) 4215.0.3 World Council of Churches: Christian Medical Commission. History of the CMC 1–9, WCC Archives (Geneva, Switzerland); '3. T. Adioya Lambo: Traditional Healing and Scientific Medicine: Some General Problems of Adjustment', Master File of Material for Consultation on Health and Salvation' (Tübingen, 1967) 4215.0.3 World Council of Churches: Christian Medical Commission. History of the CMC 1–9, WCC Archives (Geneva, Switzerland); 'John Karefa-Smart M.D. Vice-Chairman, Assistant Director-General of WHO, Evangelical and United Brethren', CMC of the WCC, 4215.1.1 World Council of Churches: Christian Medical Commission, Annual Meetings and Annual Reports 1–11, WCC Archives (Geneva, Switzerland).

37 James C. McGilvray, *The Quest for Health and Wholeness* (Gesamtherstellung: Breklumer Druckerei Manfred Siegel, German Institute for Medical Missions, Tübingen, 1981), 64–5.

38 J. Hakan Hellberg, 'Curing or Healing?' (Group 1. Art. 2.), 1–9, 4215.0.3 World Council of Churches: Christian Medical Commission. History of the CMC 1–9, WCC Archives (Geneva, Switzerland).

39 Ibid.

40 Martin H. Sharlemann, 'Health: What Is It?' (Group 1. Art. 2,), 9–13, 4215.0.3 World Council of Churches: Christian Medical Commission. History of the CMC 1–9, WCC Archives (Geneva, Switzerland).

41 G.C. Harding (possibly also with M. Sheel, and D. Jenkins), 'The Meaning of Health in the Congregation' (Group 11. Art. 2 – Consultation on Health and Salvation, Tübingen, September 1-8), 1–5, 4215.0.2 History of the CMC 1–9, WCC Archives (Geneva, Switzerland)

42 Ibid.

43 I. Ramsey, 'Summary' (Sunday 3 September 1967), 1–3, 4215.0.2. History of the CMC 1–9, WCC Archives (Geneva, Switzerland).

44 G.C. Harding and Robert A. Lambourne, 'Health and the Congregation' (Group 11. Art. 2, Consultation on Health and Salvation, Tübingen, September 1–8), 40–6. 4215.0.2. History of the CMC 1–9, WCC Archives (Geneva, Switzerland).

45 Seward Hiltner, 'The Program of the Congregation in Relation to Health' (Group 11. Art. 2), 55–8, 4215.0.2. History of the CMC 1–9, WCC Archives (Geneva, Switzerland).

46 H. Florin, Fred Sai, Anthony Bloom et. al., 'The Theological Perspective: The Role of the Church in Health and Medical Services', 28–44, 4215.1.1 World Council of Churches: Christian Medical Commission. Annual Meetings and Annual Reports 1–11, WCC Archives (Geneva, Switzerland).

47 James McGilvray, 'The Beginning of the Christian Medical Commission: Its Emphasis on Community Health Care', The Quest for Wholeness (Herausgeber: Deutsches Institut für ärztliche Mission, 1981), 63–76.

48 'Setting Our Priorities for Health: 1985 Meeting of the Christian Medical Commission', Contact: A Bimonthly Publication of the Christian Medical Commission, World Council of Churches (1985).

49 Matthew Bersagel Braley, 'The Christian Medical Commission and the World Health Organization', Religion as a Social Determinant of Public Health, ed. Ellen L. Idler (Oxford: Oxford University Press, 2014), 298–318.

50 'Non-Government Organizations and Primary Health Care', Statement Prepared for the WHO/UNICEF – Sponsored International Conference on Primary Health Care (Alma-Ata, Kazakh, S.S.R., 6–12 September 1978), 3–5, 4215.5.11 World Council of Churches: Christian Medical Commission, Other Organisations 1–12, WCC Archives (Geneva, Switzerland).

51 Socrates Litsios, 'The Christian Medical Commission and the Development of the World Health Organization's Primary Health Care Approach', American Journal of Public Health 94, no. 11 (November 2004): 1884–93.

52 M. Arole and R. Arole, 'A Comprehensive Rural Health Project in Jamkhed (India)', in Health by the People, ed. K.W. Newell (Geneva: World Health Organization, 1975), 71, http://apps.who.int/iris/.

53 Ted Karpf, 'Faith and Health: Past and Present of Relations between Faith Communities and the World Health Organization', Christian Journal of Global Health 1, no. 1 (June 2014): 16–25.

54 Fred Sai, 'Essential Aspects of Medical Work with Special Reference to Church Medical Institutions', Report of the Triennial Consultation of the Presbyterian Church of Ghana and Its Related Overseas Missionary

Societies Held at the Presbyterian Church Offices, Accra, Ghana (24–6 August 1971), 44–50, Balme Library, University of Ghana (Accra).
55 Fred Sai, *With Heart and Voice: Fred Sai Remembers* (Cambridge: Banson, 2010).
56 Frank Dimmock, Jill Olivier, and Quentin Wodon, 'Half a Century Young: The Christian Health Associations in Africa', MPRA Paper, *World Bank* (November 2012): 1–33.
57 'ICCO' (28 May 1985, DbB/ap), SOAS Library and Archives (London, UK).
58 'CHAG Relationships', *Christian Medical Commission: Programme on Getting Essential Drugs to the People through Cooperative Pharmaceutical Services* (Ghana, 15 April–11 May 1983), 25, SOAS Library and Archives (London, UK).
59 Dimmock, Olivier, and Wodon, 'Half a Century Young', 1–33.
60 'Gh.27: Ghana: CHAG's Efforts in Health Care' (August 1984), Annexes I–III SOAS Library and Archives (London, UK).
61 'CHAG Relationships', 35–8.
62 John S. Pobee, 'Religion and Politics in Ghana, 1972–1978: Some Case Studies from the Rule of General I. K. Acheampong', *Journal of Religion in Africa* 17, fasc. 1 (February 1987): 44–62.
63 Pascal Schmid, 'Mission Medicine in a Decolonising Healthcare System: Agogo Hospital, Ghana, 1945–1980', *Ghana Studies* 15/16 (2012/2013): 287–329.
64 'Medical Work', *60th Anniversary: The Salvation Army: Ghana Territory, 1922–1982*, The Salvation International Heritage Centre (London, UK).
65 'The Salvation Army Is Committed to the Total Person', Ghana Photo Collections, 6, The Salvation Army International Heritage Centre (London, UK).
66 'Notes of Paper Given by Lieutenant William Clark at the SDA/SA Conference' (16–18 March 1980), 1–2, The Salvation Army International Heritage Centre (London, UK).
67 'Memorandum: World Council of Churches', Commissioners Territorial Army (5 September 1978), The Salvation Army International Heritage Centre (London, UK); 'Council Regrets Pullout of the Salvation Army' (1978), The Salvation Army International Heritage Centre (London, UK).
68 David Maxwell, 'The Creation of Lubaland: Missionary Science and Christian Literacy in the Creation of Luba Katanga in the Belgian Congo', *Journal of Eastern African Studies* 10, no. 3 (2016): 367–92.
69 'Gh.27: Ghana: CHAG's Efforts in Health Care'.
70 Notably in relation to Ghana, see Peter A. Sarpong, 'Answering "Why" – The Ghanaian Concept of Disease', *Contact* 84 (April 1985): 5–11.

71 'Proposal Submitted Jointly to ... Misereor for support funding of the Christian Health Association of Nigeria', Other Organisations, 'Misereor' 9, 4215.5.11 World Council of Churches, Christian Medical Commission (Geneva, Switzerland).

72 'Financial Assistance for the Period Contact, 1983–4', Other Organisations, 'Misereor' 9, 4215.5.11 World Council of Churches, Christian Medical Commission, Geneva, Switzerland; Eric Ram to Misereor, Other Organisations, 'Misereor' 9, 4215.5.11 World Council of Churches Christian Medical Commission (Geneva, Switzerland).

73 'Report: Group 1: Topic: Primary Health Care', Report of the National Catholic Health Council Conference, Department of Health, National Catholic Secretariat (Nsawam, 21–4 November 1978), *Ghana – Bewilligungen 1959–1980*, Misereor-Archive (Aachen, Germany).

74 'Gh.27: Ghana: CHAG's Efforts in Health Care'.

75 Ibid.

76 Revd. Peter K. Sarpong to F.T.B. Pulis, director, Department of Overseas Personnel Service, Memisa-Medicus Mundi (12 July 1986) Collectie 999, Nummer 361, Memisa Archives, Katholiek Documentatie Centrum (Nijmegen, Netherlands).

77 Daniel Immerwahr, *Thinking Small: The United States and the Lure of Community Development* (Cambridge, MA: Harvard University Press, 2015), 88, 168.

78 For more information on how this occurred, please contact the author; thank you to the Medical Mission Sisters in Fox Chase, Philadelphia for helping me to unearth these stories and information on medical mission in Ghana more widely.

79 Primary Health Care Conference, National Women's Training Centre, Madina (18–20 October 1978), National Catholic Secretariat (Accra).

80 'Holy Family Hospital Berekum: A Report on Some Involvements in Primary Health Care Promotion', Primary Health Care Conference, National Women's Training Centre, Madina (18–20 October 1978), National Catholic Secretariat (Accra).

81 Report: Primary Health Care, Training of Trainers Workshop at Nsawam (23–27 August 1981), National Catholic Secretariat, Accra (Ghana).

82 Cueto, 'The ORIGINS of Primary Health Care and SELECTIVE Primary Health Care'.

83 Patrick A. Twumasi, *Survey Report Health Services in Ghana: National Catholic Secretariat January–April 1982* (April 1982, Department of Health, National Catholic Secretariat, Accra) 143, 146, 156, National Catholic Secretariat (Accra).

84 Ibid., 45, 51, 78, 83, 167, 171, 225, 243.

85 'Primary Health: Projects/Activities of the Members of the DHC, Diocese of Sunyani', Report of National Catholic Health Council Meeting (4–7 November 1980), *Ghana – Bewilligungen 1959–1980*, Misereor-Archive (Aachen, Germany).

86 Twumasi, *Survey Report Health Services in Ghana*, 40–1, 90–3, 172–8.

87 PHW Project Notes 7 (1966–1971), 9–15, RG15, Medical Mission Sister Archives (Philadelphia, USA).

88 Twumasi, *Survey Report Health Services in Ghana*, 162, 197, 293.

89 Annex 1, 'Emergency Assistance', K. Ward-Brew to regional director, 'AFRO – Memorandum: G-7 Primary Health Care: Catholic Relief Services' (25 August 1983), 25, 66–7, 'Economic Assistance to Ghana – Report of the Multi-Agency United Nations Mission to Ghana', G2/27/5/GHA, World Health Organization Archives (Geneva, Switzerland).

90 St Anthony's Hospital, Dzodze, Ghana: Preventative Health Scheme/ Primary Health Care Annual Report 1985 (1985), MMMP 17503, Memisa archives, Katholiek Documentatie Centrum (Nijmegen, Netherlands); St Anthony's Hospital, Dzodze, Ghana: Programme Report on Maternal and Child Care and Preventative/Primary Health Care Activities (1986), MMMP 17503, Memisa archives, Katholiek Documentatie Centrum (Nijmegen, Netherlands).

91 Sunyani District Health Services: Annual Report 1988 (1988), 2–3, MMMP 17506, Memisa archives, Katholiek Documentatie Centrum (Nijmegen, Netherlands).

92 Assin Foso Catholic Hospital and Assin District Primary Health Care: Annual Report 1984 (1985), 1–3, MMMP 17506, Memisa archives, Katholiek Documentatie Centrum (Nijmegen, Netherlands).

93 'Appendix II: Primary Health Care Strategy for Ghana', Ministry of Health, report of the National Catholic Health Council Conference, Department of Health, National Catholic Secretariat (Nsawam, 21–4 November 1978) *Ghana – Bewilligungen 1959–1980*, Misereor-Archive (Aachen, Germany).

94 'Group III: Proposal Re. Misereor Funding' Report of the National Catholic Health Council Conference, Department of Health, National Catholic Secretariat (Nsawam, 21–4 November 1978) *Ghana – Bewilligungen 1959–1980*, Misereor-Archive (Aachen, Germany).

95 Sai, 'Essential Aspects of Medical Work with Special Reference to Church Medical Institutions', 44–50.

96 Twumasi, *Survey Report Health Services in Ghana*, 25.

97 Appendix 11 - Primary Health Care Strategy For Ghana - Ministry of
Health, report on the Primary Health Care Conference: The Role and
Function of NGOs/Ghana (18–20 October 1978, Madina), sponsored by
UNICEF, 4215.5.11 Other Organisations 11–12 NGO Primary Health
Care, Christian Medical Commission, Archives of the World Council of
Churches (Geneva, Switzerland).

98 Pascal Schmid, *Medicine, Faith and Politics in Agogo: A History of Health
Care Delivery in Rural Ghana, ca. 1925 to 1980* (Vienna and Zürich: Lit
Verlag GmbH and Co. KG, 2018), 316.

99 Annual Report of the Bawku District Medical Programme 1980, Country
Files, 1–7 Ghana, 4215.3.10, Christian Medical Commission, Archives of
the World Council of Churches (Geneva, Switzerland).

100 Cueto, 'The ORIGINS of Primary Health Care and SELECTIVE Primary
Health Care'.

101 CMC/WHO Meeting on Collaboration in Strengthening District Health
Systems through PHC (23 July 1986), 4215.5.15 1–21 World Health
Organization, Christian Medical Commission, Archives of the World
Council of Churches (Geneva, Switzerland); Minutes of the WHO/CMC
Standing Committee (20 April 1990), 4215.5.15 1–21 World Health
Organization, Christian Medical Commission, Archives of the World
Council of Churches (Geneva, Switzerland).

102 WHO/CMC Standing Committee (4 March 1981), 4215.5.15 1–21 World
Health Organization, Christian Medical Commission, Archives of the
World Council of Churches (Geneva, Switzerland).

103 Minutes of the CMC/WHO Standing Committee Meeting (April 20 1982),
4215.5.15 1–21 World Health Organization, Christian Medical
Commission, Archives of the World Council of Churches (Geneva,
Switzerland).

104 Report of the Meeting between the Christian Medical Commission (CMC)
and WHO (12 March 1984), 4215.5.15 1–21 World Health Organization,
Christian Medical Commission, Archives of the World Council of
Churches (Geneva, Switzerland).

105 CMC/WHO Meeting on Collaboration in Strengthening District Health
Systems through PHC (23 July 1986), 4215.5.15 1–21 World Health
Organization, Christian Medical Commission, Archives of the World
Council of Churches (Geneva, Switzerland).

106 Agenda Item 1: CMC Standing Committee of 19 March 1987, 'Joint
Statement on the Occasion of the Meeting Between Dr Halfdan Mahler,
Director-General, WHO, and Dr Emilio Castro, Secretary-General, World
Council of Churches' (4 November 1986) 4215.5.15 1–21 World Health

Organization, Christian Medical Commission, Archives of the World Council of Churches (Geneva, Switzerland).

107 Country Files, 1–7 Ghana, 4215.3.10, Christian Medical Commission, Archives of the World Council of Churches (Geneva, Switzerland).

108 Minutes of the WHO/CMC Standing Committee (20 April 1990), 4215.5.15 1–21 World Health Organization, Christian Medical Commission, Archives of the World Council of Churches (Geneva, Switzerland).

109 4215.5.15 1–21 World Health Organization, Christian Medical Commission, Archives of the World Council of Churches (Geneva, Switzerland).

110 Jill Olivier et al., 'Understanding the Roles of Faith-Based Health-Care Providers in Africa: Review of the Evidence with a Focus on Magnitude, Reach, Cost, and Satisfaction', *The Lancet* 386, no. 10005 (July 2015): 1768.

111 Genevieve Cecilia Aryeetey et al., 'The Effect of the National Health Insurance Scheme (NHIS) on Health Service Delivery in Mission Facilities in Ghana: A Retrospective Study', *Global Health* 12, no. 32 (2016): 1–9.

112 Annabel Grieve and Jill Olivier, 'Towards Universal Health Coverage: A Mixed-Method Study Mapping the Development of Faith-Based Non-Profit Sector in the Ghanaian Health System', *International Journal for Equity in Health* 17, no. 97 (2018).

113 Grieve and Olivier (ibid.) have also shown that 123 out of 300 CHAG member facilities or institutions are Catholic, especially focused around the Upper West Region; see also Jill Olivier, Mari Shojo, and Quentin Wodon, 'Faith-inspired Health Care Provision in Ghana: Market Share, Reach to the Poor, and Performance', *MPRA Paper*, no. 45371 (November 2012).

CONCLUSION

1 James Ferguson, 'Seeing Like an Oil Company: Space, Security, and Global Capital in Neoliberal Africa', *American Anthropologist* 107, no. 3 (2005): 377–82.

2 Elisabeth Stephanie Clemens, *Civic Gifts: Voluntarism and the Making of the American Nation-State* (Chicago and London: University of Chicago Press, 2020), 264.

3 Elisabeth Stephanie Clemens, 'Delegated Governance as a Structure of Exceptions', in *States of Exception in American History*, eds. Gary Gerstle and Joel Isaac (Chicago: University of Chicago Press, 2020), 303 and 305.

4 Jean-François Bayart and Stephen Ellis, 'Africa in the World: A History of Extraversion', Centenary Issue: A Hundred Years of Africa, *African Affairs* 99, no. 395, (April 2000): 217–67.

5 Gary Gerstle and Joel Isaac, 'Afterword', in *States of Exception in American History*, 345.

6 David P. Fidler, 'The World Health Organization and Pandemic Politics: The Good, the Bad and the Ugly Future for Global Health', 10 April 2020, thinkglobalhealth.org/article/word-health- organization-and-pan- demic-politics; see also Andrew Harmer, 'The World Health Organisation and Pandemic Politics: A Reply to David Fidler', 12 April 2020, andre- wharmer.org.

7 Claire Hooker, 'Drawing the Lines: Danger and Risk in the Age of SARS', in *Medicine at the Border*, ed. Alison Bashford (London: Palgrave Macmillan, 2007), 179–95.

8 Clemens, *Civic Gifts*, 270.

9 Michael Mann, 'The Autonomous Power of the State: Its Origins, Mechanisms and Results', *European Journal of Sociology* 25, no. 2 (1984): 185–213, cited in Clemens, 'Delegated Governance as a Structure of Exceptions', in G. Gerstle and J. Isaac, eds., *States of Exception in American History*, 305.

10 Clemens, 'Delegated Governance as a Structure of Exceptions', 305.

11 There is far more to be done on the roles of countries like the Netherlands and Germany in global health, perhaps neglected because of an over-focus on Atlantic and anglo power; for a starting point, see Jesse Boardman Bump, 'The Long Road to Universal Health Coverage: Historical Analysis of Early Decisions in Germany, the United Kingdom, and the United States', *Health System Reform* 1, no. 1 (January 2015), 28–38.

12 'Deutschland: Zitate', *Der Spiegel* no. 14, Panorama (31 March 1964): 20.

13 David A. Hollinger, *Protestants Abroad: How Missionaries Tried to Change the World but Changed America* (Princeton, NJ: Princeton University Press, 2017).

14 P.W. Kok, 'Memisa: From Medical Missionary Action into a Medical Relief Organization', *Ned Tijdschr Geneeskd* 142, no. 51 (December 1998): 2800–3.

15 Harvey C. Kwiyani, 'Blessed Reflex: African Christians in Europe', *Missio Africanus: The Journal of African Missiology* 3, no. 1 (2017): 40–9; see also Harvey C. Kwiyani, 'Mission after George Floyd: On White Supremacy, Colonialism and World Christianity', *Anvil: Journal of Mission and Theology* 36, no. 3 (2020): 6–13.

16 Christopher Clark, 'Power', in *A Concise Companion to History*, ed. Ulinka Rublack (Oxford: Oxford University Press, 2011), 135.

17 Ulinka Rublack, 'Preface', in *A Concise Companion to History*, xi.

18 Katherine Marshall has shown clearly the tensions between international organisations, such as the World Bank, and the religious 'assets' with which they have been keen to work; Katherine Marshall, *Global Institutions of Religion: Ancient Movers, Moderns Shakers* (New York: Routledge, 2013). In her ethnographic analysis, Susan R. Holman has drawn out the paradoxes and hostility that exist as the relationship between the religion and global health polarizes; Susan R. Holman, *Beholden: Religion, Global Health, and Human Rights* (Oxford: Oxford University Press, 2015). As Katherine Marshall and Sally Smith experienced, clear health damage resulted from religion's neglect in the Ebola crisis in Sierra Leone, Liberia, and Guinea in 2014–16; Katherine Marshall and Sally Smith, 'Religion and Ebola: Learning from Experience', *The Lancet* 386, no. 10005 (2015): e24. By contrast, on AIDS and religion, see Marian Burchardt, *Faith in the Time of AIDS: Religion, Biopolitics and Modernity in South Africa* (London: Palgrave Macmillan, 2015); Rijk Van Dijk et al., *Religion and AIDS Treatment in Africa: Saving Souls, Prolonging Lives* (Farnham, Surrey, and Burlington, VT: Ashgate, 2014).

19 John Blevins, *Christianity's Role in United States Global Health and Development Policy: To Transfer the Empire to the World* (New York: Routledge, 2019), 5–7, 183–4.

Index